Vaccines
for the 21st Century

A TOOL FOR DECISIONMAKING

Kathleen R. Stratton, Jane S. Durch, and Robert S. Lawrence, *Editors*

Committee to Study Priorities for Vaccine Development

Division of Health Promotion and Disease Prevention

INSTITUTE OF MEDICINE

NATIONAL ACADEMY PRESS
Washington, D.C.

NATIONAL ACADEMY PRESS • 2101 Constitution Avenue, N.W. • Washington, DC 20418

NOTICE: The project that is the subject of this report was approved by the Governing Board of the National Research Council, whose members are drawn from the councils of the National Academy of Sciences, the National Academy of Engineering, and the Institute of Medicine. The members of the committee responsible for the report were chosen for their special competences and with regard for appropriate balance.

This project has been funded in whole with federal funds from the National Institutes of Allergy and Infectious Diseases, National Institutes of Health, under Contract No. N01-AI-45237. The views presented are those of the Institute of Medicine Committee to Study Priorities for Vaccine Development and are not necessarily those of the funding organization.

Library of Congress Cataloging-in-Publication Data

Institute of Medicine (U.S.). Committee to Study Priorities for Vaccine Development.
  Vaccines for the 21st century : a tool for decisionmaking / Kathleen R. Stratton, Jane S. Durch, and Robert S. Lawrence, editors ; Committee to Study Priorities for Vaccine Development, Division of Health Promotion and Disease Prevention, Institute of Medicine.
     p. ; cm.
  Includes bibliographical references and index.
  ISBN 0-309-05646-2 (hard cover)
  1. Vaccines--Research--United States--Planning. I. Stratton, Kathleen R. II. Durch, Jane. III. Lawrence, Robert S., 1938- IV. Title.
  [DNLM: 1. Vaccines. 2. Economics, Pharmaceutical. 3. Models, Theoretical. 4. Research. QW 805 I592v 2000]
  RA638 .I556 2000
  615'.372'072073--dc21

                                                                00-025528

Vaccines for the 21st Century: A Tool for Decisionmaking is available for sale from the National Academy Press, 2101 Constitution Avenue, N.W., Box 285, Washington, DC 20055. Call (800) 624-6242 or (202) 334-3313 (in the Washington metropolitan area), or visit the NAP's on-line bookstore at **www.nap.edu.** The full text of this publication is available on line at **www.nap.edu.**

For more information about the Institute of Medicine, visit the IOM home page at **www.iom.edu.**

"Knowing is not enough; we must apply.
Willing is not enough; we must do."

—Goethe

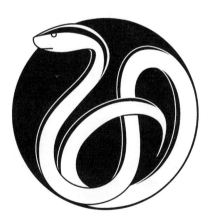

INSTITUTE OF MEDICINE

Shaping the Future for Health

THE NATIONAL ACADEMIES

National Academy of Sciences
National Academy of Engineering
Institute of Medicine
National Research Council

The **National Academy of Sciences** is a private, nonprofit, self-perpetuating society of distinguished scholars engaged in scientific and engineering research, dedicated to the furtherance of science and technology and to their use for the general welfare. Upon the authority of the charter granted to it by the Congress in 1863, the Academy has a mandate that requires it to advise the federal government on scientific and technical matters. Dr. Bruce M. Alberts is president of the National Academy of Sciences.

The **National Academy of Engineering** was established in 1964, under the charter of the National Academy of Sciences, as a parallel organization of outstanding engineers. It is autonomous in its administration and in the selection of its members, sharing with the National Academy of Sciences the responsibility for advising the federal government. The National Academy of Engineering also sponsors engineering programs aimed at meeting national needs, encourages education and research, and recognizes the superior achievements of engineers. Dr. William A. Wulf is president of the National Academy of Engineering.

The **Institute of Medicine** was established in 1970 by the National Academy of Sciences to secure the services of eminent members of appropriate professions in the examination of policy matters pertaining to the health of the public. The Institute acts under the responsibility given to the National Academy of Sciences by its congressional charter to be an adviser to the federal government and, upon its own initiative, to identify issues of medical care, research, and education. Dr. Kenneth I. Shine is president of the Institute of Medicine.

The **National Research Council** was organized by the National Academy of Sciences in 1916 to associate the broad community of science and technology with the Academy's purposes of furthering knowledge and advising the federal government. Functioning in accordance with general policies determined by the Academy, the Council has become the principal operating agency of both the National Academy of Sciences and the National Academy of Engineering in providing services to the government, the public, and the scientific and engineering communities. The Council is administered jointly by both Academies and the Institute of Medicine. Dr. Bruce M. Alberts and Dr. William A. Wulf are chairman and vice chairman, respectively, of the National Research Council.

DOROTHY MAJEWSKI, Project Assistant
HOLLY DAWKINS, Research Assistant
DONNA DUNCAN, Division Assistant
LAURIE GILL, EXCEL Consultant
ANNA MEADOWS, M.D., Scholar-in-Residence
MICHAEL A. STOTO, Ph.D., Director, Division of Health Promotion and
  Disease Prevention (until January 1, 1997)

Acknowledgments

This report has been reviewed in draft form by individuals chosen for their diverse perspectives and technical expertise, in accordance with procedures approved by the National Research Council's Report Review Committee. The purpose of this independent review is to provide candid and critical comments that will assist the institution in making the published report as sound as possible and to ensure that the report meets institutional standards for objectivity, evidence, and responsiveness to the study charge. The review comments and draft manuscript remain confidential to protect the integrity of the deliberative process. We wish to thank the following individuals for their participation in the review of this report:

Charles C.J. Carpenter, M.D., Brown University;
Gordon DeFriese, Ph.D., University of North Carolina at Chapel Hill;
Roger D. Feldman, Ph.D., University of Minnesota;
Harvey V. Fineberg, M.D., Ph.D., Harvard University;
Fernando Guerra, M.D., M.P.H., San Antonio Metropolitan Health District;
Michael Katz, M.D., March of Dimes Birth Defects Foundation;
Louis Lasagna, M.D., Tufts University School of Medicine; and
Henry W. Riecken, Ph.D., University of Pennsylvania.

While the individuals listed above have provided constructive comments and suggestions, it must be emphasized that responsibility for the final content of this report rests entirely with the authoring committee and the institution.

Contents

EXECUTIVE SUMMARY 1

1   INTRODUCTION 11
    Considerations Related to the Model and the Study, 12
    Organization of the Report, 13

2   PROGRESS IN VACCINE DEVELOPMENT 17
    Priorities of the IOM Committee in 1985, 18
    Litigation as a Barrier to Vaccine Development, 20
    A Case Study of Success, 23
    Advances in Biotechnology and Molecular Immunology and
        New Opportunities for Vaccines, 26

3   CONSIDERATIONS OF CANDIDATE VACCINES 39
    Exclusion Criteria, 39
    Additional Considerations for Inclusion, 43

4   OVERVIEW OF ANALYTIC APPROACH AND RESULTS 53
    A Cost-Effectiveness Approach, 53
    Model Overview, 61
    Examples: Hypothetical Vaccine X, 76
    Results, 86

5   REVIEW OF THE ANALYTIC MODEL 93
    Unit of Analysis, 93
    Implementing the Analysis, 94

Calculation of Health Benefits, 95
Cost Factors, 104
Vaccine Efficacy and Utilization, 107
Cost-Effectiveness Ratios, 108

6   ETHICAL CONSIDERATIONS AND CAVEATS 109
Ethical and Value Judgments Built into the Model, 111
Considerations of Justice, 116
Conclusion, 122

7   OBSERVATIONS 123
The Funding of Research, 123
Neglected Opportunities for Vaccine R&D, 126
Qualitative Judgments, 129
Vaccine Program Concerns, 130

REFERENCES 133

APPENDIXES
  1 *Borrelia burgdorferi,* 143
  2 Chlamydia, 149
  3 *Coccidioides Immitis,* 159
  4 Cytomegalovirus, 165
  5 Enterotoxigenic *E. coli,* 173
  6 Epstein-Barr Virus, 177
  7 *Helicobacter pylori,* 181
  8 Hepatitis C, 189
  9 Herpes Simplex Virus, 195
 10 *Histoplasma capsulatum,* 207
 11 Human Papillomavirus, 213
 12 Influenza A and B, 223
 13 Insulin-Dependent Diabetes Mellitus, 233
 14 Melanoma, 239
 15 Multiple Sclerosis, 245
 16 *Mycobacterium tuberculosis,* 251
 17 *Neisseria gonorrhea,* 257
 18 *Neisseria meningitidis B,* 267
 19 Parainfluenza Virus, 273
 20 Respiratory Syncytial Virus, 279
 21 Rheumatoid Arthritis, 285
 22 Rotavirus, 291
 23 *Shigella,* 295
 24 Streptococcus, Group A, 299
 25 Streptococcus, Group B, 305
 26 *Streptococcus pneumoniae,* 313

27 Information on Accessing Electronic Spreadsheets, 323

28 Summary of Workshops, 325

29 Questions Posed to Outside Experts and List of Responders, 435

INDEX 443

Executive Summary

In 1985, the Institute of Medicine (IOM) released two related reports titled *New Vaccine Development: Establishing Priorities* Vol. 1, *Diseases of Importance in the United States* and Vol. 2, *Diseases of Importance in Developing Countries* (IOM, 1985a,b). The project had been commissioned by the National Institutes of Health (NIH) as part of its planning for the future. The committee developed a quantitative model that could be used by decisionmakers to prioritize the development of vaccines against a number of disparate infectious diseases considered significant threats to public health. Data on 14 candidate vaccines against diseases of domestic importance were analyzed with the model. Several of the candidate vaccines considered in that report have in fact been licensed since its publication.

Ten years later, NIH requested that IOM convene a committee to assess the progress that has been made since publication of the reports in 1985, to discuss important barriers to vaccine research and development, and to develop another quantitative model for prioritizing vaccine development. There are several important differences between the landmark project released in 1985 and the current project.

- The current model focuses on conditions of domestic public health importance. There is no second report on international concerns.
- Candidate vaccines were to be analyzed with the model if they could be developed (achieve licensure) within the next two decades.
- The committee was explicitly asked to consider therapeutic vaccines directed against chronic conditions such as autoimmune diseases and cancers.

1

- Vaccines directed against human immunodeficiency virus are not within the scope of this project because of the rather prominent place that such vaccines already have within NIH.

THE ANALYTIC FRAMEWORK

A variety of analytic methods are available for comparative assessments to support priority-setting and resource allocation decisions. In selecting the approach to be used for this study, the committee had to have a means of comparing the anticipated health benefits and costs of vaccine use across drastically different forms of illness, ranging from pneumonia, ulcers, and cancers to temporary and long-term neurologic impairments. Furthermore, although some of the vaccines included in the study are intended to treat illness, most will be used in the more familiar role of preventing disease.

The committee adopted a cost-effectiveness approach that makes it possible to compare potential new vaccines on the basis of their anticipated impact on morbidity and mortality and on the basis of the costs for health care, use of the vaccine, and vaccine development. The analysis cannot provide the value judgments required to determine whether expected health benefits and costs justify a particular investment in vaccine development. The aim of the analysis is to clarify trade-offs in decisions to invest in the development of one vaccine as compared to another. The basis of comparison is a cost-effectiveness ratio that is expressed as cost per unit of health benefit gained. Monetary costs—the numerator of the ratio—reflect changes in the cost of health care that are expected to result from the use of an intervention such as a new vaccine plus costs associated with developing and delivering the intervention. Health benefits—the denominator of the ratio—are measured in terms of quality-adjusted life years (QALYs) gained by using the intervention under study. QALYs are a measure of health outcome that assigns to each period of time a weight, ranging from 0 to 1, corresponding to the health-related quality of life during that period, where a weight of 1 corresponds to optimal health, and a weight of 0 corresponds to a health state judged equivalent to death. These are then aggregated across time periods. The concept of QALYs, developed in the 1970s, was designed as a method that could integrate for an individual the health improvements from changes in both the quality and quantity of life, and could also aggregate these improvements across individuals. QALYs provide a summary measure of changes in morbidity and mortality that can be applied to very different health conditions and interventions. Interventions that produce both a health benefit and cost savings are inherently cost-effective, but many other interventions that do not save costs produce benefits at costs that are judged to be reasonable. An analysis such as the one performed by the present committee is a valuable tool for decisionmakers who must set priorities and allocate resources. It simplifies a complicated picture in which vastly different forms of illness and health benefits must be compared and related to a variety of costs. It cannot, however, address all of the qualitative judgments that shape policy decisions.

The cost-effectiveness approach also provides a framework within which the components of the analysis can be specified in detail and evaluated by those who use the results. This is particularly helpful for the committee's analysis, which, of necessity, rests on many estimates and assumptions about the characteristics of future vaccines and their likely impact on health and costs. The detailed specification of the components of the model also facilitates sensitivity analyses for the testing of alternative estimates and assumptions, either for individual patients or for all patients.

The cost-effectiveness analysis used by the committee can provide an estimate of the cost of achieving the anticipated health benefit for each of the vaccines studied, but it cannot determine whether that health benefit is worth the cost. That decision is a value judgment and should reflect consideration of many factors that are not included in the analysis. For example, the committee's analysis does not consider what resources will or should be available for vaccine development or how many vaccine candidates should be given priority for development. Furthermore, the analysis does not address the allocation of resources between vaccine development and the development and use of other forms of prevention or treatment. Although priority setting and resource allocation can be informed by economic analyses, they require value judgments that cannot be captured by a cost-effectiveness model.

It is also important to note that the results of the analysis depend on the accuracy and appropriateness of the data and the assumptions that are used, a point of particular relevance to the committee's work. Assumptions were necessary both to compensate for the limitations of the available data on current disease incidence and costs of care and to simplify some analytic tasks. Furthermore, the vaccines that are the focus of the study are still in development, making it necessary to rely on expert judgment for values such as costs of vaccine development and time until a vaccine will be licensed for use. Those who use the committee's analysis or similar types of studies should keep in mind that although the results are quantified they should not be treated as precise measures.

ETHICAL ISSUES

Cost-effectiveness analysis raises several ethical issues, especially in the context of priority setting. Some ethical concerns are a function of value judgments incorporated into the model, and others are related to issues that are not addressed. For example, within the model, all QALYs are considered equal without regard to the nature of the health benefit that they measure. Thus, the number of QALYs gained through many people receiving a small health benefit as a result of a reduction of a minor form of illness can be the same as the number of QALYs gained by averting a very small number of deaths.

The analysis is based on a societal perspective on health effects and costs in the United States; that is, all significant health outcomes and costs are taken into consideration, regardless of who experiences them. Thus, if use of a vaccine reduces hospital care costs, the analysis does not have to distinguish between cost savings that accrue to individuals and savings that accrue to insurers.

The societal perspective is in contrast to a more selective perspective, such as that of a particular government agency, health plan, or vaccine manufacturer used to examine these factors in other analyses. For these more selective analyses, the assessment of health effects might be limited to the members of a health plan or to a particular age group such as the Medicare population. Similarly, the costs (or savings) included in the analysis would be limited to those that would be incurred by the particular agency or organization. Costs borne by individuals or other organizations would not be considered in the analysis. A societal perspective, however, examines all costs and the health experience of the entire population.

RESULTS

The committee intends this model to be used as a dynamic instrument. The basic model and the mathematics used to create the model are described in detail in the report. In order to facilitate such use of this model, it can be accessed electronically free of charge (see the IOM home page at **www.iom.edu/vaccinepriorities** for more information). The committee developed several examples of hypothetical candidate vaccines, which are discussed in the report. These simplified examples are useful both for understanding key components of the model (and the effects of changes in those key components) and for those who wish to access and manipulate the model itself. The committee believes that this model has great utility even for those not charged with prioritizing vaccine development. Because only part of the model accounts for vaccine development time and costs, the model can be used after licensure of a vaccine to study and plan for vaccination program implementation.

The committee will *not* recommend which vaccines should be accorded research and development priority; it was not charged with doing so. In fact, the committee offers a single recommendation:

Policymakers (government agencies, research coordinators, private industry, philanthropic groups) charged with prioritizing vaccine development and vaccination program implementation should use as an aid in that prioritization process a model, such as that developed for this report, that is quantitative and relatively unbiased toward a specific vaccine candidate. Such a model should use standardly accepted data and techniques such as measures of health impact, and discounting.

The committee selected 26 candidate vaccines (in addition to the hypothetical examples) to illustrate the conceptual framework and the analytic model that it developed. The committee struggled early in its deliberations to select the candidate vaccines to be analyzed in this report. These 26 candidate vaccines are of interest to many people, could be developed within the next two decades, are directed against conditions of domestic importance, and illustrate important components of the model.

The committee was guided in their choices by a set of exclusion criteria. The following were bases for exclusion: (1) potentially vaccine-preventable conditions for which other preventive interventions were deemed more appropriate; (2) conditions for which basic science information was insufficient to predict vaccine development and licensure within 20 years; and (3) diseases of primarily non-domestic health importance. These exclusion criteria were used in the analysis undertaken for this report in order to limit the task in front of the committee. The exclusion criteria were not intended to guide public policy on vaccine R&D investments by either the public or private sector.

The primary analysis used by the committee is the annualized present value of the costs per quality-adjusted life year (QALY) gained by a vaccine strategy. The committee strongly cautions against focusing on a single ranking of candidate vaccines. In fact, the committee has deliberately chosen *not* to present a detailed ranking for the candidate vaccines. Any such ranking taken out of context of the rest of the report would assume an importance that is inappropriate given the uncertainty surrounding the data and the caveats about the modeling assumptions. The committee has placed candidate vaccines within general levels that reflect the results of the total analysis. The candidate vaccines fall into four reasonably distinct groupings or levels. That is, use of some of the candidate vaccines would save money while also saving QALYs and some of the candidate vaccination strategies would incur costs for each QALY gained. The four groups are:

Level I	Most Favorable	Saves money and QALYs
Level II	More Favorable	Costs < $10,000 per QALY saved
Level III	Favorable	Costs > $10,000 and < $100,000 per QALY saved
Level IV	Less Favorable	Costs > $100,000 per QALY saved.

Seven candidate vaccines fall into the most favorable (I) category: those with which a vaccination strategy would save money. The Level I candidate vaccines are as follows (in alphabetical order):

- cytomegalovirus (CMV) vaccine administered to 12-year-olds,
- influenza virus vaccine administered to the general population (once per person every 5 years or one-fifth of the population per year),
- insulin-dependent diabetes mellitus therapeutic vaccine,
- multiple sclerosis therapeutic vaccine,

- rheumatoid arthritis therapeutic vaccine,
- Group B streptococcus vaccine to be well-incorporated into routine pre-natal care and administered to women during first pregnancy and to high-risk adults (at age 65 years and to people less than age 65 years with serious, chronic health conditions), and
- *Streptococcus pneumoniae* vaccine to be given to infants and to 65-year-olds.

Nine candidate vaccines fall into the more favorable (II) category: those with which a vaccination strategy would incur small costs (less than $10,000) for each QALY gained. The Level II vaccine candidates are as follows (in alphabetical order):

- chlamydia vaccine to be administered to 12-year-olds,
- *Helicobacter pylori* vaccine to be administered to infants,
- hepatitis C virus vaccine to be administered to infants,
- herpes simplex virus vaccine to be administered to 12-year-olds,
- human papillomavirus vaccine to be administered to 12-year-olds,
- melanoma therapeutic vaccine,
- *Mycobacterium tuberculosis* vaccine to be administered to high-risk populations,
- *Neisseria gonorrhea* vaccine to be administered to 12-year-olds, and
- respiratory syncytial virus vaccine to be administered to infants and to 12-year-old females.

Four candidate vaccines fall into the favorable (III) category: those with which a vaccination strategy would incur moderate costs (more than $10,000 but less than $100,000) per QALY gained. The Level III vaccine candidates are as follows (in alphabetical order):

- parainfluenza virus vaccine to be given to infants and to women in their first pregnancy,
- rotavirus vaccine to be given to infants,
- Group A streptococcus vaccine to be given to infants, and
- Group B streptococcus vaccine to be given to high-risk adults and to either 12-year-old females or to women during first pregnancy (low utilization).

Seven candidate vaccines fall into the less favorable (IV) category: those with which a vaccination strategy would incur significant costs (more than $100,000 and up to well more than $1 million) per QALY gained. The Level IV vaccine candidates are as follows (in alphabetical order):

- *Borrelia burgdorferi* vaccine to be given to resident infants born in and immigrants of any age to geographically defined high-risk areas,

- *Coccidioides immitis* vaccine to be given to resident infants born in and immigrants of any age of geographically defined high-risk areas,
- enterotoxigenic *Escherichia coli* vaccine to be given to infants and travelers,
- Epstein-Barr virus vaccine to be given to 12-year-olds,
- *Histoplasma capsulatum* vaccine to be given to resident infants born in and immigrants of any age of geographically defined high-risk areas,
- *Neisseria meningitidis* type b vaccine to be given to infants, and
- Shigella vaccine to be given to infants and travelers or to travelers only.

Several of the Level I candidate vaccines were also discussed in the 1985 IOM report on vaccine prioritization. The disease burden of the four infectious conditions in Level I remains staggering due to many factors: the numbers of infected people, the seriousness of the health states caused by the infection, and the long-term sequelae (death and permanent impairment) and subsequent loss of quality of life (as measured in QALYs). The inclusion of candidate vaccines that are therapeutic suggests that vaccine strategies for noninfectious, chronic conditions holds much promise for improving health.

The inclusion in Levels I and II of candidate vaccines to be administered in puberty should serve as an indication for planning by vaccination program implementers for new approaches to encouraging the use of vaccines. The appropriate use of these candidate vaccines will require acceptance by parents, children, and health care providers that all people entering puberty are potentially sexually active. This also will require a health care milieu that is more capable than it is now of routine vaccination at puberty. Factors such as health beliefs, health care practices, performance measurements for health plans, and school entry laws have contributed to relatively successful childhood immunization efforts. These do not yet exist for the newly emerging "adolescent" or "pubertal" vaccination visits that are now recognized as important for continued protection against measles and rubella, for example.

Another challenge will be immunization of pregnant women against Group B streptococcus. The report discusses the barriers, particularly legal barriers to developing vaccines to be administered during pregnancy. The model assumes that these barrier are overcome and that immunization of pregnant women can become a standard part of prenatal care.

As stated several times in the report, the committee has not recommended which vaccines should be accorded development priority, nor will it recommend which vaccines should not be developed. Research and development of Level IV candidate vaccines can be justified on several levels. Research on these vaccines can lead to fundamental discoveries important to other candidate vaccines in the future or to other areas of basic research. Disease patterns could change and a need for these vaccines could become more compelling. These vaccines could be important due to disease burden in other countries, which is not factored in as part of this analysis. The committee argues in the report that inclusion of a candidate vaccine for malaria or dengue hemorrhagic fever in a report analyzing

U.S. public health burden was less compelling than inclusion of other candidate vaccines, and might fall into Level IV. An analysis of international disease burden for these candidate vaccines would likely lead to results that fall into more favorable levels.

OBSERVATIONS

In the course of developing and illustrating this model, the committee discussed general issues relating to the funding of research, neglected opportunities for vaccine research and development, the qualitative judgments integral to this modeling exercise, and vaccine program concerns. The committee closes the report with a series of observations that it hopes are as seriously considered as the analytic model that was the focus of this project.

Stable and sufficient funding of basic research by the federal government (which has an added benefit of recruiting young investigators from all fields of biomedical science into vaccinology), as well as creative funding mechanisms and research alliances, are crucial to assure that effective, safe, and needed vaccines will be carried through the development stage into licensure. Research and development is an expensive enterprise currently supported through a natural and fluid mix of public and private funding. New knowledge resulting from basic research funded by the federal government and private foundations is the integral first step that allows applied research and development to move forward into the private sector. Although private industry supports basic research, the most important role it plays is to assume the costs of applied research and development.

The committee can envision situations, however, where the need for a vaccine is compelling but for which the return on investment cannot be guaranteed. Examples of impediments to making a profit include possible litigation, a small target population, lack of acceptance of a vaccine strategy for a specific condition, and high costs expected of newer vaccines. Sometimes the market fails, and without subsidization candidate vaccines become neglected.

The committee discussed other barriers to achieving the maximum health benefit from the candidate vaccines. Vaccine delivery poses significant barriers to effective prevention and control of infectious disease. Children in the United States can receive up to 6 different vaccines (adding up to a maximum of 32 antigens, 6 visits to a health care provider, and 16 injections) before 2 years of age. Compliance with recommended immunizations by 2 years of age is still below that achieved by 5 years of age, primarily because of mandatory immunization for school entry. Combination vaccines promise to reduce some of the barriers to compliance but will not be a panacea. The combinations will help increase acceptance and utilization of vaccines, but clinical trial design issues are not trivial. The committee hopes that government, the medical community, the public, and vaccine manufacturers carefully think about rational approaches to combination vaccines and vaccine schedules. Furthermore, noninjection routes (e.g., oral, intranasal, or cutaneous delivery) should receive consideration. At the same time, the committee knows that market forces and corporate alliances will drive the availability of combination products.

The committee's analysis demonstrates that not all candidate vaccines will save money. Some new vaccines might be very expensive to purchase and develop. The target population might be very small. However, the health benefits for some people might still be compelling. Use of these vaccines will require a shift from an expectation that vaccines are always cost-saving to an acknowledgment that the health benefits of some vaccines might be worth the cost. Many vaccines are not covered by health care plans—neither indemnity plans nor managed care. Financial incentives to insurers or to individuals might be crucial for encouraging the use of vaccines.

However, the cost of vaccines to the individual and to insurers is not the only impediment to vaccine use. Vaccines, like other public health successes such as clean water, fluoridation to prevent caries, and food safety measures are a victim of their own success; people forget how dangerous vaccine-preventable disease can be and become complacent. This false sense of security strikes individuals, communities, health care providers, and policymakers. It is not until the system fails and illness surges (such as with antibiotic resistance, nosocomial infections, the measles outbreaks that occurred in the late 1980s, or food-borne illness) that we pay the price for interventions, such as vaccines, that are not yet developed or implemented.

The committee urges careful consideration, but not rigidity, in the use of evidence-based approaches, such as the qualitative framework and quantitative model developed for this report, for prioritization of research, development, and use of vaccines as well as other preventive and therapeutic interventions. The committee, while acknowledging the limitations of modeling exercises in general and of the one it developed and used in particular, does believe that modeling is useful and important when attempting to compare widely divergent vaccine-preventable conditions. It hopes that the inferences derived from the model will be useful to the vaccine science community, vaccine manufacturers, and research and program policymakers.

1

Introduction

In 1985, the Institute of Medicine (IOM) released two related reports titled *New Vaccine Development: Establishing Priorities* Vol. 1, *Diseases of Importance in the United States* and Vol. 2, *Diseases of Importance in Developing Countries* (IOM, 1985a,b). The project had been commissioned by the National Institutes of Health (NIH) as part of its planning for the future. The committee assembled for that project developed a quantitative model that could be used by decisionmakers to prioritize the development of vaccines against a number of disparate infectious diseases considered significant threats to public health. The variables included in that model were disease burden, costs of care, vaccine program costs, vaccine acceptance, vaccine development costs, and the likelihood of success. For volume 1, data on 14 candidate vaccines against diseases of domestic importance were analyzed with the model. Several of the candidate vaccines considered in that report have in fact been licensed since its publication. Vaccines against hepatitis B virus (recombinant), hepatitis A virus, varicella-zoster virus, *Haemophilus influenzae*, rotavirus, and pertussis acellular vaccine are all now part of the disease prevention armamentarium. The rest of the candidate vaccines are still in the pipeline.

Ten years later, NIH requested that IOM convene a new committee to assess the progress made since publication of the reports in 1985, discuss important barriers to vaccine research and development, and develop another quantitative framework for prioritizing vaccine development. There are two important differences between the landmark project completed in 1985 and the current project:

- The current analysis focuses on conditions of domestic public health importance. There is no second report on international concerns; and

• The committee was explicitly asked to consider therapeutic vaccines directed against chronic conditions such as autoimmune diseases and cancers.

CONSIDERATIONS RELATED TO THE MODEL AND THE STUDY

Before embarking on a discussion of the methods used and the results obtained, it is necessary to present several caveats, as well as an historical perspective of vaccine development since publication of the 1985 report. This report, particularly the appendixes, is not the definitive cost-effectiveness analysis of any one specific vaccine-based prevention or treatment strategy. For several of the conditions under study in this report, detailed and elaborate economic analyses have been conducted and published by other researchers. For other conditions, there are none. Published studies, however, rely on different assumptions and apply different techniques. Thus, the committee could not depend on the results in the published literature for comparable estimates of the economic burdens of the conditions to be studied.

In order to compare candidate vaccines with each other, as this committee was charged with doing, the analyses needed to be conducted in comparable ways. Resource limitations meant that the committee focused on big picture descriptions of disease burden and potential gains from vaccine use. Because fine details regarding epidemiology, clinical presentation in individuals and within a population, and costs of care are not always readily available for the 30 candidate vaccines considered, the committee necessarily made many assumptions for the data used in the model. The committee assessed the published literature and the opinions of experts in the field, and then the members of the committee used their collective scientific and clinical judgment to estimate values when there was no published consensus.

Third, the committee knows that there will be readers of this report who will object to the individual numbers used in (or omitted from) the analyses. The committee urges all readers to consider the report and its appendixes as a whole and believes the following questions can be answered in the affirmative:

• If individual values for a given parameter of a given disease seem contrary to expectation, are they relatively correct compared to the values for the other conditions?
• Do the data used as a whole represent an unbiased qualitative synthesis of the published values?
• Are all conditions being treated similarly?

The committee offers the model as a tool for decisionmakers as they assess the needs for vaccine development and the opportunities for a vaccine development strategy. An untested model would be highly suspect. Therefore, the committee used data in the model that represent the consensus of the scientific community.

The committee intends this model to be used as a dynamic instrument for the responsible prioritization of vaccine development and vaccination program implementation. The basic model and the mathematics used to create the model are described in detail in Chapter 4 and 5. Anyone with a personal computer and a spreadsheet software package could reprogram this model. Those with a mathematical understanding of modeling could do so quickly and easily. A reader could change the basic model if he or she so desired. A reader could change the data run through the model if the reader takes great exception to the data used by the committee. In order to facilitate such use of this model, it can be accessed electronically without charge (see Appendix 27). The committee also believes that this model has great utility even for those not charged with prioritizing vaccine development. Because only part of the model accounts for vaccine development time and costs, the model can be used after licensure of a vaccine to study and plan for vaccination program implementation.

ORGANIZATION OF THE REPORT

Charge to the Committee

The Committee to Study Priorities for Vaccine Development was charged with three main tasks:

1. Assessing the progress in vaccine development since publication of the 1985 IOM report.
2. Describing barriers to vaccine research and development.
3. Developing a framework by which vaccine research and development could be prioritized.

The first part of the charge is addressed in Chapter 2. The second task is addressed in part in Chapter 2 and in part in Chapter 7. The third part of the charge is addressed in Chapters 4 and 5. The application and interpretation of the analytic framework are discussed in Chapters 5 and 6 and the appendixes. It is important to discuss the specifics of the committee's third task with particular emphasis on what it does *not* entail. Specifically, the committee was asked to develop a model that could be applied to diseases affecting the U.S. population. As discussed in several places within the report, this influenced specific variables in the model and the choices of candidate vaccines to be used to illustrate the model. This restriction also caused the committee great concerns. Concerns about international health and disease burden are expressed in this chapter and in Chapter 7, Observations.

The committee was also asked to exclude vaccine candidates directed against human immunodeficiency virus (HIV), which causes acquired immunodeficiency syndrome (AIDS). Research and development (R&D) related to these vaccines is a priority of the National Institutes of Health (NIH) and many vaccine R&D companies. The rapidly changing dynamics of basic, clinical, and applied research related to HIV and AIDS could make any assumptions used in the application of the model obsolete before the report is published. The committee notes, however, that one could apply this model to HIV vaccines. The committee was also asked to consider vaccines that it thought could be licensed within the next 10 years or within the decade after that.

Committee Membership and Meetings

The committee was established in the winter of 1995. National Research Council policies on bias and conflict of interest were observed. These policies necessitated excluding from committee membership anyone employed by or with significant financial interest in any vaccine research and development company. In assembling the committee, individuals with expertise in economic modeling, public health, ethics, epidemiology, immunization policy, infectious diseases, vaccinology, immunology and pathology, and clinical medicine were sought. The committee, whose members are listed at the beginning of this volume, consisted of individuals with expertise in all of these areas. The committee met as a whole seven times. Five small-group meetings were also held throughout the deliberations. The committee also sponsored two public workshops on the science base for new vaccine development. Summaries of those workshops can be found in Appendix 28. The purpose of the workshops was to supplement the knowledge of the committee on the current science base of vaccine development as it narrowed the scope of the vaccine candidates to be included in the analysis. The committee also heard presentations from program officers at NIH, staff members responsible for federal data sources such as those managed by the National Center for Health Statistics and other components of the Centers for Disease Control and Prevention (CDC), the Food and Drug Administration, and representatives from vaccine R&D companies.

As will be described in a subsequent section of this chapter, the committee also enlisted the aid of many experts on the conditions and candidate vaccines under consideration. They did so by asking for responses to targeted questions about disease epidemiology, clinical care issues, and vaccine development issues. The questions and a list of the experts who responded can be found in Appendix 29.

Organization of the Report

The report is organized as follows: Chapter 2 describes progress in vaccine development and in basic biomedical sciences important to vaccine development since publication of the last reports in 1985. Chapter 3 describes the choice of candidate vaccines. Chapter 4 gives an overview of the analytic model and the methods used in the analysis and presents the results. Chapter 5 gives a detailed explanation of the model. Chapter 6 offers a discussion of ethical issues in modeling exercises and measures of quality of life and caveats that should be used in interpreting the results of the model. Chapter 7 concludes the report with some observations regarding vaccine research and development. The main body of the report is followed by appendixes that provide and discuss the condition-specific data used in the calculations.

2

Progress in Vaccine Development

In 1985 the Institute of Medicine (IOM) published its initial report on vaccine development: *New Vaccine Development, Establishing Priorities*, Vol. 1, *Diseases of Importance in the United States* (IOM, 1985a). This was the first report of a two-part study (IOM, 1985a,b) conducted by the Committee on Issues and Priorities for New Vaccine Development at the request of the National Institute of Allergy and Infectious Diseases (NIAID) of the National Institutes of Health (NIH). NIAID contracted with IOM for assistance in developing an approach to setting priorities for accelerated vaccine development. Committee membership embraced expertise in all those fields judged to be important to such a study, and therefore, in addition to research scientists and physicians, the committee also included economists, sociologists, ethicists, epidemiologists, industry leaders, and public health experts. As part of its charge, the committee was requested to develop a decisionmaking framework for selecting candidate vaccines of importance to the U.S. population and to use such a system to rank these candidate vaccines. A second component of the study involved prioritization of the vaccines needed by technologically less developed nations. That part of the study also modified the model to rank potential vaccines for use on an international basis. These findings were published in a second volume of the committee's report (IOM, 1985b).

The committee's analysis was based on a quantitative model in which vaccine candidates were ranked according to two principal characteristics: expected health benefits (reduction of morbidity and mortality) and expected net savings of health care resources. To compare the health impacts of disease and the potential benefits of vaccines, a measurement system based on units of infant mortality equivalents was used. The best available data were used, but where the information was incomplete, estimates and judgments by experts were used. The committee adopted a format that was flexible so that new candidate vaccines could be assessed similarly or current candidates vaccines could be reassessed with new data. A final

17

recommendation urged NIAID and other responsible agencies to improve the epidemiological data that are used to compare diseases. The variable quality of the data in some areas and the total absence of data in others were serious impediments to the development of a comprehensive prioritization scheme.

PRIORITIES OF THE IOM COMMITTEE IN 1985

Table 2-1 presents the 1985 committee's final list of pathogens for which vaccines were analyzed. For several pathogens two different forms of vaccine were considered (e.g., attenuated live virus or glycoprotein). By varying different assumptions (e.g., utilization, discount rates), vaccines against the first five pathogens retained highest priority. The committee stated that an improved pertussis vaccine (acellular antigens) merited unique treatment because of its potential for restoring public confidence in all immunization programs. Indeed, since the report was issued, a number of acellular pertussis vaccines and new combinations of acellular pertussis vaccines with other antigens have been licensed in the United States. Initially, acellular pertussis vaccines were recommended only for the fourth and fifth doses of the childhood immunization schedule, but acellular pertussis vaccines are now recommended for all doses in the immunization schedule beginning at 2 months of age. Their diminished local reactivity and systemic manifestations have rendered them highly acceptable to both health care providers and parents. This has greatly restored confidence in childhood immunizations, which had been eroded previously by concerns about whole-cell pertussis vaccines. The hepatitis B virus (HBV) vaccine, prepared by recombinant technology, has also been licensed for use and is recommended and incorporated into the infant immunization schedule. Additionally, it is widely used for various high-risk adult populations including health care workers.

Conjugate vaccines against *Haemophilus influenzae* type b (Hib) have been the remarkable success of the past 8 years. With their widespread use in infancy, the annual rates of invasive disease caused by this organism among U.S. children under 5 years of age have been reduced from 40 to 1 per 100,000 population. Varicella-zoster virus vaccine was licensed in the spring of 1995 and is recommended for infants at 1 year of age. Physicians in practice are beginning to use the vaccine, and a number of states provide it in their public health programs. Of the remaining candidate vaccines included in the 1985 analysis, only hepatitis A virus (HAV) vaccine (1995) and rotavirus vaccine (1998) have been licensed. Vaccination against HAV has been recommended for groups at special risk.

Over half of the candidate vaccines analyzed in the 1985 report on vaccine priorities have not yet been licensed. Several are still 15 years from licensure, in this committee's opinion. Although the committee did not analyze in depth each unlicensed candidate vaccine from 1985, obvious factors hindering progress

TABLE 2-1 Status of Vaccines Prioritized in 1985

Pathogen	Status
Hepatitis B virus	Recombinant hepatitis B virus surface antigen licensed and in widespread use.
Respiratory syncytial virus	Purified fusion (F) protein in phase II studies.
Haemophilus influenzae type b	Glycoconjugates licensed and in widespread use.
Influenza virus A and B	Cold-adapted live, attenuated virus vaccine in phase III trials; baculovirus-expressed recombinant HA subunit in phase III trials.
Varicella-zoster virus	Live attenuated virus licensed and in use.
Group B streptococcus	Glycoconjugates of five serotypes in phase II studies.
Parainfluenza viruses	Cold-adapted live, attenuated type 3 virus in phase II trials; bovine live, attenuated virus in phase II trials.
Cytomegalovirus	Glycoprotein subunit in phase I studies.
Rotaviruses	Attenuated live human-rhesus and bovine-human reassortants in phase III trials at beginning of project. Licensure in 1998 of one product.
Neisseria gonorrhoeae	Early basic research on various proteins.
Hepatitis A virus	Inactivated HAV particles licensed and in early use.
Coccidioides immitis	Formalin-killed spherules in phase III clinical trials.
Herpes simplex 1 and 2	Glycoprotein (D) recombinant of type 2 in phase II trials; attenuated recombinants in phase I studies.
Bordetella pertussis	Acellular products (DTaP) licensed and in widespread use.

toward licensure include unexpected obstacles in research progress (either in the more basic research phases, in clinical trials, or in scale-up processes for development and production). Alternatively, steady progress could have been made but at a much slower pace than expected. Slow progress could be attributed to either lack of scientific interest on the part of researchers or lack of adequate funding for the R&D. As discussed in Chapter 7 of the report, inadequate interest on the part of funders, such as private vaccine R&D companies, can reflect concerns about profitability because of either small market potential or possible costs due to liability for adverse events.

The committee had been told in early discussions with vaccine researchers that a primary weakness of the 1985 report was that it was overly optimistic about how long it would take for licensure of several candidates. The present analysis includes a longer time frame than the 1985 effort. Models such as that provided in 1985 and in this report do not predict which vaccines will be developed within a specific time frame. They provide comparative cost-effectiveness analyses for candidate vaccines that the committee assumes could be developed and licensed within a specific time frame.

The development of respiratory syncytial virus (RSV) vaccines has been slower than anticipated, in large part because of the extraordinarily cautious approach to the implementation of clinical trials because of the unfortunate experiences with the early inactivated RSV vaccines. The inactivated vaccines augmented clinical disease and resulted in increased rates of hospitalizations and some deaths when administered to the youngest infants, the group at highest risk from RSV disease. Clinical trials with both attenuated live virus and surface glycoprotein RSV vaccines are under way. Influenza virus vaccines consisting of both attenuated live virus variants and a number of subunit preparations are also under continuing research and development.

In contrast, the likelihood of successful licensure of parainfluenza virus vaccines, cytomegalovirus (CMV) vaccine, *Neisseria gonorrhoeae* vaccine, and *Coccidioides immitis* vaccines remain more remote. Studies of conjugate group B streptococcal (GBS) vaccines have been promising, particularly in immunization of late third-trimester pregnant women for the prevention of neonatal invasive GBS disease. However, pharmaceutical firms appear to have little enthusiasm for investing in the production of such a vaccine. Concerns regarding litigation that might ensue following unfavorable pregnancy outcomes (discussed in the following section) remain the most visible obstacle. Table 2-1 presents the current stage of development of vaccines against those pathogens assessed in 1985.

LITIGATION AS A BARRIER TO VACCINE DEVELOPMENT

The mid-1980s was a time of great struggle and even crisis for the development and manufacture of vaccines and vaccination program implementation. Public trust in vaccines was shaken and litigation concerns caused several major manufacturers to reduce or eliminate their vaccine development programs. The National Childhood Vaccine Injury Act (NCVIA; P.L. 99-660) was enacted in 1986. The legislation established a compensation fund for people who suffered specific serious adverse health effects that could potentially be attributed to vaccination with mandatory childhood vaccines (diphtheria and tetanus toxoids and pertussis vaccine, measles-mumps-rubella vaccine, oral polio vaccine, inactivated polio vaccine, and individual antigens within those vaccines). IOM embarked on two major projects to evaluate the medical and scientific literature regarding the causal association between vaccines and adverse events (IOM, 1991, 1994a,b). That body of work has been used by the U.S. Department of Health and Human Services to evaluate and refine the conditions and circumstances warranting compensation by the program. The Vaccine Injury Compensation Program (NVICP) is funded by excise taxes on the sale of vaccines covered by the program.

Although NCVIA does not protect vaccine manufacturers from all litigation, the number of suits filed against manufacturers greatly decreased, public trust in vaccines increased, and vaccine research and development returned to its previous levels. Serious litigation issues that have not been ameliorated by the 1986 legislation remain, however. Vaccines that are not mandated for use in children are not covered by NVICP. Federal vaccine advisory bodies have discussed the possibility of including influenza and pneumococcal vaccines in the program, which are aimed primarily at adults. Advocacy organizations key to the passage of the 1986 law are not supportive of that move, and no system of protection against litigation exists for these vaccines. It must be noted, however, that with the exception of year-specific concerns about a relation between influenza vaccine and Guillain-Barré syndrome, these vaccines have not caused safety concerns similar to those engendered by the childhood vaccines. This difference is probably due to differences in host reactions as well as the fact that childhood vaccines are, for the most part, mandated by the Federal government while adult vaccines are not (IOM, 1997b).

Immunization of Pregnant Women

Many researchers believe that litigation concern with regard to the immunization of pregnant women is a key factor in the slow progress in the development of a vaccine against GBS in particular. A discussion of the principles and problems surrounding immunization of pregnant women is necessary to understanding this barrier to vaccine development, which has not been resolved since the 1985 report.

Preventing infections in neonates and young infants by vaccinating pregnant women is a concept that is more than a century old. The rationale for immunization of pregnant women is based on two premises: (1) the occurrence of a substantial burden of disease from certain infectious agents during the first 3 to 6 months of life, an interval before which protection by active immunization of the infant could be achieved, and (2) the likelihood that immunization prior to or during pregnancy would induce high concentrations of specific antibodies in maternal serum that would be transferred across the placenta, thereby passively protecting the infant. This strategy has been studied extensively for the prevention of diphtheria, tetanus, and pertussis infections in infants. Worldwide, immunization of pregnant women for the prevention of infection in the infant is used routinely for neonatal tetanus, a major cause of infant mortality (Schofield, 1986). The World Health Organization (WHO) has recommended that this approach be extended for the prevention of diseases caused by other infectious agents.

The feasibility of immunizing pregnant women for the prevention of several infectious diseases whose contemporary burdens in young infants are substantial has been extensively investigated. The vaccines studied include those consisting of antigens from bacterial pathogens (GBS [Baker et al., 1988], Hib [Mulholland et al., 1996], *Neisseria meningitidis* groups A and C, *Streptococcus pneumoniae* [McCormick et al., 1980; O'Dempsey et al., 1996] and viral pathogens (HBV, influenza virus, rabies, RSV, yellow fever virus), and others have been proposed for study (CMV, herpes simplex virus, human immunodeficiency virus, rotavirus). Immunization of pregnant women is an approach that can avoid the obstacles presented by the immunologic immaturity of the neonate, has the potential to defer the need for active immunization of the infant or to decrease the number of doses needed to achieve protection during the first year of life, and may prevent the transmission of infection from the mother to the neonate. Despite considerable scientific data underscoring the feasibility, safety, and cost-effectiveness of this approach, progress in the United States has been slow or wanting. Obstacles to this approach are said to involve ethical, legal, and sociological concerns, but issues concerning the liability of vaccine manufacturers dominate the others (Insel et al., 1994; Linder and Ohel, 1994). Scientific evidence pales when concern over the liability of vaccine manufacturers arises, and vaccine manufacturers appeal to the government for indemnification before they pursue studies of existing vaccines or the development of additional reagents appropriate for immunizing pregnant women.

The committee reviewed immunization of pregnant women as a vaccination strategy in some detail, believing it to be scientifically valid for use in the United States for preventing several infectious diseases in young infants. However, this approach deserves special consideration because of the obstacles mentioned above. Thus, it is appropriate to underscore the rationale for this approach. Alternatives are discussed and critiqued in Chapter 7.

Passive immunization of the neonate and young infant depends on selective placental transfer of plasma proteins, and the transfer of immunoglobulins is limited to immunoglobulin G (IgG). Passage of antibodies is both passive (directly proportional to the maternal serum IgG concentration) and active (binding of IgG to Fc receptors, followed by receptor-mediated endocytosis). The latter accounts for the preferential transport of IgG1 and IgG3, which have greater affinities than IgG2 for binding to Fc receptors. Passage of antibodies begins at 8 weeks of gestation, but the level remains low until about 20 weeks. Neonatal cord serum IgG levels correlate with gestational age. At 32 weeks of gestation cord serum has an IgG level approximately half of that at 40 weeks, when the levels are equal to or somewhat greater than those in maternal serum. Maternal IgG has a half-life of 3 to 4 weeks, but since the duration of passive antibody protection is dictated by the actual level at birth, protection may last for 3 to 6 months.

The immune response of pregnant women is similar to that of nonpregnant women (Halsey and Klein, 1990), but there is a delay between the time of immunization and the time of fetal acquisition of maternal antibodies. This is the interval required for the mother to generate an IgG antibody response and for the antibodies to equilibrate with the circulating IgG pool and be transported across the placenta. For tetanus toxoid the optimal timing for immunization of a pregnant woman to achieve neonatal protection is 60 days before delivery (or at least 20 days after administration of the second dose) (Chen et al., 1983). The ideal vaccine should induce high maternal levels of IgG1 antibodies; the maximum response should occur after the administration of one dose, reaching its peak within 2 weeks of immunization; and protective levels should persist for several years, providing protection in subsequent pregnancies. For most vaccines, the vaccine would be given early in the third trimester (28 to 32 weeks of gestation), a time when organogenesis is complete and when most events associated with adverse pregnancy outcomes are past. Theoretically, this timing would also provide protection for many prematurely born infants.

For some diseases for which immunization of the pregnant woman has been proposed (e.g., neonatal and pregnancy-related GBS infections), active immunization of the infant would be unnecessary because susceptibility is limited to young infants, pregnant women, and adults with either defined underlying medical conditions or advanced age. For others, such as Hib and RSV infections, active immunization would also be required. Maternal antibody can interfere with infant responses to live-virus vaccines, but this has not been demonstrated for inactivated viral vaccines, such as influenza virus vaccine, or for bacterial antigens, including tetanus toxoid, serogroup A and C meningococcal polysaccharides, or Hib polysaccharide (Insel et al., 1994). While the issue of suppression, activation or priming, or alteration of the repertoire of antibody responses in the infant should be studied as vaccines are developed, the evidence to date is reassuring.

A CASE STUDY OF SUCCESS

As mentioned above, several of the vaccines recommended for accelerated development in the 1985 IOM report have been licensed for use, and several vaccines now in the development pipeline were not even contemplated in 1985. Rapid advances in the biomedical sciences and new knowledge about disease etiology and epidemiology can quickly change priorities. Before reviewing some of the major biomedical advances that are allowing vaccine development to proceed in ways not previously imagined, it will be useful to take a look at one of the vaccine successes known to all—the development of polio vaccines and the near eradication of a dreaded disease.

Disease Burden

Poliomyelitis was a relatively insignificant disease in the United States before 1900, when epidemics of increasing severity began to appear in different parts of the country. The average annual incidence of the disease for the years

1910 to 1914 was about 6 cases per 100,000 population. The frequency of paralytic polio continued to increase during the subsequent decades, and the rate for 1952 was approximately 37 cases per 100,000 population.

In the early 1900s most deaths due to poliomyelitis were observed in infants under 1 year of age and in children 1 to 4 years of age. The death rate declined sharply in cases occurring at older ages (Health Information Foundation, 1959). However, by the early 1950s, poliomyelitis was observed with increasing frequency in school-age children and young adults. Around this period, sanitation and community conditions of hygiene began to improve significantly largely due to the efforts begun in the 1930s and 1940s. As living conditions improved, a good proportion of the population probably was not exposed to the virus until an older age. These observations may explain the apparent shift in the age of susceptibility to the development of paralytic disease between the 1900s and the 1950s (Health Information Foundation, 1959).

Polio Vaccine Development

Efforts to develop immunoprophylaxis against polioviruses began immediately after the isolation of the virus. Both killed and live virus candidate vaccines were developed as early as 1910, although at that time knowledge of the existence of three distinct poliovirus types was not available, and the fact that paralytic cases of polio represented only a tiny fraction of the total number of infections was not appreciated (Harrington, 1932; The National Foundation, 1961, 1962). For every known patient with paralysis, there may be as many as 100 to 1,000 patients who have subclinical infections (Harrington, 1932). During the early 1930s, studies were undertaken to vaccinate humans with infected monkey spinal cord suspensions inactivated with formalin or sodium ricinoleate (Brodie and Park, 1936; Kolmer et al., 1935). However, those trials failed because of a lack of adequate controls, the failure or inability to standardize vaccine preparations, and a lack of reproducible quantitative methods for virus titration.

The battle against polio began seriously at the national level with the establishment of the National Foundation for Infantile Paralysis-March of Dimes organization in 1938. During World War II, information became available regarding the distinct antigenic types of the virus, their ability to induce specific antibody responses after inactivation, the ability of inactivated virus to induce protection against intracerebral challenge (Bodian, 1949; Morgan, 1948), and the capacity of polioviruses to replicate in vitro in human and primate tissue culture cells (Enders, 1952; Enders et al., 1949). Other wartime efforts directed toward the control of epidemics of influenza with an inactivated vaccine resulted by 1953 in a renewed interest in the development of formalin-inactivated poliovirus vaccines (Salk, 1953). The introduction of tissue culture techniques and the characterization of poliovirus passage in tissue culture were breakthroughs, and represent the cornerstone of current knowledge of cell-virus interaction. These observations significantly facilitated the development of other live attenuated or inactivated candidate vaccines (Koprowski et al., 1952; Sabin, 1955). The inactivated type of poliovirus vaccine (IPV, also known as the "Salk vaccine") was licensed in April 1955, and the oral, live-attenuated polio vaccine (OPV, also known as the "Sabin vaccine") was licensed for human use in 1961–1962 (Commission on the Cost of Medical Care, 1964).

With the introduction of polio vaccines, the incidence of poliomyelitis declined sharply. In 1965, only 59 cases of poliomyelitis were reported in the United States, and continued widespread use of OPV alone has essentially eliminated polio in the Americas. The last case of indigenously acquired wild-type poliovirus infection reported in the United States occurred in 1979 (Hinman et al., 1987). In 1985, the Pan-American Health Organization (PAHO) established the goal of eliminating poliomyelitis from the Western Hemisphere. The subsequent success of their efforts is best exemplified by the fact that the last confirmed case of paralytic poliomyelitis associated with wild-type virus infection occurred in Peru in 1991.

The worldwide rate of routine immunization for polio increased from about 47% in 1985 to 80% in 1994. The annual number of cases of polio reported decreased from 39,361 in 1985 to about 6,241 in 1990, a decline of nearly 85%. Encouraged by these dramatic results, WHO established the goal of the global eradication of poliomyelitis by the year 2000 (CDC, 1995c). The worldwide eradication campaign is relying on use of OPV, but several countries in Europe successfully eradicated poliovirus with IPV only.

Advantages of Evolving Vaccine Strategies

As pointed out earlier, the large-scale use of IPV reduced the annual reported worldwide incidence of paralytic polio to about 0.8 cases per 100,000 population (about 900 cases) by 1961. At that time, more than 485 million doses of the vaccine had been distributed in the United States. Occasional cases of disease were reported in fully vaccinated subjects in the early phases of the vaccination program, so continued efforts in vaccine development led to improvements in its biologic activity and the introduction of enhanced-potency IPV (eIPV). Vaccine failures with eIPV are much reduced from the earlier version of the vaccine. No cases of paralytic disease have been reported in subjects successfully immunized with eIPV, which is extensively used as the vaccine of choice in many parts of the world.

Since 1962, the United States had depended primarily on OPV in its polio eradication efforts. Between 1969 and 1983, however, about 225 cases of paralytic poliomyelitis associated with OPV were identified in the United States. An average of 8 to 10 cases of vaccine-associated paralytic polio continued to be reported in the United States each year. Despite the success and the benefits achieved with OPV and the continued absence of wild-type virus-associated disease, the rare occurrence of vaccine-associated paralytic disease has resulted in a change in societal and individual perspectives on the overall risk-to-benefit assessment for OPV in the United States (Plotkin, 1995). The availability of two complementary vaccines for the same disease allowed for a change in national recommendations in 1996: eIPV is now recommended for at least the first two of the four polio immunizations in the United States. This policy assures the protection of the population against natural infection of those immunized against the rare but real possibility of adverse effects of vaccination.

As the polio success story demonstrates, active vaccine development efforts in the face of changing epidemiology, scientific advances in basic virology, licensure of more than one polio vaccine, improvements in existing polio vaccines, worldwide efforts at eradication, and re-evaluation of domestic vaccination policies have all been necessary to give the U.S. population nearly complete protection from the threat of poliovirus at the close of the 20th century.

ADVANCES IN BIOTECHNOLOGY AND MOLECULAR IMMUNOLOGY AND NEW OPPORTUNITIES FOR VACCINES

As illustrated in the previous section, rapid scientific advances, changes in disease epidemiology, and development prioritization fueled the successful development of two different polio vaccines and the near eradication of a feared disease. Science has developed in an extraordinary fashion since the publication of 1985 IOM reports on vaccine development priorities (IOM, 1985a,b). These advances have occurred because of the development of molecular approaches to the cloning and characterization of virulence determinants of specific viral, bacterial, and parasitic organisms and because there is a better understanding of the cellular and molecular interactions that follow host responses to deliberate immunization or infection with a specific pathogen. This section presents a brief summary of some of the major scientific successes so that their contribution to the development of specific vaccines can be more fully appreciated.

Fundamental Understanding of Helper T Cells for Antibody Versus CMI Responses, and for Cytotoxicity

It may be useful to describe the development of regulatory T cells by simply considering mature T cells that are recent emigrants from the thymus and are naïve (e.g., they have not yet encountered an antigen as precursor T-helper cells). Note that precursors of Th cells normally recognize foreign peptides in association with major histocompatability complex (MHC) class II on antigen-presenting cells (APCs) and express the $\alpha{:}\beta$ T-cell receptor with a $CD3^+$, $CD4^+$, $CD8^-$ phenotype. On the other hand, precursors of cytotoxic T lymphocytes (pCTLs) express the $\alpha{:}\beta$ TCR. These pCTLs usually recognize foreign peptide in the context of MHC class I on target cells and normally exhibit a $CD3^+$ $CD4^-$,

CD8$^+$ phenotype. Thus, encounters with foreign antigens (peptides) result in the development of effector T cells that are either T-helper cell types for cell-mediated immunity (CMI), delayed-type hypersensitivity (DTH), or antibody responses that lyse infected target cells (cytotoxic T lymphocytes [CTLs]).

As T-helper cells mature in response to foreign antigens, they take on unique characteristics normally manifested by the production of distinct cytokine arrays. (Cytokines are nonantibody proteins released by a cell population, such as primal T lymphocytes, on contact with a specific antigen. They act as intercellular mediators, such as in the generation of an immune response.) Of great interest has been the finding that the environment and cytokine milieu greatly influence the further differentiation of T-helper cells. For example, stimulation by certain pathogens such as intracellular bacteria often leads to the formation of T-helper type (Th1) cells producing gamma interferon, interluken 2 (IL-2) and tumor necrosis factor beta, and these T cells often develop following the production of IL-12 by activated macrophages (Hsieh et al., 1993), presumably following ingestion of the particular intracellular pathogen or viral pathogen. In vivo, Th1-type immune responses are associated with the development of CMI and DTH responses and B-cell responses characterized by IgG2a antibody synthesis. On the other hand, exogenous antigen can also induce a unique CD4$^+$ T-cell subset to produce IL-4 (Seder and Paul, 1994), which can trigger the formation of Th2-type cells that produce IL-4, IL-5, IL-6, IL-9, IL-10, and IL-13 (Coffman et al., 1991; Mosmann and Coffman, 1989; Seder and Paul, 1994). This latter array of cytokines is conducive to B-cell switches from secretary IgM (sIgM) expression to certain IgG subclasses and IgE. Furthermore, Th2 cells are considered to be the major helper cell phenotype for support of IgGl, IgG2b, IgE, and IgA responses in mice.

CTLs have been shown to be important for eliminating virus-infected cells for clearing of infection (Taylor and Askonas, 1986; Yap et al., 1978; Zinkernagel and Doherty, 1979; Zweerink et al., 1977). It is generally accepted that the endogenous viral peptide processing that occurs during natural infection is a major pathway for the induction of effector CTLs. Most virus-specific CTLs are CD4$^-$, CD8$^+$ and recognize viralus peptides in association with MHC class I expressed on infected target cells. Since CTLs have been shown to be important effector cells for eliminating virus-infected cells, it will be of considerable importance to continue to determine the significance of antigen-specific CTL responses in mucosa-associated tissue, where most virus infections actually occur (see below). In this regard, several studies have shown that cell-mediated cytotoxicity, antibody-dependent cytotoxicity, and natural killer cell activity can be found in mucosa-associated tissues for immunity at sites of initial infection (Davies and Parrott, 1981; Ernst et al., 1985).

Major Advances in Mucosal Immunity

The mammalian mucosal immune system is an integrated network of tissues, lymphoid and constitutive cells, and effector molecules that protect the host from infection of the mucous membrane surfaces. This signifies a major difference from the peripheral immune system, where lymphoid cells and effector molecules are confined to individual lymph nodes, and intercommunication occurs by cell trafficking through the lymphatic and blood circulations. The induction of peripheral immune responses by parenteral vaccination does not result in significant mucosal immunity; however, the reverse is not true. Induction of mucosal immune responses can result in protective immunity in the peripheral immune compartment as well.

The mucosal immune system is anatomically and functionally divided into sites where foreign antigens are encountered and selectively taken up for the initiation of an immune response and the more diffuse collection of B and T lymphocytes, differentiated plasma cells, macrophages, and other antigen-presenting cells, as well as mast cells that comprise effector tissues for mucosal immunity. This network is highly integrated and tightly regulated. The outcome of mucosal tissue encounters with foreign antigens and pathogens can range from mucosal and serum antibody responses and T-cell-mediated immunity to systemic anergy to oral or intranasal antigen, a response that is now termed *mucosal tolerance*. The separation between the mucosal immune system and the peripheral immune system has evolved as a major host defense mechanism. Mucosal surfaces are enormous, approximately 300 to 400 m^2 and as such they require a significant expenditure of lymphoid cell elements for immunity. In this regard, the major antibody isotype in external secretions is IgA, and approximately 40 mg of IgA per kg of body weight is made in mucosal effector tissues each day, especially in the gastrointestinal tract (Conley and Delacroix, 1987). When this output of IgA is combined with its synthesis in bone marrow and peripheral lymphoid tissues, this isotype represents twice the amount of other isotypes combined, including the IgG subclasses, which are produced in higher mammals. Despite this propensity to produce IgA, the major effector cells in the mucosal immune system are T lymphocytes of both $CD4^+$ and $CD8^+$ phenotypes, and in some cases they can represent up to 80% of the entire cell population, clearly indicating their importance in mucosal immunity.

The use of vaccines that induce protective mucosal immunity thus becomes attractive when one considers that most infectious agents come into contact with the host at mucosal surfaces. Induction of mucosal immune responses may not only protect the host from morbidity and mortality due to infection but may possibly prevent infection altogether. The childhood immunization schedule recommended by the Centers for Disease Control and Prevention (CDC, 1999) lists seven vaccines that children should receive: (1) HBV; (2) diphtheria and tetanus toxoids and pertussis (DPT); (3) Hib; (4) poliovirus; (5) measles, mumps, rubella; (6) varicella; and (7) rotavirus. Of those vaccines, OPV and rotavirus are administered by the mucosal route. In fact, of 30 classes of vaccines, toxoids, and proteins currently licensed for use in the United States, only 4 (OPV, rotavirus, adenovirus, and typhoid) are administered orally (CDC, 1994b) and none are given intranasally. Although parenterally administered vaccines induce protective immune responses, they rarely, if ever, induce mucosal immune responses that may prevent infection at the site of initial contact between the host and the infectious agent. The following sections describe some of the cellular and molecular components of the mucosal immune system of relevance to current mucosal vaccine strategies.

Mucosal Immune System Organization

Generally, foreign antigens and pathogens are encountered through ingestion or by inhalation, and the host has evolved in these regions organized lymphoid tissues that facilitate their uptake. These inductive sites contain B and T lymphocytes that in the presence of appropriate antigen-presenting cells, respond to the encountered antigen by developing into effector and memory B and T cells. These antigen-specific B- and T-cell populations then emigrate from the inductive environment via lymphatic drainage, circulate through the bloodstream, and home to mucosal effector regions using distinct homing receptors that recognize mucosal addressins. Thus, mucosal effector sites include these more diffuse tissues where antigen-specific T and B lymphocytes ultimately reside and perform their respective functions (i.e., cytokine and antibody synthesis, respectively) to protect mucosal surfaces.

After the initial exposure to antigen in mucosal inductive sites, mucosal lymphocytes leave the inductive sites and home to mucosal effector tissues. Antigen-specific mucosal effector cells include IgA-producing plasma cells as well as B and T lymphocytes. Polymeric, usually dimeric, IgA is the primary immunoglobulin involved in the protection of mucosal surfaces and is locally produced in the gastrointestinal and upper respiratory tracts, nose, middle ear, gall bladder, uterine mucosa, and biliary tree as well as glandular tissues such as salivary, lactating mammary, prostate, and lacrimal glands (Phillips-Quagliata et al., 1994). The observation that antigen-specific S-IgA responses may be detected at mucosal surfaces other than the inductive site where antigen uptake initially occurred led to the discovery of the common mucosal immune system. Studies to elucidate the common mucosal immune system pathway showed that immunization of one mucosal inductive site could induce mucosal immune responses in all mucosal effector tissues. The common mucosal immune system provides a unique opportunity to develop mucosal vaccines that can be delivered orally or intranasally but that subsequently result in mucosal immunity at sites where immune protection is most desirable.

One major hallmark of the mucosal immune response is the presence of IgA antibodies at mucosal surfaces. The importance of IgA transport across epithelial surfaces to external secretions should be considered when vaccines are being designed to prevent infections that occur at mucosal surfaces. Passive transfer studies with antigen-specific monoclonal IgA antibodies have provided evidence that antigen-specific IgA alone was able to protect against intranasal influenza virus infection (Renegar and Small, 1991), intestinal infection with *Vibrio cholerae* or *S. typhi* (Winner et al., 1991; Michetti et al., 1992), and gastric infection with *Helicobacter felis* (Czinn et al., 1993). Antigen-specific IgA presumably forms immune complexes with the colonizing pathogen and thereby inhibits the interaction of the pathogen with host epithelial cells, a protective mechanism known as immune exclusion (Mestecky and McGhee, 1987). In fact, passive transfer of monoclonal IgA antibodies by a backpack hybridoma method provided protection against mucosal challenge with virulent organisms but was generally unable to prevent infection when the organisms were introduced parenterally, suggesting that mechanisms for protection at a mucosal surface do not correlate with protection from systemic challenge (Michetti et al., 1992). Therefore, induction of antigen-specific IgA responses may provide a means of totally preventing bacterial infections or at least greatly reducing the size of the infectious inoculum at the sites of initial contact between most infectious agents and the host, the mucosal surfaces.

Molecular Aspects of Virulence and Design of Recombinant Protein Vaccines

The use of recombinant techniques for the production of protein-based vaccines as well as three-dimensional immunogenic structures is well exemplified by the safe and effective recombinant HBV vaccine. Even though an effective plasma-derived vaccine for HBV has been available for many years, the recombinant DNA-derived vaccine has resulted in two licensed vaccines, the baculovirus- and yeast-derived HBV vaccines. This example can be extended to virtually all current killed or partially purified bacterial or viral vaccines. Improvements in DPT involve the use of recombinant partial structures for diphtheria (CRM 197) and tetanus (fragment C) toxoids as well as partially purified proteins from *Bordetella pertussis,* the so-called acellular pertussis vaccine. The acellular pertussis vaccines were found to be effective following several trials in Italy, Sweden, and Germany during the past 3 years. This new generation rDaPrT vaccine should be followed by a completely recombinant form of pertussis vaccine in the next few years.

Another important feature of new, recombinant vaccines involve the use of the insert baculovirus system to express genes for several proteins that comprise the virus capsid, which encloses the nucleic acid. The nucleic acid-free, viruslike particles (VLPs) represent important structures for vaccine development. For example, most pathogenic viruses express ligands in capsid proteins for receptors on host epithelial cells, which are the major initial site for virus entry into the host.

In many instances, the VLPs also retain the receptor binding ligand that allows their uptake into a mucosal inductive site. As discussed above, the mucosal and systemic lymphoid cell systems are distinct and exhibit separate modes for the induction of immunity. The use of particulate VLPs that bind epithelial cells and M cells of mucosal sites such as the Peyer's patches or GALTs may represent ideal modes for the induction of mucosal immunity to viruses.

Although polysaccharide vaccines are usually not very immunogenic in infants, the titers of antibodies are increased by covalent coupling to protein carriers such as tetanus or diphtheria toxoid. Studies indicate that conjugates elicit T-cell-dependent antibody responses characterized by higher titers and switching to non-IgM isotypes. The current major conjugate vaccines have been developed to Hib or to several different capsular polysaccharide types of *Streptococcus pneumoniae,* and these represent important advances that have used molecular immunology, chemistry, and infectious disease expertise.

Novel Vaccine Delivery Systems

A number of major breakthroughs have occurred in the development of particulate vaccines. These range from lipid- or detergent-based enclosures; for example, liposomes (Gregoriadis, 1990) and immune-stimulating complexes (ISCOMS) (Morein et al., 1984; Claassen and Osterhaus, 1992), to chemical polymers, for example, microspheres (Eldridge et al., 1990; O'Hagan et al., 1993). Microphages are briefly described here to illustrate the promise of inert particles for vaccine delivery. Several types of microspheres have been used. The coating material is usually a biodegradable polymer, and methods for microencapsulation usually involve the separation of two-phase polymers. Emulsions from solvent evaporation-extraction are common. The microspheres produced in this way are spherical. Those ranging from 1 to 10 g are most effectively taken up by antigen-presenting cells as well as M cells in mucosal inductive sites (Eldridge et al., 1990). In general, the copolymer poly (dl-lactide-coglycolide) has been more extensively studied, and variations in polymer ratios can affect the rate of hydrolysis and antigen release. Other promising microspheres involve the polyphosphacenes-polyalignates. Because of their hydration properties, they are amenable to encapsulation of proteins in physiologic buffers, which avoid denaturation.

Salmonella strains were the first to be used to investigate the potential for expression and delivery of recombinant vaccine proteins to the host immune system. This approach has been elegantly extended to other enteric gram-negative organisms, that is, recombinant *V. cholerae* and *Shigella*—as well as to recombinant bovine growth hormones, and to commensal bacteria—for example, oral streptococci and *Lactobacillus,* which is present in yogurt. However, recombinant *Salmonella* has remained the prototype for this approach and can be used to illustrate the principle (Hone et al., 1991; Chatfield et al., 1992; Tackett et al., 1992; Roberts et al., 1994). An important benefit of using recombinant *Salmonella* is that it remains an enteric bacterium that, following oral administration, colonizes and penetrates the mucosal inductive tissues via the M cell and presumably delivers recombinant proteins to elicit mucosal immunity (see below). Current attenuation mutations involve deletions of two or more genes and are designed to avoid complementation by the host or other indigenous flora. A major advantage of this approach is that oral immunization with recombinant *Salmonella* can elicit protection from *S. typhi,* and at present several vaccines relying on recombinant *Salmonella* strains are in human phase I and phase II trials.

Major breakthroughs have also been made in the development and use of former viral pathogens for the delivery of foreign antigens. Vaccinia virus has been used successfully for several antigens and cytokines. However, since most viruses impinge on the epithelium, which lines the mucosal immune system, more attention has been paid to the development of mucosal virus delivery. Two examples will suffice: recombinant poliovirus, since this has been a successful oral vaccine; and recombinant adenovirus (also a successful respiratory pathogen) for delivery to the mucosal tissues of the gastrointestinal tract as well as to the upper respiratory tract and lungs.

The success and efficacy of OPV make it an attractive vector for the delivery of mucosal vaccines, particularly when immunity to enteric pathogens is desired. This vaccine induces both mucosal and systemic immune responses and offers protection from infection. Polio-virus-specific MHC class II-restricted $CD4^+$ T cells in peripheral blood mononuclear cells from orally vaccinated individuals have also been detected. This finding suggests that poliovirus can be used as an antigen delivery vehicle to induce $CD4^+$ T-helper cells that can regulate mucosal IgA B-cell responses, in addition to the typical virus-induced CTL type of immunity.

Recently, investigators have used chimeric poliovirus genomes in which *gag* and *pol* genes of human immunodeficiency virus type 1 were substituted for the VP2 and VP3 outer capsid genes of poliovirus (Porter et al., 1993; 1995). Transfection of the minireplicon genomes containing the *gag* or *pol* gene into cells produced the appropriate fusion protein. These minireplicons were then encapsulated and amplified by transfecting them into cells previously infected with a recombinant vaccinia virus that expresses poliovirus capsid precursor protein Pl. For immunization studies, the encapsulated replicons were passaged in the presence of poliovirus type 2 Lansing, which again resulted in encapsidation of the replicons by the capsid proteins provided by poliovirus. These replicons were then given to mice by the intramuscular, intrarectal, or oral routes, and the mice were later boosted by the same route. Results from these studies indicated an increased production of antipoliovirus antibodies in serum and increased virus-specific IgA antibodies in saliva and in gastrointestinal tract secretions. In addition, the detection of anti-Gag and anti-Env antibodies in serum after intramuscular immunization and in external secretions (Moldoveanu et al., 1995) following mucosal delivery has clearly established the immunogenicities of the minireplicons.

Delivery of vaccines by intranasal immunization has shown that this is a very effective route for the induction of respiratory and parenteral immune responses. However, few recombinant, avirulent viruses and no bacteria are available to take advantage of this novel mode of immunization. One major exception is the adenovirus vectors, which have generated interest not only as a means for mucosal immunization but also as potential vectors to transfer the corrective *CFTR* gene for the treatment of cystic fibrosis. The major advantages of adenovirus are its cloning efficiency and its ability to accommodate large foreign DNA sequences. In this regard, most adenovirus-based vectors have been derived from group C adenoviruses, and the first generation of adenovirus vectors were made replication-defective by deletion of the viral one region (Yang et al., 1994). This region encodes the immediate-early gene products and is required for the initiation of viral replication. Although adenovirus vectors were rendered replication defective, a number of studies have shown that these vectors can induce unwanted inflammatory responses (Yang et al., 1994). Second-generation vaccines with additional deletions should obviate some side effects. It should be noted that an adenovirus vaccine has been given by the oral route to military recruits and has been successful. The next challenge will be to use the attenuated adenoviruses as vectors for effective intranasal immunization.

Recent studies have shown the feasibility of using recombinant plants for the generation of vaccines. Initial work with the tobacco plant showed that foreign gene expression could be accomplished. However, of more importance, it has now been shown that potato tubers may be used to express proteins including *Escherichia coli* labile toxin B subunit, rotavirus VLPs and HBV antigen (Haq et al., 1995; Thanavala et al., 1995). At present, the level of expression of recombinant protein is relatively low; however, it is anticipated that much higher levels can be achieved, making this approach one of the most promising ways of devising and producing an oral vaccine. Another interesting benefit from transgenic plant technology has been the production of a functional IgA antibody molecule (Ma et al., 1995), which again offers an alternative approach to the production of vaccines for passive mucosal immunity.

It has been known for a long time that the use of live, attenuated vaccines results in more appropriate and protective immune responses than does the use of inactivated vaccines. Expression of antigens in the host results in the correct protein conformation and glycosylation patterns. Even more important, intracellular protein processing can allow presentation by the class I MHC for effective CTL responses. A limitation to the development of vaccines against viruses such as the influenza virus is the diversity of viral envelope proteins among different strains. Therefore, efforts in vaccine development have focused on induction of memory CTLs that react to epitopes shared by different strains of virus. Most efforts to generate CTL responses have used replicating vectors to either produce the antigen in the host cell or to deliver peptides into the cytoplasm. However, the selection of peptide epitopes presented by MHC molecules is dependent on the structure of individual MHC molecules, and the peptide approach has been shown to have some limitations in humans.

As an alternate method of immunization against influenza virus (e.g., use of a plasmid), DNA vaccines have become promising approaches for the protection of mucosal surfaces. Like recombinant vectors, the transfected DNA results in the presentation of antigenic epitopes in association with the class I MHC. In addition, the significant advantages of using gene transfer technology for mucosal immunization against a pathogen such as the influenza virus are that (1) no infectious agents are being used, (2) combined vaccines are easily and rapidly made, and (3) DNA stability is not affected by high temperatures and therefore is more suitable as a vaccine in less developed countries.

The feasibility of polynucleotide vaccines was first shown in studies in which plasmid DNA was directly injected into the quadriceps of mice. Many recent studies have shown that protection against mucosal pathogens may be achieved by DNA immunization. Most DNA immunization protocols performed so far have used inoculation of the DNA into muscle cells or particle bombardment into dermal or epidermal cells. However, in nature, most foreign antigens are first confronted by the mucosa. Thus, gene administration to the mucosal surfaces would mimic exposure to most pathogens and may more efficiently induce a protective immune response. In this regard, it has been shown in mice that intranasal inoculation of a plasmid expression system for influenza virus hemagglutinin induces resistance to lethal challenge with live influenza viruses.

This technology has more recently been extended to other viruses including antigen components of human immunodeficiency virus, simian immunodeficiency virus, and rabies virus, among others. Thus far, most preclinical results have been promising, and phase I trials with DNA vaccines are now under way.

Recent Advances in Development of Novel Adjuvants

Most vaccine antigens yield only weak immune responses when given by themselves either parenterally or orally. Thus, the generation of an effective immune response usually requires the addition of an adjuvant, which is a substance that enhances the immune response. Adjuvants have been shown to affect virtually every measurable aspect of antibody responses, including the kinetics, duration, quantity, isotype, avidity, and generation of neutralizing or protective antibodies.

Certain adjuvants can enhance T-cell-mediated immunity, including both delayed-type hypersensitivity mediated by $CD4^+$ cells and CTL responses mediated by $CD8^+$ cells. However, fewer adjuvants tend to stimulate cell-mediated immune responses than to stimulate antibody formation.

Although adjuvants have been used empirically for many years, the mechanisms by which they act are not well understood, partly because the adjuvants themselves have been very complex, making such evaluations difficult (Waksman, 1979). The best-understood adjuvants have a multiplicity of effects on immune cells, and different adjutants have very divergent effects on the same cells. Waksman (1979) made the point that one must define the target cell affected by the adjuvant and the cellular and molecular modes of action of the adjuvant on the target cell. This information is either rudimentary or nonexistent for most adjuvants. Recently, more highly purified molecules have been isolated from traditional adjuvants, such as muramyl dipeptide from mycobacteria and monophosphoryl lipid A from endotoxin. This may simplify the dissection of their effects.

Although many if not all of these mechanisms are likely to apply to mucosal adjuvants as well, there is little information on agents with mucosal adjuvanticity, despite a great need for such agents. Mucosal immunization is the route of choice for protection from many pathogens, but the development of effective mucosal vaccines has lagged, in part due to a lack of suitable mucosal adjuvants. Most protein antigens are not only poor immunogens when given mucosally but also induce tolerance instead of immunity. Mucosal adjuvants are needed to overcome this potential outcome of mucosal antigen exposure. Cholera toxin has been shown to enhance the immunogenicity of relatively poor mucosal immunogens when it is mixed or conjugated together and given orally; thus, cholera toxin and its B subunit have generated a great deal of interest as potential adjuvants for vaccines.

Scientific Rationale for Vaccines against Autoimmune Diseases

During this past century, the number of diseases attributable to the body's own self-reactivity has risen, so that now it is recognized that there are autoimmune diseases directed against every organ, as well as systemic diseases affecting a broad range of systems. Examples of these diseases include diabetes, rheumatoid arthritis, multiple sclerosis, thyroiditis, myocarditis, and systemic lupus erythematosus.

Within the last 15 years, the subfield of autoimmunotherapy within immunology has made impressive strides, along with the detailed knowledge of the initiation and propagation of autoimmune diseases. Nevertheless, almost to the present, the major treatments have been (1) generic anti-inflammatory agents such as steroids, which have well-known, serious side effects; or (2) cytostatic and cytotoxic drugs whose nonspecific effects on unrelated systems lead to additional morbidity and mortality. In model animal systems, a wide variety of specific therapies in combination with the above general agents have been explored successfully with the aim of transferring this technology to human use.

Several general approaches have been attempted in the effort to either prevent or to alter the course of autoimmune diseases. One strategy is to employ specific antigens or peptides for the induction of immune tolerance among the relevant cells. This approach requires that the antigen or peptide can be defined, although more recently it has been clear that bystander regulation induced by a specific agent could be successful in preventing initiation of other immunospecific clones. A second strategy is through affecting T-cell subset choice by deviation of the T-cell system from one differentiation arm to another, such as Th1 to Th2 or Th3. The change in cytokine pattern produced by the same clone might be able to prevent specific damage, as well as provide protection by bystander suppression. A third strategy is the use of regulatory peptides derived from the T-cell receptors themselves, which are employed by the organism to bring about homeostasis through suppression of unwanted reactivity. Fourth, treatments directed against an important receptor or its mediator can have a curative effect in some cases. Finally, viral vectors carrying genes coding for specific antigen products, and/or ameliorating agents such as cytokines and chemokines have been shown to be potent response modifiers. Each of these classes of agents will now be considered in greater detail.

Immune Tolerance Induction

If immune tolerance is defined as the state in which response to a particular immunogen is absent, this would include cases in which the specific precursor T or B cell is deleted/anergized, or exhausted through chronic expansion of precursors. It would also include immune deviation where the cell in question does not become immunologically silent but rather follows a different functional program. In fact, systemic introduction of a native antigen or peptide, or one that has been modified to increase its affinity for the MHC or TcR, can induce deletion of clones with the highest affinity for the antigen. A feature of self-antigens is that under usual conditions, the B and especially the T cells directed against the most dominant self determinants will have been removed owing to deletional mechanisms in the thymus and periphery, leaving a rather large assemblage of lymphocytes directed against subdominant and cryptic determinants. This protected repertoire can be engaged under highly inflammatory conditions. The secondary determinants, which appear to then be the dominant ones, and which can activate this protected repertoire, can be removed by appropriate antigenic administration, and this may suffice to prevent autoimmunity. Another mechanism of T-cell deletion is brought about by apoptosis of specific lymphocytes, via antigen-induced T-cell death. Apoptosis can represent the final mechanism of both exhaustion and deletion.

One important feature of autoimmune pathology is that the initial response, which may be directed against a single or small number of antigenic determinants, then diversifies to include many more determinants and a broader repertoire of T cells, in what has been termed intramolecular and intermolecular determinant spreading. Thus, it appears to be important to regulate T cells directed against the initiating determinant. It has also been shown that tolerance induction to the secondary determinants plays a role in the prevention of spreading. It becomes necessary to consider how the response that has been established can be diverted effectively, and this will be the most difficult aspect of therapeutic vaccines. So far, even in model systems, the best results have been obtained by treatments close to the beginning of the appearance of symptoms.

Oral and nasal tolerance induction are very effective in regulating autoimmune diseases in animal models, and show some promise in human trials. Administration of antigen by these routes leads to a combination of effects, including deletional and anergic consequences as well as immune deviation. A deviated response that is often curative in animal models of diabetes and multiple sclerosis, for example, involves a switch from a Th1 to a Th2 direction, and will be discussed below. Much of the benefit from the tolerance induced through the mucosal route may occur by deviation. It can be hoped that for clinical purposes, when the inciting antigen(s) is (are) known, tolerance induction may lead to a broadened effect via bystander suppression or regulatory spreading.

Immune Deviation

It is evident from model systems that the induction of a Th2 (anti-inflammatory) or a Th3 (regulatory cytokine) state of differentiation can prevent or down-regulate an autoimmune disease course. One of the favored ways of accomplishing this is through mucosal introduction of antigen, which generally deviates responses in a Th2 or Th3 direction. In the type I diabetes of the non-obese diabetic (NOD) mouse, treatment involving deviation has been shown to prevent the disease at a time well after its initiation, in the midst of increasing insulitis. This occurs in what is conceived to be a Th1 mouse strain, particularly disposed towards inflammatory induction; in other strains of mice of the Th2 type, such as the BALB/c, certain autoimmune diseases are difficult to induce. The nature of the peptide chosen for therapy is an important ingredient: for example, determinants with high affinity for the MHC tend to induce Th1 responses. On the other hand, altered peptide ligands may be designed so as to induce a Th2 or regulatory response. In allergic individuals, the reverse deviation, from Th2 to Th1, may be an effective route to therapy.

Receptor-Centered Regulation

The intrinsic regulatory properties of T- and B-cell circuits can be employed in vaccines. Accordingly, it has been shown in lupus that T cells that modulate B-cell activation can be induced with peptides derived from the B-cell receptor. Likewise, in such diseases as multiple sclerosis and its animal equivalent, experimental autoimmune encephalomyelitis (EAE), or collagen arthritis, regulatory T cells specific for antigenic determinants on the aggressive T-cells receptor have been shown to exert a curative effect. In the B10.PL mouse strain, which demonstrates a single spike transient EAE, such TcR-specific regulatory T cells can be demonstrated when disease disappears, and not earlier. Recently it has been shown that the consequence of these regulatory circuits is to divert the effector population from the dangerous Th1 state to a protective Th2 direction.

Targeting Cytokines or Their Receptors

Antibodies directed against cytokines or their receptors may appear to be just one step removed from the generic type of steroid therapy. Nevertheless, applied at the right time, an agent such as anti-TNF (tumor necrosis factor) antiserum can exert a remarkable effect on patients with rheumatoid arthritis. The success of this treatment has led to more efficacious approaches now in clinical trials that counteract the effects of TNF, such as ligands that bind preferentially to the TNFa receptor.

Viral Vectors in Autoimmune Therapy

Gene therapy using viral vectors can be used to modulate autoimmune disease, not in an effort to permanently alter the recipient, but rather to provide a localized, potent, short-acting agent—more like a molecular medicine. For example, treatment with an adenovirus bearing IL-12 genes can serve as a protective vaccine for a Th2 mouse, which is unable to raise a strong, protective Th1 response against a microorganism. Such animal experiments suggest that in treatments of the near future, combinations of agents provided through genetic alteration of a viral vector will be used as prime modifiers of disease.

Preventive Vaccines for Autoimmune Diseases

Preventive vaccines for autoimmune diseases are also on the near horizon. Individuals who are genetically susceptible to type I diabetes can be identified now, and quite early in the disease course, when diagnostic antibodies appear to antigens of the islets of Langerhans, tolerance-inducing therapy to insulin or glutamic acid decarboxylase, two major candidate diabetogens, can be introduced. In other diseases in which the inciting antigens are known, immune deviation may be started at the very first signs of disease.

3

Considerations of Candidate Vaccines

The committee was charged with considering up to 30 candidate vaccines using analytic model that it developed. Far more than 30 candidate vaccines are in the research and development (R&D) pipeline. The committee struggled early in its deliberations to select the candidate vaccines to be analyzed for this report. The committee followed a modified delphi approach and winnowed a very long list of candidates into a manageable and meaningful list of 26 candidate vaccines (see Table 3-1). The committee was guided in their final decisions by its charge to consider vaccines directed against conditions of domestic health importance that could be licensed within 20 years. The committee was further guided by a set of rather firm exclusion criteria, additional considerations of a qualitative nature regarding the benefits of certain vaccines and avenues of R&D, and finally, by considerations of vaccine program implementation and utilization. Each of these points will be discussed in turn.

EXCLUSION CRITERIA

The committee was guided in their choices by a set of exclusion criteria. The following were bases for exclusion: (1) conditions for which basic science information was insufficient to predict vaccine development and licensure within 20 years; (2) potentially vaccine-preventable conditions for which other preventive interventions were deemed more appropriate; and (3) diseases of primarily non-domestic health importance. These exclusion criteria were used in the analysis undertaken for this report in order to establish a more manageable task for the committee. The exclusion criteria were not intended to guide public policy on vaccine R&D investments by either the public or private sector.

TABLE 3-1 Candidate Vaccines Included for Full Analysis*

Borrelia burgdorferi
Chlamydia
Coccidioides immites
Cytomegalovirus
Enterotoxigenic E. coli
Epstein-Barr virus
Helicobacter pylori
Hepatitis C virus
Herpes simplex virus
Histoplasma capsulatum
Human *papillomavirus*
Influenza
Insulin-dependent diabetes mellitus (therapeutic)
Melanoma (therapeutic)
Multiple sclerosis (therapeutic)
Mycobacterium tuberculosis
Neisseria gonorrhea
Neisseria meningitidis B
Parainfluenza
Respiratory syncytial virus
Rheumatoid arthritis (therapeutic)
Rotavirus
Shigella
Streptococcus, group A
Streptococcus, group B
Streptococcus pneumoniae

---

*Candidate vaccines are preventive unless indicated as (therapeutic).

Insufficient Basic Science Information

The Committee judged that a vaccine approach to control a number of diseases caused by microorganisms was not attainable within the next 20 years. In some instances not enough information was available concerning the antigens that stimulate protective immune response or the host responses necessary to provide protection. In other cases, a class of infectious agents are known to cause disease (e.g., periodontal disease), but the major contributors to disease within that class are not yet identified. In other cases, knowledge of the natural history of the infection was inadequate. Some of these infectious diseases against which vaccines were not yet considered feasible occur in healthy hosts who experience the loss of integrity of the skin or the disruption of normal intestinal barriers to microorganisms, which permits the development of secondary infections (e.g., infections caused by *Clostridium perfringens* or *Bacteroides fragilis*). Other diseases are the result of intimate exposure of healthy hosts to others who harbor certain pathogens (e.g., *Treponema pallidum* and *Mycobacte-*

riun leprae). Still others occur in individuals with underlying medical conditions that impair host defenses, allowing an opportunistic agent to become invasive (e.g., *enterococci*) or the acquisition of nosocomial agents (e.g., *Serratia marcescens*). Innovative or expanded methods for preventing nosocomial infections, with their multitude of potential specific etiologic agents, make immunization an inferior option. This list of pathogenic microorganisms excluded from consideration due to lack of scientific knowledge is not intended to be exhaustive, and the following illustration for one agent is intended to provide a rationale that would be common to several others.

Syphilis is a prominent example of an infection in the immunocompetent host that poses both a substantial disease burden and a substantial expenditure of public health resources in the United States, and against which the development of a vaccine seems unlikely in the near future. The late 1980s saw a dramatic resurgence of syphilis, especially among women (with a parallel increase in congenitally acquired infections) and among ethnic minority groups in urban areas. At least 20,000 cases of primary or secondary syphilis are reported each year, but it is estimated that only one in three or four cases is reported. Because this is a sexually transmitted infection, both the infected individual and the exposed sexual partner require counseling, diagnostic testing, treatment, and follow-up testing.

The causative agent, *T. pallidum,* has a complex morphology and composition. An outer membrane surrounds the endoflagella, cytoplasmic membrane, and the protoplasmic cylinder. It also is believed that *T. pallidum* has a glycosaminoglycan surface layer that is antiphagocytic. The organism also has more than 15 major protein constituents, some of which are covalently linked to fatty acids. The outer membrane consists of a lipid bilayer, presumably with few proteins. However, the precise cellular locations of these antigens and the identities of nonprotein constituents remain controversial.

Humoral immunity in syphilis has been studied for nearly a century. Human infection uniformly invokes immunoglobulin G (IgG) and IgM antibodies to a wide variety of *T. pallidum* proteins, but that infection progresses to secondary and eventually tertiary manifestations unless specific therapy is administered. Passive administration of serum from rabbits recovering from experimental infection attenuates but does not prevent infection. This finding and other evidence suggest that humoral immunity is not sufficient for the prevention of infection, and recent data indicate that cellular immune mechanisms are considerably more important. Thus, most experts conclude that despite the impressive disease burden attributable to syphilis, there is insufficient knowledge concerning mechanisms of protective immunity to *T. pallidum* to propose that a vaccine be developed in the near future.

Existence of Appropriate Prevention Interventions

For a number of important diseases caused by microorganisms, the committee judged a vaccine approach to be secondary compared to other public health measures for disease prevention and control. Most important among these were the great number of nosocomial infections that occur annually in the United States. These result from contamination or other conditions of hospital care that lend themselves to prevention through improved adherence to infection control procedures and universal precautions.

Prominent offending organisms in this category include *Pseudomonas aeruginosa*, enterococci, and *Staphylococcus aureus*. Of these, only *P. aeruginosa* is responsible for a significant disease burden in other contexts, such as cystic fibrosis, and even in patients with cystic fibrosis, new and innovative approaches to treating/managing the pathophysiology of the underlying disease make specific immunization a secondary option.

Another example of candidate vaccines that the committee chose not to include are waterborne pathogens. Again, this exclusion is not meant to discount the disease burden imposed by such agents but rather to emphasize that well-established and validated public health principles are available to meet the challenge of contaminated water supplies.

A third transmission mode that can be better approached by strategies other than direct immunization involves vector-borne microbial agents. In almost all instances in the United States in which vectors are involved in the transmission of serious infectious diseases, vector control is a more appropriate public health option than large-scale immunization efforts.

Finally, a number of infections of increasing importance in the United States occur in immunocompromised hosts. With the continuing HIV epidemic, the size of the susceptible immunocompromised population is increasing, and so the numbers of infections are growing among such individuals. Nevertheless, vaccine strategies are not viewed as a high priority in that setting, if only because the underlying condition that renders the host susceptible makes immunization unlikely to provide protection. That is not to say that anticipatory immunization with some of the established vaccines cannot play an important role in early intervention; rather, the range of infections caused by organisms against which new vaccines would be needed are unpredictable in a given host and occur only when the immune response is already deeply impaired.

International Burden of Disease

Without question, the great unsolved "giant" problems of global infectious disease (see Murray and Lopez, 1996) are very different from the list of priority problems that the committee has developed for the United States. Although malaria was of tremendous importance during the early history of this country, it currently occurs only sporadically among travelers returning from areas where the disease is endemic and/or rarely in limited local outbreaks secondary to their return. With such infrequent and narrow threats, efforts at vector control have proved adequate U.S. public health responses.

However, malaria is an enormous problem elsewhere, with a high morbidity and mortality burden (3 million deaths per year). The emergence of multiple-drug-resistant variants of *Plasmodium*, along with insecticide resistance among the vectors of malaria coupled with environmental impediments to vector control, are all factors that make a vaccine approach to malaria control a matter of high priority when assessed from a global perspective. Furthermore, the scientific status of malaria vaccine research promises that exciting progress may be at hand (IOM, 1996b). Therefore, although the mandated U.S. focus of the project does not include malaria, a global overview would surely place it at a high level in a list of priorities—not only malaria but, indeed, all parasitic diseases (e.g., schistosomiasis, leishmaniasis, and Chagas disease) were excluded from the committee's analysis despite their high global toll on health. Finally, some diseases are of marginal importance to U.S. citizens except during military service.

The committee has included in its analysis candidate vaccines that would be of great international benefit in addition to that gained with domestic use. Its analysis, however, does not include benefits to be gained by such international use. An analysis that included international disease burden might well have significant impact on the results (ranking or grouping into broad categories of benefits) of the modeling. For example, the resurgence of tuberculosis in the United States, and especially the emergence of multiple-drug-resistant strains, is of sufficient concern to raise it to a high level of concern even in U.S. terms. Globally, however, it dwarfs all other pathogens, causing 3 million deaths per year. It is the proximate cause of approximately half of AIDS deaths in Africa. Along with the emergence of HIV in Asia, where tuberculosis is highly prevalent, it is likely to assume even greater dominance as the most lethal infectious pathogen of humans.

Similar changes in priority might be seen for viral and bacterial respiratory infectious diseases. Improved vaccines against RSV, *Streptococcus pneumoniae,* and group A streptococci, among other agents, would also be included on a global priority ranking. Likewise, enteric viruses such as rotavirus and bacteria such as *Shigella* are important contributors to mortality worldwide.

ADDITIONAL CONSIDERATIONS FOR INCLUSION

In addition to the explicit inclusion criteria based on the charge to discuss candidate vaccines of domestic health importance and feasibility of licensure, the committee seriously considered candidate vaccines for reasons other than judgment about disease burden and likelihood of development within 20 years.

The committee notes that a policymaker concerned with decisions about investing in vaccine R&D might consider on an ad hoc basis a candidate vaccine that precipitously emerges in importance for any of several reasons (e.g., sudden shift in disease epidemiology, genetic variations, or new information linking an infectious agent to serious and chronic disease). Obviously, the committee could not second-guess such a situation and include an example.

The committee included three candidate vaccines of primary importance to a geographically restricted target population. These candidate vaccines are directed against *Coccidioides immitis, Histoplasma capsulatum,* and *Borrelia burgdorferi.* The analysis of these candidate vaccines illustrates how regionally important candidate vaccines stand in a ranking based on national importance. If one assessed the potential benefit of these vaccines compared to other candidate vaccines for those regions alone, the benefits might be quite large and apparent. The committee's model could also be used for such an assessment of regional vaccine programs.

The committee made an explicit decision to include in its analysis two candidate vaccines that were very far along in the development process. The committee knew that vaccines for both rotavirus and *Borrelia burgdorferi* could be licensed before the report was completed. In fact, vaccines for these pathogens were licensed in August 1998 and December 1998, respectively. The committee believed that readers of the report might wish to know how these vaccines compare to others in an analysis such as that performed for this report. In addition, it should be noted that the newly licensed vaccine for *Borrelia burgdorferi* is currently approved by the Food and Drug Administration for use only in people between 15 and 70 years of age. The analysis in the report is for a vaccine licensed for use in infancy. The rotavirus vaccine recently licensed matches the candidate vaccine analyzed in the report.

Other important reasons considered by the committee for including a candidate vaccine were that the population most at risk for the disease is very vulnerable. The committee ultimately decided not to include in its analysis a candidate vaccine against *Pseudomonas aeruginosa.* This infection is an important source of morbidity and mortality in persons with cystic fibrosis. It was not, however, felt to be a significant source of disease in otherwise healthy individuals. Other examples of vulnerable populations considered by the committee include organ transplant patients and persons otherwise immunocompromised, such as those with AIDS. Such populations are sometimes quite small, but the potential reductions in health care costs and improvements in health status by preventing infections make development of certain candidate vaccines worth considering.

Finally, vaccine development efforts for some diseases that impose relatively little disease burden can lead to scientific advances that will be influential for vaccine R&D years later for candidate vaccines for other diseases. For example, the committee believed that research into a vaccine against *Streptococcus mutans* will lead to benefits far beyond those achieved by prevention of dental caries. The basic and applied science of mucosal immunity will influence vaccine research for many candidate vaccines in the future. The committee did not include candidate vaccine for *S. mutans* in its analysis, but recognizes the incalculable benefit to basic science of current vaccine research in the area.

Therapeutic Vaccines

The inclusion of therapeutic vaccines directed against autoimmune diseases such as rheumatoid arthritis or multiple sclerosis is a departure from a traditional array of candidate vaccines. Because there are no licensed therapeutic vaccines, understanding of when health benefits could be realized in the course of disease with a vaccine strategy is incomplete. The varied pathophysiology of such diseases also leads to varying expectations regarding when they can be used effectively in the course of disease. It is possible that some therapeutic vaccines would provide effective treatment at later stages of disease, whereas other vaccines would be effective only in early stages. The committee assumed in its analysis that such vaccines are given near to the time of diagnosis; that is, in early disease stages.

Programmatic Considerations

An influential factor in the committee's deliberations about the qualitative inclusion criteria, and in the analytic model, concerns implementation and utilization issues. The committee expects that the report can be useful to vaccine program implementers and policymakers, as well as for the research and development community. The committee has only included vaccines it believes can be important medical and public health tools. However, the committee is cognizant of the concerns of those who will need to plan for the use of the many vaccines that could be licensed in the next 20 years. The chapter concludes with a discussion of implementation issues for children, adults, and pregnant women.

Delivery of Vaccines to Children

The use of vaccines for infant and childhood immunization in the United States is a complex issue, with multiple factors influencing the success of the implementation of the schedules recommended by the Federal Advisory Committee on Immunization Practices and the Committee on Infectious Diseases ("Redbook Committee") of the American Academy of Pediatrics (AAP). Many studies have investigated the reasons for poor compliance with these schedules and have provided greatly varying conclusions. Issues that are repeatedly encountered include the complexity of the vaccination schedule, the costs of the vaccines, problems with access to health care services, the need for multiple injections at a single visit, lack of parental awareness, competing parental priorities, parental complacency, long waiting times in public clinics, lack of reliable transportation, inappropriate interpretation by physicians and other health care workers of contraindications to immunization, missed opportunities for vaccination (at acute care or emergency room visits), poor record keeping, or the unavailability of records, and concerns regarding adverse reactions to vaccines. The single most important determinant of up-to-date vaccination status by the age of 2 years is the presence of an effective primary care system (Guyer et al., 1994).

Children should receive the majority of the recommended immunizations by age 2. In the 1970s, low rates of immunization among 4- to 6-year-old children who were entering school became a concern. Several efforts contributed to increasing immunization rates to well over 95% among this age group. Specifically, all 50 states instituted the requirement that all children must have received all of the recommended immunizations before entering the public school system. In addition, CDC, AAP, and many nongovernmental community-based organizations undertook major efforts to improve immunization rates.

In the 1990s, concern shifted to improving immunization rates among preschool-age children. Coverage rates for some specific vaccines have now risen to over 90% for 2-year-olds, but rates of completion of the full set of recommended immunizations remain below 80% (CDC, 1998). A number of imaginative programs have been undertaken to improve this rate of coverage. Some of the steps include opening public health clinics in the evening and on Saturdays to accommodate families in which both parents are employed or to accommodate single-parent families. Immunization clinics have been established in or near the offices of various federal entitlement programs such as those for the Aid to Families with Dependent Children program and the Supplemental Food Program for Women, Infants and Children. The requirement that an immunization visit include a full health examination has been abandoned in public clinics. Illinois established a program that provided public clinics with a $10 bonus for each child who was up-to-date on the recommended schedule by age 2 years and a $15 bonus for each child if the overall rate of immunization coverage at the clinics was greater than 85%. With this type of stimulation, coverage rates in Illinois have improved markedly (from 75% to 89%) despite the introduction of new vaccines that have further complicated the immunization schedules. Finally, to help make the receipt of multiple immunizations more convenient, some public schools have incorporated immunizations into their school health programs so that preschool-age infants and children may attend neighborhood-school health clinics where school health nurses or other personnel immunize younger cohorts who are not yet attending school.

In attempts to reduce the numbers of required injections, pharmaceutical firms have accelerated R&D on products that combine multiple antigens (diphtheria and tetanus toxoids and acellular pertussis vaccine plus Hib, Hib plus hepatitis B [HBV], and others yet to come). The increased costs of some of these combination products will be balanced by the eventual reduction in the number of visits required to receive immunizations.

Investments are continuing to be made in the development of vaccines that can be administered by mucosal routes (gastrointestinal or respiratory tract) obviating the need for injections. Although the oral poliovirus vaccine remains the only mucosal vaccine in widespread use, licensed vaccines against typhoid and cholera, not to mention the newly licensed vaccine for rotavirus, exemplify the potential of these routes.

In the era of managed care, reimbursement for vaccines and vaccine administration follows a number of different pathways. For some families, health insurance pays. The Vaccines for Children Program provides vaccines for nearly 60% of the nation's children. More than a dozen states provide free vaccines for all children, whatever their family's income may be.

In an attempt to overcome the problem of inadequate record keeping, immunization registries have been initiated by a number of states and communities. The registries initially covered public health clinics but have also provided the opportunity for the participation of private providers. It is hoped that registries will help overcome the major problem of a lack of availability of up-to-date immunization records during clinic and office visits. Although concerns regarding the confidentiality of records have been raised, such problems should be amenable to solution. As quality assessment programs are instituted for managed care, the provision of immunization (and other preventive medicine measures) should become a hallmark of quality performance. This too should further ease the problem of families whose current insurance coverage does not include immunization.

Delivery of Vaccines to Adults

The primary care setting is an important site for adult immunizations. In 1992, 85% of influenza immunizations in the United States were administered by private physicians to patients who paid for the vaccine themselves (Fedson, 1995). On the whole, relatively few patients received influenza vaccine from state or local health departments. Several studies have shown that high rates of immunization occur in the office setting whenever patients are offered vaccines during office visits (ACP, 1990). In one study, patient acceptance of vaccination increased 11- to 12-fold when it was recommended by health professionals (Siegel et al., 1990).

Despite the generally favorable attitudes of physicians toward vaccines for adults and evidence that vaccines are cost-effective, major gaps in adult immunization still exist. Although rates of influenza immunization for elderly people have increased nationally, with coverage rates now above 50%, pneumococcal and HBV vaccines are underused (General Accounting Office, 1995; Williams et al., 1988). Only about one-quarter of high-risk persons have ever received pneumococcal vaccine.

Physician reminders have been shown to be successful in increasing rates of immunization; physicians who received computer-generated reminders vaccinated their eligible high-risk patients twice as often as they vaccinated patients in a control group (McDonald, 1992). A simple reminder sheet completed by the clinician and detailing vaccine eligibility, patient status, and reasons for refusal of the vaccine was successful in significantly increasing the rate of influenza immunization for high-risk outpatients (Merkel, 1994).

An increasing fraction of physicians' offices in the United States are becoming computerized, and most physicians' offices are now capable of creating an electronic database for the patients they treat. These systems were originally introduced largely to improve office administration and billing practices, and their role in enhancing the delivery of preventive services has not been well developed.

Such an approach has been tested and has been shown to enhance the delivery of influenza vaccine to elderly people (Bennett et al., 1994). From 1988 to 1991 internists and family practitioners in private practices in Monroe County, New York, participated in a series of demonstration studies to determine whether a target-based approach could increase the rate of influenza immunizations among elderly people. These studies indicate that the rate of immunization can be increased substantially after physicians are made aware of target groups within their practices and are given a simple means of monitoring their rate of coverage (Buffington et al., 1991).

One important logistic hurdle in the comprehensive delivery of influenza vaccine in the office setting is that this vaccine is given during a 3-month period each fall, and eligible patients may not be scheduled to see their physicians during that time. To achieve high immunization rates, physicians must develop initiatives to immunize all eligible patients, not just those who have a visit scheduled during the period when the influenza vaccine is being given.

Hospitals are also important sites for immunization. One of the most effective interventions appears to be the implementation of standing orders for vaccination. This consists of an institutional policy stating that everyone eligible for vaccination is to be vaccinated. Under this protocol, nurses can initiate immunizations without specific orders. Perhaps the best-documented multifactorial hospital-based interventions are those described by Nichol and coworkers (1990) at the Minneapolis Veterans Affairs Medical Center. Programs that ensure that hospitalized patients are immunized with influenza and pneumococcal vaccines are particularly important because two-thirds of the patients hospitalized for pneumococcal infections had been hospitalized within the previous 5 years, and 25% or more of elderly patients admitted for influenza-associated respiratory conditions had been discharged during the immunization season immediately preceding the outbreak period (Fedson, 1987).

Emergency departments can also play an important role in providing influenza and pneumococcal immunizations, especially for people who have no other source of routine medical care. In two studies of emergency departments in university-affiliated hospitals, relatively little effort was required to raise the immunization rates. In one study of emergency department patients, 54% of unvaccinated patients were willing to be immunized when asked (Wrenn et al., 1994). In a second study, about half of elderly patients who were not vaccinated against influenza were vaccinated in the emergency department after receiving information about the vaccine (Rodriguez and Baroff, 1993).

Additional strategies for increasing vaccine use include community-based strategies. Compulsory immunization linked to school attendance has been the single most important strategy for ensuring high rates of childhood immunization among school-age children. School-based programs are also important for the delivery of adult vaccines. The American College Health Association now recommends that all students show records of receipt of vaccinations against measles, mumps, rubella, tetanus, and diphtheria. Some colleges have successfully implemented these recommendations by requiring such evidence before students enroll, before they are given grade reports, or before the transcripts of their records are issued.

Mass immunizations in settings where high-risk patients live have been particularly effective at delivering annual influenza immunizations. An underused approach is the use of Visiting Nurse Associations. Because of their contact with homebound elderly people, these nurses can effectively promote and administer the influenza vaccine. In one Canadian community-based study, public health nurses provided influenza vaccine to elderly people in their homes, at residences for senior citizens, and at well-advertised clinics (Sadoway et al., 1994). They accounted for 69% of the immunizations against influenza that were given, with an overall increase of 26% over the prior year. Potential immunization partnerships that have not been well studied include collaborations with pharmacists, chiropractors, and other health care providers who are outside the more traditional health care delivery systems.

Local health departments can play a major role in coordinating comprehensive efforts at immunizing at-risk populations. During the Medicare Influenza Demonstration Project in Rochester, New York, the Monroe County Health Department (MCHD) took responsibility for coordinating all aspects of vaccine distribution, promotion, and Medicare reimbursement (Bennett et al., 1994). For the duration of the project, proprietary nursing homes were given the option of holding open clinics, and vaccine was released to neighborhood health centers. Special urban outreach clinics were organized in churches, activity centers, and shopping malls. The coordinating role played by MCHD helped ensure that underserved and more vulnerable populations would have access to immunizations.

Encouraging Medicare beneficiaries to take advantage of preventive services is another important strategy. The most effective measures are personalized ones, such as a postcard reminder, particularly if the reminder is followed up with a telephone call (Pearson and Thompson, 1994). In the Monroe County demonstration, all Medicare beneficiaries received a letter from the Health Care Financing Administration, the federal agency that manages the Medicare program, encouraging all Part B recipients to get a free influenza immunization from their physicians. Other promotional and public health educational efforts have included television, radio, brochures, newspapers, public appearances, and press conferences.

National Health Interview Survey data indicate that African Americans and Hispanics are less likely than whites to have received pneumococcal or influenza vaccine (Centers for Disease Control and Prevention, 1995a). During the Monroe County demonstration, investigators noted low rates of immunization with the influenza vaccine among urban, nonwhite elderly people (Bennett et al., 1994). In response to this problem, MCHD convened a task force composed of representatives from urban churches, health centers, and community-based organizations to develop an action plan to increase the rates of immunization among individuals in this group of underserved Medicare beneficiaries. Partnerships were formed with organizations that could influence members of minority populations who were not receiving vaccination services. Media efforts were targeted toward this underserved population, and special outreach clinics were staffed by members of the African-American senior citizen community. Partnerships were formed with church leaders, who publicly encouraged immunization with the influenza vaccine, distributed educational materials in church bulletins, and assisted in transporting their church members to special clinics located throughout the inner city. The processes used to improve the rates of immunization among individuals in underserved groups are the same as those used among well-served groups in the population. The key difference is the selection of appropriate partners in the immunization outreach effort and ensuring that information is channeled through sources that are used by individuals in the underserved groups.

The examples described above and many others not included here provide convincing evidence that adult immunization programs can be successful if they are well organized and efficiently administered. Nonetheless, such "model" programs are in the minority. Improved immunization strategies, not simply better vaccines, will be required if substantial improvements in adult immunization rates are to be made.

Delivery of Vaccines to Pregnant Women

Immunization of pregnant women against conditions such as neonatal and pregnancy-related group B streptococcal infections has been proposed. Such efforts would eliminate the need for active immunization of infants against some diseases for which susceptibility is limited to young infants, pregnant women, and adults with either defined underlying medical conditions or advanced age.

For most vaccines targeted to pregnant women, vaccination would be given early in the third trimester (28–32 weeks of gestation), a time when organogenesis is complete and when most events associated with adverse pregnancy outcomes have passed. This timing would also theoretically provide protection for many prematurely born infants. Early in the third trimester is also a period when most pregnant women encounter the health care system. Preconceptional or adolescent encounters with the health care system are far less frequent, and efforts targeted at nonpregnancy-related health care visits would result in much lower rates of immunization than efforts targeted at pregnant women in the third trimester.

Because of the exaggerated concerns about the use of vaccines during pregnancy, the most frequent suggestion is to provide immunizations prior to childbearing. This approach requires special access to the health care system, whereas immunization during the third trimester would use existing access mechanisms and assumes that the antibody response would persist for several years at levels ensuring protection for the infant. Many experts have suggested vaccine administration around the age of puberty, and with the recommendation for booster doses of vaccines, including those for measles, mumps, rubella, and tetanus. At this age, an existing medical access system could be used. However, if a girl was immunized at age 12 years with a quadravalent group B streptococcal glycoconjugate vaccine, for example, and had her first pregnancy at age 32 years, several problems would be expected. First, it is unlikely that 20 years later levels of antibodies to this pathogen would be sufficiently high to ensure protection of the infant. Second, a small number of girls would become pregnant before the "adolescent" or "puberty" immunization visits. Third, if proof of vaccine efficacy were to require testing of adolescents and observation through the first pregnancy, the logistics and expense of such a study would likely be an even greater deterrent to the pharmaceutical industry than considering a trial that would immunize women in the third trimester.

4

Overview of Analytic
Approach and Results

The committee was charged with developing an analytic framework and an associated quantitative model that can aid in setting priorities for vaccine research and development. The committee sought an approach that makes it possible to compare the different potential new vaccines on the basis of their anticipated impact on both costs and benefits. The committee has used a cost-effectiveness model adapted from the model developed for the previous Institute of Medicine (IOM) study of priorities for vaccine development (IOM, 1985a). The model was implemented with spreadsheet software run on a personal computer. This chapter reviews key strengths and limitations of cost-effectiveness models, provides an overview of key components of the committee's analysis, illustrates certain features of the model with hypothetical vaccine examples, and describes the results obtained by the committee when the model was applied. The committee examined 27 separate cases, each representing a specific combination of pathogen or condition, a candidate vaccine, and a population targeted to receive the vaccine. The committee examined 26 candidate vaccines, but included two distinct target populations for one candidate, thus 27 separate cases (see Table 4-1). The specifics of the calculations are described in Chapter 5 for those readers who desire more detailed explanations.

A COST-EFFECTIVENESS APPROACH

A variety of analytic methods are available for comparative assessments to support priority-setting and resource allocation decisions. In selecting the approach to be used for this study, the committee had to have a means of

54

Table 4-1 Vaccine Candidates

Vaccine	Target Population	Utilization (%)	Purchase $ (per dose)	Time to Licensure	Development $ (millions)
BORRELIA					
	Infants (restricted geography)	90	100	3	120
	Migrants (restricted geography)	10	100	3	120
CHLAMYDIA					
	12-year-olds	50	50	15	360
COCCIDIOIDES IMMITIS					
	Infants (restricted geography)	90	50	15	360
	Migrants (restricted geography)	10	50	15	360
CYTOMEGALOVIRUS					
	12-year-olds	50	50	7	360
ENTEROTOXIGENIC E. COLI					
	Infants	90	50	7	240
	Travelers	30	50	7	240
EPSTEIN-BARR VIRUS					
	12-year-olds	50	50	15	390
HELICOBACTER PYLORI					
	Infants	30	50	7	240
HEPATITIS C					
	Infants	90	50	15	360
HERPES SIMPLEX VIRUS					
	12-year-olds	50	50	7	240
HISTOPLASMA CAPSULATUM					
	Infants (restricted geography)	90	50	15	360
	Migrants (restricted geography)	10	50	15	360
HUMAN PAPILLOMAVIRUS					
	12-year-olds	50	100	7	360
INFLUENZA					
	Universal (every 5 years)	30	50	7	360
INSULIN-DEPENDENT DIABETES MELLITUS (therapeutic)					
	Early-stage patients	90	500	15	360

MELANOMA				
Patients	90	500	7	360
MULTIPLE SCLEROSIS				
Patients	90	500	15	360
MYCOBACTERIUM TUBERCULOSIS				
High-risk populations	90	50	15	360
Universal in multidrug-resistant areas	60	50	15	360
NEISSERIA GONORRHEA				
12-year-olds	50	50	15	360
NEISSERIA MENINGITIDIS B				
Infants	90	50	7	300
PARAINFLUENZA				
Infants	90	50	7	300
12-year-old females	90 or 10	50	7	360
RESPIRATORY SYNCTIAL VIRUS				
Infants	90	50	7	360
12-year-old females	50	50	7	360
RHEUMATOID ARTHRITIS				
Patients	90	500	15	360
ROTAVIRUS				
Infants	90	50	3	120
SHIGELLA				
Infants	90	50	7	240
Travelers	30	50	7	240
STREPTOCOCCUS GROUP A				
Infants	90	50	15	400
STREPTOCOCCUS GROUP B				
High-risk people, and either:	30	50	7	See below
12-year-old females or	50	50	7	300
Women in their first pregnancy	10 or 90	50	7	400
STREPTOCOCCUS PNEUMONIA				
Infants	90	50	3	240
65-year-olds	60	50	3	240

comparing the anticipated health benefits and costs of vaccine use across drastically different forms of illness, ranging from pneumonia, ulcers, and cancers to temporary and long-term neurologic impairments. Furthermore, some of the vaccines included in the study are intended to treat illness, while most will be used in the more familiar role of preventing disease.

Cost-effectiveness analysis was judged to be the most satisfactory way to make these comparisons. The basis of comparison typically is a cost-effectiveness ratio that is expressed as cost per unit of health benefit gained. Monetary costs—the numerator of the ratio—reflect changes in the cost of health care that are expected to result from the use of an intervention such as a new vaccine plus costs associated with developing and delivering the intervention. Health benefits—the denominator of the ratio—increasingly are measured in terms of quality-adjusted life years (QALYs) gained by using the intervention under study. QALYs are a measure of health outcome that assigns to each period of time a weight, ranging from 0 to 1, corresponding to the health-related quality of life during that period, where a weight of 1 corresponds to optimal health, and a weight of 0 corresponds to a health state judged equivalent to death; these are then aggregated across time periods (Gold et al., 1996). The concept of QALYs, developed in the 1970s, was designed as a method that could integrate the health improvements for an individual from changes in both the quality and quantity of life, and could also aggregate these improvements across individuals (Torrance and Feeny, 1989). QALYs provide a summary measure of changes in morbidity and mortality that can be applied to very different health conditions and interventions. Interventions that produce both a health benefit and cost savings are inherently cost-effective, but many other interventions that do not save costs produce benefits at costs that are judged to be reasonable.

Although cost-effectiveness analysis facilitates comparisons among interventions, comparisons across studies are often undermined by critical differences in assumptions and analytic techniques. A report by the Panel on Cost-Effectiveness in Health and Medicine (Gold et al., 1996), convened by the U.S. Public Health Service, reviews the field and provides recommendations intended to improve the quality and comparability of studies. In its assessment of potential new vaccines, the committee has generally followed the recommendations of that panel. An analysis such as the one performed by the present committee is a valuable tool in a variety of contexts for decisionmakers who must set priorities and allocate resources. It simplifies a complicated picture in which vastly different forms of illness and health benefit must be compared and related to a variety of costs. It cannot, however, address all of the qualitative judgments that shape policy decisions. The analysis cannot provide the value judgments required to determine whether expected health benefits and costs justify a particular investment in vaccine development. The aim of the analysis is to clarify trade-offs in decisions to invest in the development of one vaccine as compared to another.

Reasons for Using Cost-Effectiveness Analysis

Several factors make cost-effectiveness analysis particularly well-suited to the committee's assessment of vaccine development priorities. It is a well-established tool for informing decisions regarding the allocation of resources related to health and health care. Comparisons of the benefits of preventing or treating very different forms of illness are made possible by measuring all health benefits in terms of QALYs. Cost-benefit analysis is similar in many respects to cost-effectiveness analysis but relies on valuing benefits in monetary terms. Cost-effectiveness analysis values health consequences in terms of their impact on the health of a community, while cost-benefit analysis values those consequences in terms of the monetary willingness of citizens to pay for them. Cost-effectiveness analysis is generally preferred for health-related studies because many health policymakers and analysts question the appropriateness of measuring the value of additional life expectancy or other health benefits in monetary terms, and because they have ethical qualms about using willingness to pay (and, implicitly, ability to pay) as a basis for guiding resource allocation.

The cost-effectiveness approach also provides a framework within which the components of the analysis can be specified in detail and evaluated by those who use the results. This is particularly helpful for the committee's analysis, which, of necessity, rests on many estimates and assumptions about the characteristics of future vaccines and their likely impact on health and costs. The detailed specification of the components of the model also facilitates sensitivity analyses for the testing of alternative estimates and assumptions, either for individual patients or for a population. Sensitivity analyses are discussed later in the chapter.

Limits of Cost-Effectiveness Analysis

The cost-effectiveness analysis used by the committee can provide an estimate of the cost of achieving the anticipated health benefit for each of the vaccines studied, but it cannot determine whether that health benefit is worth the cost. That decision is a value judgment and should reflect consideration of many factors that are not included in the analysis. For example, the committee's analysis does not consider what resources will or should be available for vaccine development or how many vaccine candidates should be given priority for development. Moreover, the analysis does not address the allocation of resources between vaccine development and the development and use of other forms of prevention or treatment. Although priority setting and resource allocation can be informed by economic analyses, they require value judgments that cannot be captured by a cost-effectiveness model.

It is also important to note that the results of the analysis depend on the accuracy and appropriateness of the data and the assumptions that are used, a point of particular relevance to the committee's work. Assumptions were necessary both to compensate for the limitations of the available data on current disease incidence and costs of care and to simplify some analytic tasks. Moreover, the vaccines that are the focus of the study are still in development, making it necessary to rely on expert judgment for values such as costs of vaccine development and time until a vaccine will be licensed for use. Those who use the committee's analysis or similar studies should keep in mind that although the results are quantified, they should not be treated as precise measures.

Ethical Issues

Cost-effectiveness analysis raises several ethical issues, especially in the context of priority setting. Although ethical issues are discussed in greater detail in Chapter 6, a few ethical concerns should be mentioned here in the context of cost-effectiveness analyses. Some of these concerns are a function of value judgments incorporated into the model, and others are related to issues that are not addressed. For example, within the model, all QALYs are considered equal without regard to the nature of the health benefit that they measure. Thus, the number of QALYs for many people receiving a small health benefit as a result of a reduction of a minor form of illness can be the same as the number of QALYs achieved by averting a very small number of deaths. Some question the appropriateness of using such trade-offs. (See Chapter 6 for additional discussion.)

Whether these quality-adjusted years of life should be counted equally across all ages is a separate concern. The committee specifically chose not to follow the practice of some analysts who have assigned a greater value to the economically productive adult years than to years at younger or older ages (Murray and Lopez, 1996). The committee's principal analysis follows the standard practice for QALY-based analysis of assuming that a QALY, once calculated, is not directly affected by age. The structure of the model, however, would permit others to perform analyses that incorporate age- or condition-specific weighting of QALYs.

Not addressed by the model are issues of equity in the allocation of resources. Some might argue that the needs of specific populations such as those defined by race, ethnicity, socioeconomic status, or health status should be given a higher priority than would be suggested by a strict ranking of cost-effectiveness ratios. The responsibility for judging what constitutes an equitable allocation should lie with accountable policymakers.

Analytic Perspectives

The analysis reflects several decisions by the committee regarding the approach to be used. These decisions resulted in the adoption of a societal perspective for measuring health effects and costs; a domestic perspective for identifying diseases of significance; an incremental perspective regarding the benefits that the vaccines under study would bring in comparison to current forms of care; and a steady-state perspective for assessing likely levels of vaccine use.

A societal perspective for measuring health effects and costs in the United States means that all significant health outcomes and costs are taken into consideration, regardless of who experiences them. Thus, if use of a vaccine reduces hospital care costs, the analysis does not have to distinguish between cost savings that accrue to individuals and savings that accrue to insurers.

The societal perspective can be contrasted with a more selective perspective, such as that of a particular government agency, health plan, or vaccine manufacturer, that might be used to examine these factors in other analyses. For these more selective analyses, the assessment of health effects might be limited to the members of a health plan or to a particular age group such as the Medicare population. Similarly, the costs (or savings) included in the analysis would be limited to those that would be incurred by the particular agency or organization. Costs borne by individuals or other organizations would not be considered in the analysis. A societal perspective, however, examines all costs and the health experience of the entire population.

The analysis also reflects the domestic perspective in the charge to the committee. The vaccine candidates analyzed in depth were selected on the basis of their relevance to health status in the United States, not globally. Thus, for the vaccines that are likely to be used in many countries in addition to the United States, the analysis includes only a portion of the total health benefits and savings in costs of care that can be expected for relatively little additional investment in vaccine development. Excluded from the analysis are other vaccines that would be valuable for conditions that are important health problems in other countries, such as malaria and schistosomiasis, but that pose little threat in the United States. The committee would have liked to have examined the effect of a global perspective on the results of the analysis. To do so would have greatly increased the committee's task and would have introduced sufficient uncertainties into the estimates that their relevance for domestic policy would be greatly undermined. Additional discussions of conditions of particular importance outside of the United States appear in Chapters 3 and 7.

The cost-effectiveness ratios calculated for this study represent the estimated incremental changes in costs and health effects that can be expected with the use of a new vaccine compared to those from the use of current forms of prevention and treatment. For the vaccines against influenza and *Streptococcus pneumoniae*, the analysis must also consider the costs and health effects associated with the use of existing vaccines.

The committee has based its analysis on the patterns of annual vaccine use that are expected at the point at which a "steady-state" of usage has been achieved. When a vaccine is first introduced, initial patterns of use can be expected to be unstable and to differ from those that will be seen in later years when a more stable level of use has been reached. During this period of instability, both costs and health benefits will vary from year to year in ways that are difficult to estimate and that will differ from the typical costs and health benefits expected at steady-state levels of use. Several factors are likely to contribute to the early variation and instability in patterns of use. As the health care system and the public become more familiar with a vaccine, levels of use in a vaccine's planned target population are likely to increase over time. The initial period of vaccine use is also likely to be affected by efforts to "catch up" on coverage. For preventive vaccines, this would involve administering additional doses of vaccines to groups beyond the target population, thus increasing the cost of vaccine delivery and altering the assumptions regarding the timing of health benefits relative to vaccination. Similarly, for some therapeutic vaccines, a catch-up effort might include administering the vaccine to a portion of the population of patients who already have a condition in addition to newly diagnosed cases. Treating these patients might contribute some added health benefits in the early years of vaccine use, as well as added costs, that would not match the levels associated with what the committee's analysis has assumed to be a typical level of vaccine use. (In the case of diabetes and perhaps other therapeutic vaccines, however, such catch-up vaccination efforts will not be effective in treating established cases of illness.)

Time Horizon and Discounting

The conditions that the committee studied have different time lines for development of a vaccine, the age at which the vaccine would be given, and the age at which health effects and related costs would be experienced. For example, one vaccine might be available in 3 years for use in infants to prevent a condition that usually occurs within the first 2 years of life. Another vaccine might require 15 years in development for use in adolescents to prevent a condition that usually occurs at about age 50. For the first vaccine, benefits might be observable within 5 years, but for the second one, more than 50 years would be needed to realize the benefits of the vaccine.

To provide a common point of comparison for the analysis, the health effects and costs for each case are calculated on an "annualized" basis and are discounted to their present values. The annualized estimates reflect the lifetime stream of health effects and costs that result from cases occurring during 1 year. The costs of vaccine development, which are assumed to be independent of the number of people who will use the vaccine, are prorated, or "amortized," to produce an estimate of annual costs.

Determining the "present value" of these health effects and costs requires the use of discounting to adjust their value on the basis of the interval between the present and the time at which the health effect or the cost will occur in the future. A standard assumption in cost-effectiveness analysis is that future dollars and health benefits have a lower value than dollars and health benefits available in the present. The scale of this "time preference" for present over future consumption is captured by the discount rate, which has been set at 3% for the committee's basic analysis, as recommended in the review of cost-effectiveness methods (Gold et al., 1996). The discount rate is also used to amortize the fixed expenditure for vaccine development. Because some analysts question the appropriateness of discounting health effects (for a discussion of the issue, see Gold et al., 1996), the committee tested the impacts of using no discounting in its sensitivity analyses, which are reviewed later in this chapter.

MODEL OVERVIEW

The essential calculation for the cost-effectiveness ratio for each candidate vaccine is the net cost (i.e., the costs of vaccine development plus the costs of administering the vaccine to the target population, minus the saving in cost of care expected with the use of the vaccine) divided by the expected gain in health benefits. Interested readers are referred to several recent publications (e.g., Gold et al. 1996, Russell et al., 1996).

Health Benefits: The Denominator

Measuring the health benefits of vaccine use requires a quantitative assessment of a condition's "burden of illness" in terms of both morbidity and mortality. The difference between the current burden of illness associated with each condition and the level that would be expected if a vaccine were in use represents the health benefit attributable to the vaccine. To compare the vaccines under study, the measure of the burden of illness must be applicable to widely varied conditions (e.g., pneumonia, meningitis, diarrhea, urethritis, melanoma, diabetes). The committee made this comparison using QALYs, a standard measure of burden of illness and health benefits for cost-effectiveness analyses (Gold et al., 1996).[*] QALYs reflect the combined impact of morbidity and mortality on the health-related quality of years of life lived. The measure can be applied to the total lifetime or to a specified interval such as the time spent with a temporary disability. The key steps in calculating health benefits are briefly reviewed here and illustrated further in Box 4-1. The entire process is reviewed in greater detail in Chapter 5 and summarized in Box 5-1.

---

[*]A substantial literature exists on the theory and practice of quantifying health status and the burden of illness. Key issues include defining the domains of health status, developing instruments to measure health status, determining preferences for health states, and applying health status measures to quality of life adjustments. Some sources that readers may wish to consult include Bergner et al., 1981; Drummond et al., 1987; Kaplan and Anderson, 1988; Ware and Sherbourne, 1992; Patrick and Erickson, 1993; McDowell and Newell, 1996; IOM, 1998.

BOX 4-1 Illustrating the Calculation of a Vaccine's Health Benefits

The basic features of the calculation of QALYs can be illustrated with a simple scenario. Assume 100,000 cases of an illness X, occurring at an equal rate at all ages and no deaths. Half of the cases of disease result in a mild illness determined to have an HUI-based quality-adjustment weight of .90 and half in a moderate illness with a quality adjustment weight of .70. Either form of illness is assumed to last 2 weeks (.0384 years).

The quality-adjustment weights for illness X must be adjusted for the underlying health status of the population. Using survey-based data on general health status, the average quality–adjustment weight for the health status of the population without this illness is .896. Thus the adjustment weight for the mild form of illness becomes .806 (.90 • .896) and the weight for the moderate form of illness becomes .627 (.70 • .896).

To calculate QALYs, these adjustment weights are multiplied by the time spent with the illness. With a 2-week duration, a case of mild illness occurring in a given year accounts for .031 QALYs (.806 • .0384). With the same 2-week duration, a case of moderate illness accounts for .024 QALYs (.627 • .0384). For an individual in the general population not experiencing this illness, the same 2-week period would represent .034 QALYs (.896 • .0384).

Use of a vaccine that prevents illness X would result in a gain of .003 QALYs for a case of mild illness (.034 – .031) and .010 QALYs for a case of moderate illness (.034 – .024). With cases distributed evenly between mild and moderate illness, the average gain would be .007 QALYs [(.5 • .003) + (.5 • .010)]. With 100,000 cases per year, the annual gain for the population would amount to 700 QALYs (.007 • 100,000). (The complete analysis would also require discounting QALYs for the interval between age at vaccination and average age of onset of illness X.)

Quality Adjustments: Weighting

To calculate QALYs, a quality-adjustment weight is applied to each period of time during which a person experiences a changed health state due to a particular condition, and these quality-adjusted time periods are added together. In theory, "perfect health" carries a weight of 1.0, giving full value to periods to which it applies. Death carries a weight of 0.0. A health state judged to be equivalent in quality to death would also have a weight of 0.0, meaning that time spent in that health state would have a QALY value of 0.0. A condition considered worse than death can be assigned a negative weight. These quality-adjusted periods can be summed over a person's expected lifetime (or some other specified period of time).

Several methods are available for determining the quality-adjustment weights to be applied to calculate QALYs. For this purpose, the committee selected the Health Utilities Index (HUI) Mark II (see, e.g., Patrick and Erickson, 1993; Feeny et al., 1995; Torrance et al., 1995; McDowell and Newell, 1996). The HUI Mark II characterizes morbidity by using seven health attributes (sensation, mobility, emotion, cognition, self-care, pain, and fertility), each of which is divided into three, four, or five levels. Each level has a fixed quantitative score representing the "preference" for that level relative to full health or death. For the HUI Mark II, these preferences are derived from analyses of responses of a random sample of parents in a Canadian community (Torrance et al., 1995). As illustrated in Box 4-2, the score for normal function in any attribute is 1.0. Deviations from that level of functioning are scored somewhere between 0 (death) and 1. The score for limitations in sensory functions even with equipment (e.g., glasses or hearing aids) is 0.86. The score for severe pain not relieved by drugs and leading to constant disruption of normal activities is 0.38.

Other quality-adjustment systems considered by the committee include the Disability-Distress Index (DDI) (Rosser, 1987; Rosser, et al., 1992; Kind and Gudex, 1994), the Quality of Well-Being Scale (QWB) (Kaplan and Anderson, 1988), and the World Bank/World Health Organization disability used to calculate disability-adjusted life years (DALYs) (Murray and Lopez, 1996). The HUI Mark II system was preferred to these alternatives because the multiple levels of its seven component attributes provided an explicit and flexible framework for the committee to use in characterizing the morbidity associated with diverse conditions included in the analysis. The HUI Mark II permits the identification of 24,000 unique health states versus 29 for DDI and 6 for DALYs. The QWB was not chosen because its weights tend to overvalue mild health problems. Some authors have attributed this problem with the QWB to the fact that the weights were obtained by rating scale methods rather than explicit tradeoff elicitation (Eddy, 1991). The HUI Mark II system was favored over DALYs because its weights are derived from community-based health-state preferences rather than expert judgment and are determined without regard to age. Another factor in the committee's decision to use the HUI Mark II was the availability from the Canadian National Population Health Survey of age-specific health status weights for a general population (Wolfson, 1996). Although the committee found the HUI to be the most suitable instrument for its purposes, the model can accommodate quality-adjustment weights derived in other ways.

Morbidity Scenarios

The committee, with the advice of outside experts, developed morbidity scenarios to describe the characteristic patterns of illness associated with each condition under study. A scenario consists of a sequence of acute or chronic health states of specified duration that are experienced by a specified proportion of patients. The scenarios also capture the premature mortality associated with a condition, but is delayed 1 or more years beyond the onset of the condition. For example, some infants infected with group B streptococcus at birth survive with neurologic impairment for several years but die by about age 10.

BOX 4-2 HUI-based Quality-adjustment Weight for Ectopic Pregnancy				
Attribute	Description		Utility Function	
1. Sensory	1. Able to see, hear, and speak normally for age	√	1.00	
	2. Requires equipment to see or hear or speak		0.95	
	3. See, hears, or speaks with limitations, even with equipment		0.86	
	4. Blind, deaf, or mute		0.61	
1. Sensory Total				b1 = 1.0
2. Mobility	1. Able to walk, bend, lift, jump and run normally for age		1.00	
	2. Walks, bends, lifts, jumps, or runs with some limitations, but does not require help		0.97	
	3. Requires mechanical equipment (such as canes, crutches, braces, or wheelchair) to walk or get around independently		0.84	
	4. Requires the help of another person to walk or get around and requires mechanical equipment as well	√	0.73	
	5. Unable to control or use arms and legs		0.58	
2. Mobility Total				b2 = .73
3. Emotion	1. Generally happy and free from worry		1.00	
	2. Occasionally fretful, angry, irritable, anxious, or depressed (or suffering night terrors—for children)		0.93	
	3. Often fretful, angry, irritable, anxious, depressed, (or suffering night terrors—for children)		0.81	
	4. Almost always fretful, angry, irritable, anxious, or depressed	√	0.70	
	5. Extremely fretful, angry, irritable, or depressed, usually requiring hospitalization or psychiatric institutional care		0.53	
3. Emotion Total				b3 = .7
4. Cognitive	1. Learns and remembers normally for age (e.g. schoolwork—for children)		1.00	
	2. Learns and remembers more slowly than normally for age (e.g. schoolwork, for children)	√	0.95	

BOX 4-2 *Continued*				
	3. Learns and remembers very slowly and usually requires special assistance in learning situations		0.88	
	4. Unable to learn and remember		0.65	
4. Cognitive Total				b4 = .95
5. Self-care	1. Eats, bathes, dresses, and uses the toilet normally for age		1.00	
	2. Eats, bathes, dresses, or uses the toilet independently with difficulty		0.97	
	3. Requires mechanical equipment to eat, bathe dress, or use the toilet independently	√	0.91	
	4. Requires the help of another person to eat, bathe, dress, or use the toilet		0.80	
5. Self-care Total				b5 = .91
6. Pain	1. Free of pain and discomfort		1.00	
	2. Occasional pain; discomfort relieved by nonprescription drugs or self-control activity without disruption of normal activities		0.97	
	3. Frequent pain; discomfort relieved by oral medicines with occasional disruption of normal activities		0.85	
	4. Frequent pain; frequent disruption of normal activities; discomfort requires prescription narcotics for relief	√	0.64	
	5. Severe pain; pain not relieved by drugs and constantly disrupts normal activities		0.38	
Pain Total				b6 = .64
7. Fertility	1. Able to have children with a fertile spouse		1.00	
	2. Difficulty in having children with a fertile spouse	√	0.97	
	3. Unable to have children with a fertile spouse		0.88	
Fertility Total				b7 = .97
Health State: Utility Function	$1.06 \cdot (b1 \cdot b2 \cdot b3 \cdot b4 \cdot b5 \cdot b6 \cdot b7) - .06$			
	$[1.06 \cdot (1.0 \cdot .73 \cdot .70 \cdot .95 \cdot .91 \cdot .64 \cdot .97) - .06 = .23]$			HUI = .23

For most of the conditions included in the committee's analysis, several scenarios were required to depict the associated morbidity. To illustrate some of the features of these scenarios, the scenarios developed for *Neisseria meningitidis* B are presented in Box 4-3.

BOX 4-3 Morbidity Scenarios: *Neisseria meningitidis* B

	Duration	HUI		Duration	HUI
Meningitis (ICU)			**Bacteremia/ Sepsis**		
ICU	2 days	0.24	ICU (Waterhouse Friederichsen)	4 days	0.16
Inpatient after ICU	5 days	0.28	Inpatient after ICU	10 days	0.44
Meningitis (no ICU)			**Bacteremia/Sepsis (no ICU)**		
Inpatient	5 days	0.39	Inpatient	5 days	0.71
Meningitis complications			**Bacteremia/Sepsis—complications**		
Acute complications (gangrene, arthritis, heart failure, etc.)	10 days	0.27	Acute complications (cardiac, DIC, pneumonia, etc.)	10 days	0.59
Meningitis sequelae			**Bacteremia/Sepsis—sequelae**		
Neurologic sequelae (cranial nerve damage, deafness, etc.)	(remaining lifetime)	0.60	Amputation, etc.	(remaining lifetime)	0.63

NOTE: ICU = intensive care unit; DIC = disseminated intravascular coagulation.

Once the morbidity scenarios were developed, the committee reviewed each health state and assigned a level in each of the seven attributes of the HUI Mark II. Box 4-2 shows the committee's attribute scoring for one health state (ectopic pregnancy). The quality-adjustment weight for the health state was obtained by combining the scores for each attribute using the multiplicative HUI Mark II formula. Box 4-4 shows examples of the quality adjustment weights obtained for several health states.

Quality Adjustments for Average Population Health States

To measure the health benefits associated with an intervention such as the use of a new vaccine, it is necessary to compare health status with and without the intervention. The quality-adjustment weights for each condition's morbidity scenarios (described above) are used to calculate QALYs lived without the intervention. Quality-adjustment weights reflecting the average health status of the population are used to calculate QALYs lived with the intervention. To measure the impact of mortality and lifetime impairment, life-expectancy was "quality adjusted" for the average health status of the population and discounted to its present value. For example, the life expectancy at birth is 75.5 years in the 1993 life tables used in the committee's analysis. The discounted quality-adjusted present value of that life expectancy is 26.8 years. For a person 50 years old

---

BOX 4-4 Examples of Quality-Adjustment Weights Obtained
Using the Health Utility Index

HUI Range	Disease	Health State	HUI
≥.90	Epstein-Barr virus	Uncomplicated mononucleosis	
	Histoplasma	Flu-like illness	0.90
	Insulin-dependent diabetes	Uncomplicated (first 20 years)	0.90
>.50, <.90	Neisseria gonorrhea	Urethritis	0.84
	Coccidioides immitis	Pneumonia (outpatient)	0.75
	Enterotoxigenic E. coli	Prolonged diarrhea	0.75
	Rheumatoid arthritis	Moderate joint pain	0.72
	Chlamydia	Chronic pelvic pain	0.60
	Influenza	Pneumonia (hospitalization)	0.52
≤.50	Cytomegalovirus	Severe CNS sequelae	0.48
	Helicobacter pylori	Complications of peptic ulcer disease	0.40
	Streptococcus, Group B	Meningitis	0.27
	Herpes Simplex Virus	acute encephalitis	0.19
	Streptococcus, Group A	toxic shock or severe necrotizing fasciitis	0.16

NOTE: CNS, central nervous system.

---

today, the life-expectancy is 29.2 years; the discounted quality-adjusted present value of that life expectancy is 15.7 years.

The average health status in the population represents the maximum level of health that can be achieved by use of the vaccines under study. Although an individual might be considered to experience periods of perfect health, represented by a quality-adjustment weight of 1.0, the health status of a population will reflect a range of individual quality levels and should not be represented by a quality-adjustment weight set at 1.0. The committee adopted HUI Mark II-based age- and sex-specific health status results from the Canadian NPHS (Wolfson, 1996) to serve as the quality-adjustment weights for the health status of the U.S. population. The weighted average of the population HUI ranges from 0.92 for people 44 years of age and under to 0.66 for people 85 years of age and older.

Disease Incidence and Death Rates

Estimates of current age-specific incidence and mortality for each condition were assembled on the basis of the published literature, the advice of experts in clinical medicine and epidemiology, and the judgment of committee members. Although data are available from surveillance systems for some of the conditions included in the analysis, the completeness of reporting varies by condition. Some estimates are based on data from state- or community-level studies. Others rest largely on expert judgment. The specific sources of data for each condition are described in the Appendixes. For all conditions, the analysis uses incidence data, that is, the number (or rate) of new cases that would be expected during 1 year. For chronic illnesses such as multiple sclerosis, these data will differ from the estimates of prevalence that are often reported.

Time Intervals

As described in a previous section, discounting is applied to future health benefits as well as costs. The timing of the health benefits expected from the use of the potential new vaccines included in the committee's analysis will vary depending on the intervals between the typical age at immunization and the age at onset of an illness or the age at death. The intervals calculated for the analysis are the following: the time from vaccination to the average age at onset of illness, and the difference between the average age at onset of illness and average age at the time of illness-related death. The latter is of interest for those acute conditions for which the age at death from the condition differs markedly from the overall age of patients with that condition. The time interval related to premature death following a period of chronic illness is accounted for separately.

Age at vaccination was determined by the vaccination strategy, as reflected by the target population. Most cases fall into one of the following categories:

Target Population	**Age at Vaccination**
Infants	6 months
Adolescents	12 years
Pregnant women	Average age of mothers at first births, minus 2 months (24.7 years)
New cases (therapeutic vaccines)	Age at diagnosis (assumed to equal average age at onset)

See Table 4-1 for information on the designated target population for each candidate vaccine.

QALYs Gained with Vaccine Use

To calculate health benefits anticipated with vaccine use, the QALYs associated with each health state were combined. First, the state-specific QALYs were summed for each morbidity scenario. By using the scenario totals, the QALYs lived with the condition under study were subtracted from the QALYs for the general population without the condition. This provides an estimate of the QALYs that could be gained in each scenario with vaccine use.

The scenario-specific QALYs to be gained were multiplied by the proportion of cases of illness experiencing that scenario and were summed across all scenarios. This total was multiplied by the number of cases, or by the number of deaths for the QALYs associated with mortality, to calculate the overall benefit that the use of a vaccine for the condition under study would be expected to have in the population. If subpopulations were used in the analysis, the results were calculated for each subpopulation, and the subpopulation results were summed to produce an estimate of the total health benefit.

Costs: The Numerator

Costs associated with the development and use of a vaccine provide the numerator of the cost-effectiveness ratio for each of the cases considered by the committee. The cost components include the costs of vaccine development, the cost of vaccine use, and the reduction in health care and related costs that would be expected with vaccine use. All cost estimates are presented in constant dollars.

Cost of Research and Development

The costs of future research and clinical trials needed to complete development of a vaccine and have it licensed are a mix of public- and private-sector expenditures, of which the private-sector component is especially difficult to estimate. In the absence of real data regarding these development costs, they were assumed to fall at one of six levels: $120 million, $240 million, $300 million, $360 million, $390 million, or $400 million. The committee assigned each candidate vaccine to one of these cost levels on the basis of its assessment of the current stage of the vaccine's development (see Table 4-1). For many conditions under study, work is being done on more than one type of candidate vaccine. The committee did not think that differences among the candidate vaccines in terms of development costs (or cost per dose or effectiveness) were likely to be significant enough to warrant separate analysis.

The committee also considered the time required to achieve licensure of a vaccine. Since specific evidence on which to base fine distinctions among the candidate vaccines was not available, the committee assigned each candidate vaccine to one of three development intervals: 3, 7, or 15 years. Discounting incorporated this development interval to adjust for the differences in when the associated costs and benefits of the vaccines will be realized.

Cost of Vaccine Use

The cost of vaccine use is a function of the cost per dose of the vaccine, the cost to administer the vaccine, the number of doses each person must receive to be fully immunized, and the size of the population targeted to receive the vaccine.

A vaccine's cost per dose is represented in this analysis by an estimated purchase price rather than the marginal cost of producing a single dose. Because the committee felt that it could not accurately predict detailed differences in the price of future vaccines, it chose to assume that the cost of prophylactic vaccines would be either $50 or $100. It was assumed that the cost of therapeutic vaccines would be significantly higher and was set at $500 (see Table 4-1). The marginal cost of administering a dose of vaccine was assumed to be small and was set at $10. For most vaccines, it was assumed that three doses would be needed to achieve full immunity.

The cost of vaccine use is also influenced by the size and nature of the population targeted to receive the vaccine. As the size of the target population increases, costs increase because more doses of vaccine must be administered.

Health Care Costs

In much the same way that it was necessary to establish a common measure of health effects that could be used to compare very different conditions, it was also necessary to establish a common basis for comparing the costs of care associated with those conditions. Costs for specific services are represented in the committee's analysis by charges for those services. Charges vary regionally and among health care providers within a region. Published cost-effectiveness studies on some of the conditions were reviewed by the committee, but because those studies draw their cost data from a variety of sources, they were not always consistent and could not be directly compared. Furthermore, such studies were not available for every condition under consideration, making it necessary for the committee to assemble those cost data in any case.

The morbidity scenarios developed for use in the calculation of health benefits associated with a vaccine also provided the basic framework for the calculation of health care costs that would be averted with vaccine use. For each morbidity scenario, the committee developed a companion "clinical scenario" that specified the health services required, including hospitalizations, procedures, medications, office visits, rehabilitation services, and long-term institutional care. An appropriate unit of service (e.g., hospital days or doses of medication) was specified and the amount of care received was defined in terms of those units. Costs also were specified in terms of units of service. In addition, for each form of care, the committee specified the proportion of patients within the scenario that received that form of care. It was assumed that all costs of care associated with the condition under study would be averted with vaccine use.

For all conditions, the committee estimated cost of care on the basis of national data. For inpatient hospitalizations, hospital costs were estimated by using average national diagnosis-related group payments by the Health Care Financing Administration (HCFA) (St. Anthony's DRG Guidebook, 1995). Outpatient costs and inpatient physician visits were also estimated from HCFA data (HCFA, 1995). For these costs, the committee estimated general categories of costs (outpatient physician visit with and without tests, etc.) and applied these to the morbidity scenarios. See Box 4-5 for examples of unit costs.

Vaccine Efficacy and Utilization

An additional component of the committee's analysis took into account assumptions about the efficacy of each vaccine under study and the extent to which the target population would use the vaccine. An efficacy or utilization

---

BOX 4-5 Examples of Health Care Cost Estimates Used

Outpatient Costs

Physician A	$50
Physician B (specialist)	$100
Physician C (in hospital)	$150
Medication A (non-prescription)	$10
Medication B (inexpensive prescription)	$50
Medication C (expensive prescription)	$150
Diagnostic A	$50
Diagnostic B	$100
Diagnostic C	$500

Hospitalization Costs (per admission; based on hospitalization)

Complicated delivery (additional cost)	$1,000
Gastroenteritis	$2,000
Multiple sclerosis	$3,000
Cellulitis	$3,000
Ectopic pregnancies	$3,000
Ulcer	$3,000
Infectious myocarditis	$3,000
Diabetic complications	$3,000
Pneumonia	$4,000
Digestive malignancy	$4,000
Melanoma	$4,000
Cirrhosis	$5,000
Viral meningitis	$6,000
Tuberculosis	$6,000
Amputation	$7,000

rate of less than 100% will reduce the health benefits and savings in the cost of care that can be expected. A lower utilization rate will also have the effect of reducing the costs associated with vaccinating the target population.

With regard to efficacy, it was assumed that preventive vaccines would achieve an efficacy level of 75%. The efficacy of therapeutic vaccines was assumed to be 40%. This lower estimate reflected the committee's belief that therapeutic vaccines would be expected to achieve a lower threshold of efficacy than for preventive vaccines for both licensure approval by the FDA and for acceptance by patients and medical care providers. In fact, many therapeutic drugs are approved for licensure or for new indications with an efficacy of 40% or lower.

Each candidate vaccine was also assigned a utilization rate of 10, 30, 50, 60, or 90% (see Table 4-1). The committee's utilization rate assignments were guided by an examination of the coverage rates achieved for existing vaccines, which were assumed to suggest rates that could be anticipated for new vaccines. Also considered were specific factors that might influence the rate at which a particular vaccine would be used. For example, a 50% utilization rate by an adolescent target population for a vaccine for a sexually transmitted disease (STD) reflects the committee's assessment of the difficulty in reaching this population and possible reluctance of parents to acknowledge a child's risk and therefore the potential benefit of a vaccine. For vaccines targeted to pregnant women, two alternatives were considered plausible: the utilization rate would stabilize at 10% due, in part, to persistent concerns about potential adverse effects on the fetus, or the utilization rate would reach 90% because use of the vaccine becomes an accepted element of good prenatal care.

In the past, more extensive use of some vaccines has been hindered by an inadequate supply. For this analysis, however, it was assumed that adequate supplies would be available to meet the demand for all vaccines.

Cost-Effectiveness Ratios

The final stage/step of the analysis is the calculation of the cost-effectiveness ratio for each candidate vaccine, the basis for comparisons among the vaccines. Three sets of cost-effectiveness ratios were calculated. The first ratio examines the potential impact of the vaccine on morbidity and costs under the assumption that the vaccines are available immediately without any additional cost or time for development and that they are fully efficacious and are used by the entire target population. This comparison focuses attention on what might be considered an ideal vaccine benefit. The second cost-effectiveness ratio factors in the adjustments for incomplete efficacy and use, which tend to increase the cost of achieving the anticipated health benefit. The final ratio shows the impact of the time and money needed to develop these vaccines. Some vaccines that promise substantial benefit require a longer and more expensive period of development, whereas others that offer smaller benefits are expected to be available more quickly and cheaply. In general, the committee found that the adjustments for efficacy and utilization had a more substantial impact on a vaccine's cost-effectiveness than the additional time and cost needed for development. Although these adjustments changed the cost-effectiveness ratios, only a few vaccines shifted in their cost-effectiveness relative to the other vaccines.

For each of the conditions included in the study, multiple sensitivity analyses could be performed to test alternative assumptions regarding the morbidity scenarios, the quality-adjustment weights, the costs of care and vaccine development, utilization rates, and numerous other factors. Because 26 conditions were considered, however, the committee was not able to undertake a detailed case-by-case approach to sensitivity analysis. As an alternative, a series of hypothetical cases for *vaccine x* were developed to illustrate the effects that changes in various factors (e.g., numbers of cases, age distribution of patients, severity of illness, unit costs of care, and so on) would produce in the cost-effectiveness ratio.

The committee chose to perform sensitivity analyses for *vaccine x* with limited set of factors of significance across all conditions. One of these analyses addressed the debate within the committee and in the cost-effectiveness literature over the appropriateness of discounting future health benefits. The basic analysis used a 3% discount rate for both health benefits and costs. Two sensitivity analyses were performed: (1) the discount rate for health benefits was set at zero, whereas the rate for costs was maintained at 3% and (2) the discount rate was set at zero for both health benefits and costs. The results of these analyses are discussed later in this chapter.

Exclusions from the Analysis

Several factors excluded from the committee's analysis are reviewed briefly. In theory, the analysis should also consider the impact of vaccine use on the time costs borne by patients in obtaining treatment or vaccination for any of the conditions studied and by parents, spouses, or other unpaid caregivers who provide care to individuals who experience any of these conditions. For some conditions, these costs could be substantial. For example, an analysis of the cost-effectiveness of a varicella vaccination program estimated an annual savings of $325 million (discounted 1990 dollars) in parents' time lost from work (Lieu et al., 1994).

The committee felt, however, that it lacked adequate information to make a consistent assessment across the various conditions of the time involved in obtaining treatment or of the extent of care from unpaid caregivers. It is readily apparent that sick children will require care from parents or other adult caregivers, but it is less clear whether adults who are ill routinely receive similar unpaid care from others and, if they do, how much care they receive. Therefore, the committee chose not to include these costs in its analysis. If suitable time cost estimates were to become available, however, they could readily be incorporated into the model.

The committee also excluded from the analysis the possible impact of vaccine use on the cost of current public health services such as disease surveillance or contact-tracing programs. A reduction in the number of cases of a single condition may not translate into a direct proportional change in the cost of public health services, which may be used in conjunction with a variety of other conditions as well. For example, a vaccine that prevents one type of STD will tend to reduce the burden on some services, but those services will continue to be needed in connection with other STDs.

It should also be noted that the committee's analysis does not include as a cost factor a monetary value for changes in income associated with time lost to illness or use of a vaccine. This feature of the model reflects a widely accepted assumption in cost-effectiveness analysis (see Gold et al., 1996) that this opportunity cost of illness, in terms of both lost wages and time lost from unpaid work or leisure, is captured by the quality adjustment weights assigned to periods with and without illness. Thus, the cost of lost work is accounted for in nonmonetary terms rather than being excluded from the analysis.

This analysis could also include the impacts of the possible adverse effects of a vaccine, but the committee made an explicit decision not to incorporate this component. Adverse effects would generally result in a reduction in the health benefits produced by vaccine use and an increase in the costs of care. They could also limit the public's acceptance of a vaccine. Estimating the magnitudes of these factors for each vaccine candidate would require assessments of the frequency of adverse effects, their nature and severity, the kinds of care required, and public reaction to them. The committee agreed that making meaningful predictions regarding any aspect of possible adverse effects of future vaccines would be very problematic and that there was no basis for distinguishing differences among the vaccines included in the study.

There is a reasonable basis for concluding that exclusion of adverse effects from the analysis has not altered the results in any meaningful way. Evidence regarding existing vaccines (IOM, 1991, 1994a, 1996a) suggests that adverse effects are infrequent and that very few are severe. This is consistent with preliminary analyses performed for the 1985 IOM report on the development of new vaccines, which found that estimated numbers of adverse effects produced minimal changes in the measures of disease burden and cost and did not alter the relative rankings of candidate vaccines. That committee also decided not to include estimates of adverse effects in the final analyses for its report. Although the present committee chose not to incorporate an estimate of adverse effects in its quantitative analysis, the issue of vaccine safety is of serious concern and is discussed further in several publications by other committees and forums held by the IOM (IOM, 1991; 1994a,b; 1996a; 1997a,b).

It is likely that some of the vaccines considered by the committee will become components of combination vaccine products similar to the familiar DTP products currently in general use. For vaccines intended for universal use, especially among infants and children, combination products have the advantage of reducing the number of separate vaccine doses that must be administered, which can aid efforts to achieve desired levels of vaccine utilization. Including combination vaccines in the analysis is not difficult in principle, but would add to the burden of assessing expert judgment on utilization, costs, and effectiveness of the vaccines if available in combination forms. Many vaccine combinations might be possible, and the committee had no basis for selecting any specific combinations as more or less likely. Therefore, combination products were not included in the analysis.

The committee was originally asked to include in its analysis the contraceptive vaccines that are in development. Although the scientific foundation for research and development of a contraceptive vaccine is clear and such vaccines are being studied and can be expected to provide a needed addition to the array of contraceptive options that are currently available, an analysis of their anticipated cost-effectiveness within the framework adopted for this study poses particularly difficult ethical and philosophical problems that the committee felt unqualified to address.

Trying to measure the health benefits produced by a contraceptive vaccine would require a determination of whose health is affected by an unintended pregnancy (the mother's health, the child's health, or the health of others in the family), what those effects are (psychological distress or a normal life expectancy), and how long they last. For the most part, the benefits of contraceptive vaccines are not health-related but relate instead to the economic and psychological well-being of the mother. Therefore, societal priorities for such vaccines should be based on a broader concept of benefit than quality-adjusted life years. For the other vaccines in the study, there is little question that the prevention or treatment of an illness is a desirable outcome. For a contraceptive vaccine, however, it is not clear whether prevention of a pregnancy can always be viewed as completely desirable. For a woman who does not wish to become pregnant, the outcome can be considered positive, but a concern is how to assess the health effects that result if a contraceptive vaccine prevents a desired pregnancy. Questions also arise regarding the costs to be considered in the analysis. For example, should the vaccine be credited with saving the cost of raising a child or with having prevented the productivity of that child? Until a clearer consensus is established regarding the answers to questions such as these, it seems inappropriate to include a contraceptive vaccine in a cost-effectiveness model.

EXAMPLES: HYPOTHETICAL VACCINE X

Before discussing the results obtained by applying the model developed for this report to the selected candidate vaccines, the committee provides some examples of results obtained from an analysis of a hypothetical candidate vaccine X directed for use for the prevention of disease X.

The characteristics of a base case scenario (Case 1) for vaccine X-1 are presented in Table 4-2. Candidate vaccine X-1 is under development and would be directed against disease X-1, which affects 100,000 people annually. Disease X-1 has a 1% case fatality rate (CFR). All age groups are affected equally. Half of the people experience a mild illness (2-week duration; HUI = .90) and half experience a moderate illness (2-week duration; HUI = .70). The health care costs include a physician visit for patients with mild cases and more extensive and more expensive treatment (including a brief hospitalization) for patients with moderate illness. The candidate vaccine will be licensed within 7 years, after expenditures of $240 million in additional research and development costs. The vaccine will cost $50 for each dose of the 3-dose series, which will be given in infancy. The vaccine will be 75% effective, and 90% of the target population (i.e., infants) will be vaccinated.

In such a hypothetical scenario, the cost per QALY gained by use of the vaccine is approximately $125,000. The number of QALYs lost to disease X-1 is 7,000, almost 6,800 of which are due to the effects of mortality. With the specified assumptions regarding effectiveness and utilization, only 4,700 QALYs would be gained if the vaccine were available immediately. Discounting to allow for the time needed for vaccine development reduces the annualized present value of the QALYs gained to 3,300.

The discounted cost of care saved by this vaccine strategy is approximately $43 million. Program costs for vaccinating all infants with three doses of the $50 vaccine amount to $720 million; adjustments for the rate of utilization and discounting for vaccine development time reduces the annualized present value of those costs to approximately $450 million. Although the investment required to bring this vaccine to licensure is estimated to be $240 million, the amortized amount attributed to a single year is $7.2 million. The net cost (development cost plus delivery costs minus health care savings) is approximately $420 million.

The following examples (Table 4-3) are based on modifications of Case 1 and will demonstrate the effects of changes in target population, program considerations, disease severity, and discounting. This section closes with a description and example of how the cost-effectiveness model developed for research and development prioritization can be used by other policymakers to plan vaccine programs, for example. The chapter then closes with the results obtained for the 26 candidate vaccines chosen by the committee for further illustration.

Target Population

If the disease only affects children under 5 years of age (Case 2), the cost per QALY gained by vaccination drops to less than $30,000. Key factors influencing this dramatic difference between the two examples are the greater number of QALYs gained in Case 2 (12,000 in Case 2 compared with 3,300 in Case 1) and the cost of care saved ($114 million in Case 2 compared to $43 million in Case 1). The gain in QALYs is higher in Case 2 for two main reasons. First, averting deaths of 1,000 infants and children "recovers" or "saves" many more years of future life than does averting the same number of deaths at older ages. Second, the vaccine benefits are realized much sooner after immunization in Case 2 than in Case 1, in which some of the vaccinees will not benefit from the vaccine until decades after their immunization as an infant. The model assumes that costs and health benefits in the present are more highly valued than those accrued in the future.

If Case 2 is changed such that the disease strikes only those older than 65 years of age, the cost per QALY gained by vaccination increases to more than$1 million (Case 3). However, that scenario assumes that the affected people are vaccinated during infancy and will not reap the benefits of the vaccine for more than six decades. A more reasonable vaccination strategy might be to vaccinate people much closer to the time that they might experience the disease. In such a scenario (Case 4), 100,000 cases of disease still occur each year. Because there are far fewer people 60 years of age than there are infants, the costs of an adult immunization program are lower than those of a program aimed at infants. Thus, by this adult immunization strategy, the cost per QALY gained drops to approximately $70,000.

There are two key factors that explain why, if in both examples the vaccine is administered to the vulnerable age group, the cost per QALY gained in Case 4 is more than twice that in Case 2. First, the maximum interval between vaccination and time to benefit in Case 2 is less than 5 years. In Case 4, some vaccinees experience the benefit in 5 years, but other vaccinees will not realize the benefit until 20 years after the vaccination. The second factor is that the number of QALYs saved by vaccination against a disease that affects those under 5 years of age exceeds the QALYs saved by a vaccination against the same number of people 60 years of age or older. This is explained by the effect of age on baseline health status, as discussed in an earlier section of this chapter.

Program Considerations

Case 4 illustrates the selection of a target population based on age-related risk. Other important bases for selection of a target population (and tailoring of a vaccine program) are geography or preexisting condition. If disease X-5 affects 100,000 people of all ages each year and has a 1% case fatality rate, and if the cases are restricted in some identifiable manner (e.g., geographic area), a vacci-

Table 4-2 Vaccine X-1: Mild/Moderate Illness with Deaths, Uniform Ages (cases: 100,000/year)

Deaths (from acute infection)	1%			

Morbidity scenarios	Distribution of Cases	Duration	HUI	Health Care Costs
Mild	50%	2 weeks	0.90	1 MD visit = $50
Moderate	50%	2 weeks	0.70	1 MD visit = $50
Severe[a]	0%	4 weeks	0.40	Brief hospitalization = $5,000; 3 MD visits = $150
Permanent impairment[a]	0%	Remaining lifetime		Brief hospitalization = $5,000; ICU hospitalization = $4,500

Characteristics of Vaccine Use and Development

Target population for vaccination	4 million infants
Cost of vaccine per dose	$50
Doses required	3
Vaccine effectiveness	75%
Utilization of vaccine	90%
Time to adoption at anticipated utilization	5 years
Cost for vaccine development	$240 million
Time for vaccine development	7 years
Discount Rates (r)	
Health benefits	3%
Costs	3%

Cost per QALY gained with vaccine

a. Immediately available vaccine (100% efficacy and use, no development cost or time) $89,660

b. Immediately available vaccine with likely effect and use (no development cost or time) $123,816

c. Vaccine available with addition of development cost and time $125,980

	QALYs to Be Gained	Net Cost	Cost of Care Saved	Delivery Costs	Development Costs
a. *Baseline*					
Immediately available vaccine (100% efficacy and use, no development cost or time)	7,026.64	$630,009,848	$89,990,152	$720,000,000	$240,000,000
b. *Adjustments for Vaccine Efficacy and Utilization*					
Anticipated vaccine efficacy: 75%	5,269.98		$67,492,614	N/A	N/A
Anticipated vaccine utilization: 90%	4,742.98	$587,256,647	$60,743,353	$648,000,000	N/A
c. *Adjustment for Vaccine Development Costs and Time*					
Vaccine available with addition of development cost and time	3,326.63[b]	$419,089,997	$42,604,166[b]	$454,494,162[b]	$7,200,000[c]

[a]Not applicable for Vaccine X-1; relevant for other Vaccine X examples.

[b]Annualize present value = (adjusted baseline) $/ (1 + r)^{T_{use}}$, where T_{use} is the time to adoption at the anticipated utilization rate plus time to vaccine licensure.

[c]Amortized development cost = Development costs $\times r$.

nation strategy that targets 500,000 high-risk infants leads to a cost per QALY gained of $6,000 (Case 5). This change can be attributed entirely to the reduction in the cost of the delivery program. The number of vaccinees and, therefore, the delivery costs in Case 5 are one-eighth those in Case 1.

Another vaccine program component of great interest to readers of the report is the cost of the vaccine itself. If the cost per dose of the vaccine is assumed to be twice the cost estimated for Case 1, the program costs almost double to $110 million versus $60 million in Case 1 (the $10 added per dose for administration of the vaccine does not change) and the cost per QALY saved increases from approximately $125,000 to approximately $240,000 (Case 6).

Disease Severity

Several other scenarios are instructive. Consider Case 7, which differs from Case 1 only in that there are no deaths. If the disease X-7 results in the mild and moderate illnesses described for Case 1, the cost per QALY gained with a vaccine is well in excess of $3 million. The program costs and costs of care are the same as those for Case 1, but only a small number of QALYs are gained when no deaths result. If, however, disease X-8 has a 100-fold higher incidence than X-7, then a vaccine X-8 strategy becomes cost saving. The number of QALYs saved with a vaccine strategy increase by 100 fold. Vaccine delivery and development costs remain the same, and the health care costs increase 100 fold. The net cost of a vaccine strategy changes from a cost of over $400 million to a savings of almost $4 billion.

Another instructive example is the role that long-term disability plays in cost-effectiveness applications. If instead of the mild/moderate disease and CFR of 1% associated with disease X-1, there is severe disease and a 1% rate of long-term, serious sequelae (instead of a 1% CFR), the cost per QALY gained by vaccination is $80,000 (Case 9). In this scenario, use of the vaccine results in a moderate gain in QALYs and a substantial savings in the costs of care.

Discounting

As discussed in the beginning of this chapter, the committee followed the recommendations of the Panel on Cost-Effectiveness in Health and Medicine and applied a 3% discount rate for both costs and health benefits. Because discounting is a difficult concept for some readers, the committee has modified Case 1 to show the effects of discounting for costs only and of discounting for neither costs nor health benefits. The numbers of QALYs to be gained under Case 1 increase significantly absent discounting for health benefits: from approximately 3,300 QALYs (with a 3% discount rate applied) to 25,500 QALYs with no discounting. This approximately 8-fold difference in the denominator of the cost-effectiveness ratio leads to a proportional decrease in the cost per

TABLE 4-3 Assumptions and Results of "Vaccine X" Analyses

Vaccine X	Case 1: Mild/Moderate Illness with Deaths, Uni- form Ages	Case 2: Mild/Moderate Illness with Deaths, in Children	Case 3: Mild/Moderate Illness with Deaths, in the Elderly
Cases	100,000/yr	100,000/yr	100,000/yr
Age-specific incidence	uniform	all <5	all 65+
Deaths (from acute infection)	1%	1%	1%
Morbidity scenarios			
Mild scenario	50%	50%	50%
Moderate scenario	50%	50%	50%
Severe scenario	0%	0%	0%
Permanent impairment	0%	0%	0%
Target Population	infants	infants	infants
(infants, adolescents, etc.)	4,000,000	4,000,000	4,000,000
Cost of Vaccine/dose	$50	$50	$50
Discount Rates			
Health benefits	3%	3%	3%
Costs	3%	3%	3%

a. Immediately available vaccine (100% efficacy and use, no development cost or time)

$/QALY	$89,660	$18,580	$837,629
QALYs to be gained	7,027	25,826	826
Net cost	$630,009,848	$479,838,815	$692,003,742
Cost of care saved	$89,990,152	$240,161,185	$27,996,258
Delivery costs	$720,000,000	$720,000,000	$720,000,000
Development costs	$0	$0	$0

b. Immediately available vaccine with likely effect and use (no development cost or time)

$/QALY	$123,816	$27,873	$1,128,135
Net cost	$587,256,647	$485,891,200	($608,845,879)
Cost of care saved	$60,743,353	$162,108,800	$18,897,474
Delivery costs	$648,000,000	$648,000,000	$648,000,000
Development costs	$0	$0	$0

c. Vaccine available, expected use, and effectiveness with addition of development cost and time

$/QALY	$125,980	$28,462	$1,146,543
QALYs to be gained	3,327	12,227	391
Net cost	$419,089,997	$347,994,312	$448,439,854
Cost of care saved	$42,604,166	$113,699,851	$13,254,308
Delivery costs	$454,494,162	$454,494,162	$454,494,162
Development costs	$7,200,000	$7,200,000	$7,200,000

Continued

NOTE: "C" is the primary analysis reported in the results section

TABLE 4-3 *Continued*

Vaccine X	Case 4: Mild/Moderate Illness with Deaths, in the Elderly	Case 5: High-Risk Infant Target Population	Case 6 High Cost Vaccine ($100)
Cases	100,000 / yr	100,000 / yr	100,000 / yr
Age-specific incidence	all 65+	uniform	uniform
Deaths (from acute infection)	1%	1%	1%
Morbidity scenarios			
Mild scenario	50%	50%	50%
Moderate scenario	50%	50%	50%
Severe scenario	0%	0%	0%
Permanent impairment	0%	0%	0%
Target Population	60 years of age	high risk infants	infants
(infants, adolescents, etc)	2,000,000	500,000	4,000,000
Cost of Vaccine / dose	$50	$50	$100
Discount Rates			
Health benefits	3%	3%	3%
Costs	3%	3%	3%

a. Immediately available vaccine (100% efficacy and use, no development cost or time)

$/QALY	$41,176	$1	$175,049
QALYs to be gained	4,796	7,027	7,027
Net cost	$197,476,989	$9,848	$1,230,009,848
Cost of care saved	$162,523,011	$89,990,152	$89,990,152
Delivery costs	$360,000,000	$90,000,000	$1,320,000,000
Development costs	$0	$0	$0

b. Immediately available vaccine with likely effect and use (no development cost or time)

$/QALY	$66,197	$4,271	$237,668
Net cost	$629,102,526	$20,256,647	$1,127,256,647
Cost of care saved	$18,897,474	$60,743,353	$60,743,353
Delivery costs	$648,000,000	$81,000,000	$1,188,000,000
Development costs	$0	$0	$0

c. Vaccine available, expected use, and effectiveness with addition of development cost and time

$/QALY	$69,368	$6,435	$239,833
QALYs to be gained	2,271	3,327	3,327
Net cost	$157,503,581	$21,407,605	$797,835,132
Cost of care saved	$76,943,500	$42,604,166	$42,604,166
Delivery costs	$227,247,081	$56,811,770	$833,239,298
Development costs	$7,200,000	$7,200,000	$7,200,000

Continued

NOTE: "C" is the primary analysis reported in the results section

TABLE 4-3 *Continued*

Vaccine X	Case 7: Mild/Moderate Illness, No Deaths, Uniform Ages		Case 8: Mild/Moderate Illness, No Deaths, Uniform Ages, High Incidence	Case 9: No Deaths with Moderate/ Severe Disease, Impairment
Cases	100,000 / yr		10,000,000 / yr	100,000 / yr
Age-specific incidence	uniform		uniform	uniform
Deaths (from acute infection)	none		none	none
Morbidity scenarios				
Mild scenario		50%	50%	0%
Moderate scenario		50%	50%	50%
Severe scenario		0%	0%	50%
Permanent impairment		0%	0%	1%
Target Population	infants		infants	infants
(infants, adolescents, etc)		4,000,000	4,000,000	4,000,000
Cost of Vaccine / dose		$50	$50	$50
Discount Rates				
Health benefits		3%	3%	3%
Costs		3%	3%	3%

a. Immediately available vaccine (100% efficacy and use, no development cost or time)

$/QALY		$2,597,233	($341,305)	$10,174
QALYs to be gained		$243	$24,257	$3,623
Net cost		$630,009,848	($8,279,015,232)	$36,857,314
Cost of care saved		$89,990,152	$8,999,015,232	$683,142,686
Delivery costs		$720,000,000	$720,000,000	$720,000,000
Development costs		$0	$0	$0

b. Immediately available vaccine with likely effect and use (no development cost or time)

$/QALY		$3,586,639	($331,411)	$76,420
Net cost		$587,256,647	($5,426,335,282)	$186,878,687
Cost of care saved		$60,743,353	$6,074,335,282	$461,121,313
Delivery costs		$648,000,000	$648,000,000	$648,000,000
Development costs		$0	$0	$0

c. Vaccine available, expected use, and effectiveness with addition of development cost and time

$/QALY		$3,649,335	($330,784)	$80,618
QALYs to be gained		115	11,484	1,715
Net cost		$419,089,997	($3,798,722,390)	$138,272,951
Cost of care saved		$42,604,166	$4,260,416,552	$323,421,211
Delivery costs		$454,494,162	$454,494,162	$454,494,162
Development costs		$7,200,000	$7,200,000	$7,200,000

Continued

NOTE: "C" is the primary analysis reported in the results section

TABLE 4-3 *Continued*

Vaccine X	Case 10: Discounting for Costs Only		Case 11: No Discounting	
Cases	100,000 / yr		100,000 / yr	
Age-specific incidence	uniform		uniform	
Deaths (from acute infection)		1%		1%
Morbidity scenarios				
Mild scenario		50%		50%
Moderate scenario		50%		50%
Severe scenario		0%		0%
Permanent impairment		0%		0%
Target Population	infants		infants	
(infants, adolescents, etc)		4,000,000		4,000,000
Cost of Vaccine / dose		$50		$50
Discount Rates				
Health benefits		0%		0%
Costs		3%		0%

a. Immediately available vaccine (100% efficacy and use, no development cost or time)

$/QALY	$16,671	$12,305
QALYs to be gained	$37,790	$37,790
Net cost	$630,009,848	$465,000,000
Cost of care saved	$89,990,152	$255,000,000
Delivery costs	$720,000,000	$720,000,000
Development costs	$0	$0

b. Immediately available vaccine with likely effect and use (no development cost or time)

$/QALY	$23,022	$18,656
Net cost	$587,256,647	$475,875,000
Cost of care saved	$60,743,353	$172,125,000
Delivery costs	$648,000,000	$648,000,000
Development costs	$0	$0

c. Vaccine available, expected use, and effectiveness with addition of development cost and time

$/QALY	$16,430	$18,656
QALYs to be gained	25,508	25,508
Net cost	$419,089,997	$475,875,000
Cost of care saved	$42,604,166	$172,125,000
Delivery costs	$454,494,162	$648,000,000
Development costs	$7,200,000	$0

NOTE: "C" is the primary analysis reported in the results section

QALY saved to $16,000. If the model includes no discounting for either costs or health benefits, the cost per QALY saved (compared to case 1) is approximately $19,000 (see Cases 10 and 11). The committee reiterates, however, that both costs and benefits should be discounted.

An Idealized Scenario

The committee believes that the model it recommends can and should have far more utility beyond informing research and development priority considerations. For example, a policymaker might want to evaluate and inform decisions about the value of investments in new vaccine delivery programs. Such a policymaker might also wish to evaluate those options in an idealized scenario. Therefore, the committee offers several examples, using the Vaccine X scenarios described above, of results obtained in the idealized scenario; that is, vaccines against disease X-1 through X-9 have just become available, they are all 100% effective, and there is a means to ensure that the entire target population is vaccinated immediately. The following discussion illustrates results that might be important if there is now a desire to find out the cost-effectiveness of an investment in a vaccine program against one of these nine diseases, if that program were to begin today. Because the model includes discounting for both costs and benefits, components of the model with a time factor are particularly affected by this change in analysis.

The cost-effectiveness ratios for vaccines X-1 through X-9 in the idealized scenario change in some fairly predictable ways. Vaccine strategies appear more cost-effective when analyzing this "idealized scenario" compared to the primary analysis reported by the committee (less-than-perfect utilization and efficacy, including development costs and time until program is stabilized). The denominator (health benefits) is higher (approximately two-fold) compared to the standard analysis in every case. The factors responsible for this are the positive change by increasing utilization and effectiveness and the absence of the negative impact of discounting the health benefits during the 12 years until the vaccine program is fully implemented (7 years for vaccine licensure and another 5 years for vaccine use to stabilize).

The numerator of the cost-effectiveness ratio is changed in the idealized scenario in several ways, and not always in ways that will be intuitively obvious. Costs for vaccine development ($7,200,000 for these vaccines) are zero in this analysis. Delivery costs increase in the idealized scenario because utilization is 100% and, therefore, 10% more vaccine needs to be purchased. Delivery costs are also increased because they do not need to be discounted to account for the time for vaccine licensure and for usage to stabilize. The cost of care saved with a vaccine strategy is higher in the idealized scenario because more people experience health benefits due to higher efficacy and utilization. In addition, the discounting is not applied for the 12-year lag required for licensure and for usage to stabilize. The net costs can be higher or lower in this scenario compared to the standard analysis depending on the change in delivery costs relative to the change in health care costs saved.

Summary

In summary, the hypothetical cases discussed above illustrate key factors that influence the cost per QALY gained with a new vaccine. These include the following:

- the number of vaccinees compared to the number of cases,
- the interval between the time of vaccination and the time at which disease is averted (i.e., the time at which the vaccinee experiences health benefits and savings in costs of care are realized),
- the number of QALYs to be gained by protection from disease for one age group compared with that for another age group (for the same number of calendar years), and
- mortality or long periods spent in a disabled state.

RESULTS

The committee was not charged to recommend which candidate vaccines should be developed. It has focused on developing a conceptual framework and a quantitative model for that framework to aid researchers and policymakers in planning research and development efforts for the plethora of candidate vaccines that have emerged over the last 10 years. As described in a preceding section, this model can aid policymakers in planning for use of new vaccines once licensed.

The primary measure used to report these results is a cost-effectiveness ratio of cost per QALY gained based on the annualized present value of the component costs and QALYs. As described in Chapter 3, there were many considerations in choosing these 26 diseases for which a vaccination strategy was considered feasible and appropriate. The committee chose a range of conditions (in terms of factors such as target populations, incidence of disease, and health states) for which a vaccination strategy might be used. The committee expected that the final results of the exercise would range widely.

The candidate vaccines fall into four reasonably distinct groupings or levels: candidate vaccines that would save money and QALYs; candidate vaccines that would require small costs (<$10,000) for each QALY gained; candidate vaccines that would require modest yet reasonable costs (<$100,000) for each QALY gained; and candidate vaccines that would require large costs (more than and much more than $100,000) per QALY gained.

Level I	Most favorable	Saves money and QALYs
Level II	More favorable	Costs < $10,000 per QALY saved
Level III	Favorable	Costs > $10,000 and <$100,000 per QALY saved
Level IV	Less favorable	Costs >$100,000 per QALY saved.

Seven candidate vaccines fall into the most favorable (I) category: those with which a vaccination strategy would save money. The Level I candidate vaccines are as follows (in alphabetical order):

- cytomegalovirus (CMV) vaccine administered to 12-year-olds,
- Group B streptococcus vaccine to be well-incorporated into routine prenatal care and administered to women during first pregnancy and to high-risk adults (at age 65 years and to people less than age 65 years with serious, chronic health conditions),
- influenza virus vaccine administered to the general population (once per person every 5 years, or one-fifth of the population per year),
- insulin-dependent diabetes mellitus therapeutic vaccine,
- multiple sclerosis therapeutic vaccine,
- rheumatoid arthritis therapeutic vaccine, and
- *Streptococcus pneumoniae* vaccine to be given to infants and to 65-year-olds.

Nine candidate vaccines fall into the more favorable (II) category: those with which a vaccination strategy would incur small costs (less than $10,000) for each QALY gained. The Level II candidate vaccines are as follows (in alphabetical order):

- chlamydia vaccine to be administered to 12-year-olds,
- *Helicobacter pylori* vaccine to be administered to infants,
- hepatitis C virus vaccine to be administered to infants,
- herpes simplex virus vaccine to be administered to 12-year-olds,
- human papillomavirus vaccine to be administered to 12-year-olds,
- melanoma therapeutic vaccine,
- *Mycobacterium tuberculosis* vaccine to be administered to high-risk populations,
- *Neisseria gonorrhea* vaccine to be administered to 12-year-olds, and
- respiratory syncytial virus vaccine to be administered to infants and to 12-year-old females.

Four candidate vaccines fall into the favorable (III) category: those with which a vaccination strategy would incur moderate costs (more than $10,000 but less than $100,000) per QALY gained. The Level III vaccine candidates are as follows (in alphabetical order):

- Group A streptococcus vaccine to be given to infants,
- Group B streptococcus vaccine to be given to high-risk adults and to either 12-year-old females or to women during first pregnancy (low utilization)
- parainfluenza virus vaccine to be given to infants and to women in their first pregnancy, and
- rotavirus vaccine to be given to infants.

Seven candidate vaccines fall into the less favorable (IV) category: those with which a vaccination strategy would incur significant costs (more than $100,000 and up to well more than $1 million) per QALY gained. The Level IV vaccine candidates are as follows (in alphabetical order):

- *Borrelia burgdorferi* vaccine to be given to resident infants born in and immigrants of any age into geographically defined high-risk areas,
- *Coccidioides immitis* vaccine to be given to resident infants born in and immigrants of any age into geographically defined high-risk areas,
- enterotoxigenic *Escherichia coli* vaccine to be given to infants and travelers,
- Epstein-Barr virus vaccine to be given to 12-year-olds,
- *Histoplasma capsulatum* vaccine to be given to resident infants born in and immigrants of any age into geographically defined high-risk areas,
- *Neisseria meningitidis* type B vaccine to be given to infants, and
- *Shigella* vaccine to be given to infants and travelers or to travelers only.

The application of the committee's framework and model are both predictable and surprising. On a pragmatic and qualitative level, the framework developed for the assessment of these vaccines is an advance from that developed in 1985. The spreadsheets will be available for anyone who wishes to experiment with the model and change assumptions or data. The measure of health benefits, QALYs, is being used by many in the health field, so it is a much more familiar concept than that used in 1985.

The Level I candidate vaccines include several that were discussed in the 1985 IOM report on vaccine priorities. The four infectious diseases (cytomegalovirus, influenza A/B, Group B streptococcus, and streptococcus pneumoniae) with Level I candidate vaccines continue to have a staggering burden of disease for many reasons: the numbers of infected people, the seriousness of the health states caused by the infection, and the incidence of long-term sequelae (death and permanent impairment) and subsequent loss of quality of life (as measured in QALYs). A common factor in the analysis for these four vaccine strategies is the relatively short interval between vaccine administration and realization of health benefits for many of the affected people.

The inclusion in Level I of candidate therapeutic vaccines suggests that vaccine strategies for noninfectious, chronic conditions hold much promise. These results are seen even though the estimated efficacy (40%) is much less than that for the preventive candidate vaccines (75%). The acceptance, however, was estimated to be very high, and the interval from vaccination to realization of health benefits is very short. In the absence of experience with therapeutic vaccine strategies, it is not clear that the results obtained were predictable at the outset of this analysis. The committee hopes that the results will encourage continued research into the use and benefits of this relatively new class of vaccine strategies.

As mentioned, the results presented above are based on the full analysis described at the beginning of the chapter. Readers might question the effects of changing certain assumptions or components of the model, and the committee tested the effects of changing certain assumptions. To illustrate how the model could be used by vaccine program planners, the committee assumed that the vaccines are currently available (i.e., requiring no more time or costs for development). There was no change in the assignment of vaccines to Levels I-IV. When the committee further assumed that the vaccines are currently available, 100% effective, and utilized by 100% of the target population (i.e., the ideal scenario; an analysis requested of the committee by the project sponsor, NIH), five vaccines shifted into an adjacent category. Specifically, four vaccines in Level II—chlamydia, melanoma (therapeutic), mycobacterium tuberculosis, and respiratory syncytial virus—moved into Level I. A fifth vaccine, against *Coccidioides immitis*, moved from Level IV to Level III.

Challenges

Licensure of the Level I candidate vaccines poses several challenges for vaccination programs and health care providers. For example, the committee believes that a CMV vaccine would best be administered during puberty to protect neonates from CMV infection. This would require acceptance by parents, children, and health care providers that the potential for sexual activity among young adolescents argues for ensuring that the vaccine is administered to 12-year-olds (the proxy age used in the modeling). This also will require a health care milieu that is more capable than it is now of routine vaccination at ages other than infancy. Factors such as health beliefs, health care practices, performance measurements for health plans, and school entry laws have contributed to relatively successful childhood immunization efforts. Similar incentives are not yet as widespread for the newly emerging "adolescent" or "pubertal" vaccination visits that are now recognized as being important for protection against measles and rubella, for example.

Another challenge will be immunization of pregnant women against Group B streptococcus. Previous chapters discussed the barriers, particularly the legal barriers, to the development of vaccines to be administered during pregnancy. The committee's analysis assumes that these barriers have been overcome. The analysis also assumes that immunization of pregnant women can become a standard part of prenatal care. With an alternative assumption that few pregnant women will be immunized, the development of a Group B streptococcus vaccine becomes much less favorable (see Level III).

A third challenge will be acceptance of vaccines using DNA-based technologies. The committee has not factored into the analysis the effect that fear or reluctance might have on the extent to which this emerging technology might be used. The final challenge relates to therapeutic vaccines. Their effectiveness will depend on the early detection of an incipient disease; the committee has not envisioned how this might be done, especially for the therapeutic vaccine for insulin-dependent diabetes mellitus (IDDM). The committee assumes that, during the 15 years of development that remain until the expected licensure of these candidate vaccines, clinical research will provide a better understanding of the population at risk of IDDM and a means of screening for early signs of pancreatic ϑ-cell destruction.

The Level II candidate vaccines include many of the candidate vaccines from the 1985 IOM report on vaccine priorities. This set includes candidate vaccines for sexually transmitted diseases, important pediatric viral infections, bacterial and viral infections associated with long-term chronic disease states, and a therapeutic vaccine directed against a cancer, melanoma. The challenges posed by the licensure of these candidate vaccines are similar to those discussed above for the most favorable set. Vaccines to be administered during puberty require health care delivery systems and practices not yet adequately developed.

The placement in Level II of a vaccine directed against tuberculosis illustrates an interesting point. Although tuberculosis is a very serious disease with high associated health care costs, the number of new cases of tuberculosis is much lower than the number of new cases of many of the other diseases considered in the committee's analysis. However, the assumption by the committee that the vaccine would be given to high-risk populations in a very targeted manner means that program costs are low compared with the cost of annual immunization of the birth cohort of almost 4 million infants.

The Level III candidate vaccines include vaccines to be given during puberty (or during pregnancy, but with a low utilization rate) to protect newborns and infants and vaccines to be administered during infancy to prevent diseases in infants and all others. Challenges related to immunization of pregnant women and of adolescents were discussed above. The committee has assumed that utilization of all vaccines during puberty will be in a midrange of approximately 50%. A Group B streptococcus vaccination strategy that targets girls during puberty or pregnant women with an assumption of a 10% utilization rate falls into Level III. An assumption of a high rate of utilization during pregnancy moves the Group B streptococcus vaccination strategy into the cost-saving set (Level I) of candidate vaccines, as discussed above.

The committee began its deliberations before the licensure of a rotavirus vaccine in 1998. The committee finalized its analysis of rotavirus vaccine with two separate assumptions. One analysis assumed that licensure was imminent in 3 years and required development costs. The other analysis assumed that licensure had occurred and that there were no more development costs. Both analyses place rotavirus vaccine in Level III.

The Level IV candidate vaccines include those whose development might seem less compelling because of limited disease burden, primarily because of low numbers of cases. Several of the candidate vaccines in this category would be used by restricted populations. These populations are limited by geography (e.g., *Borrelia burgdorferi, Histoplasma capsulatum,* and *Coccidioides immitis* vaccines) or by occupation or activity. For example, the shigella and enterotoxigenic *Escherichia coli* vaccines are targeted to overseas travelers, including members of the military.

As stated several times in the report, the committee has not recommended which vaccines should be accorded development priority, nor will it recommend which vaccines should not be developed. Research and development efforts related to Level IV candidate vaccines can be justified in several ways. Research on these vaccines can lead to fundamental discoveries important to other candidate vaccines in the future or to other areas of basic research. Disease patterns could change, increasing the disease burden and making the need for these vaccines more compelling. The discussion of the development of the polio vaccine (Chapter 2) demonstrates that disease epidemiology can indeed change in a relatively short time, making what once seemed like a minor disease a much bigger concern; in this case, ongoing research on poliovirus and poliovirus vaccines contributed greatly to the speedy development of two complementary vaccine strategies once the need was recognized. These Level IV candidate vaccines could also be important due to the burden of disease in other countries, which is not factored into this analysis. The committee argued in Chapter 3 that the inclusion of a candidate vaccine for malaria or for dengue hemorrhagic fever in a report focused on U.S. public health problems was less compelling than inclusion of other candidate vaccines. An analysis of international disease burden would be likely to result in a more favorable cost-effectiveness result for such candidate vaccines.

As this chapter illustrates, a cost-effective analysis is an important tool available to policymakers concerned with vaccine research and development, as well as with vaccine program implementation. Not every scenario could be analyzed and presented, but an important tool has been developed and recommended for use. Prominent candidate vaccines have been used to illustrate the model. The availability of the software and spreadsheets used in the analysis of Vaccine X and of the 26 candidate vaccines means that dialogue around vaccine research and development priorities can continue with a common tool and a common language.

5

Review of the Analytic Model

This chapter reviews in greater detail the components of the committee's analytic model, which were outlined in Chapter 4.

UNIT OF ANALYSIS

The basic analysis included 27 separate cases. Each case represents a specific combination of pathogen or condition, a vaccine candidate, and a population targeted to receive the vaccine. The committee examined 26 candidate vaccines, but included two distinct and alternative target populations for one candidate, thus 27 separate cases. As explained previously, the conditions selected for analysis are a mix of infectious diseases, cancers, and autoimmune disorders of health significance in the United States, and are conditions for which the committee judged that an adequate science base for vaccine development existed. Targeted populations were defined on the basis of factors such as age, health status, or risk of exposure (e.g., geographic region). Among the target populations are infants, adolescents, pregnant women, travelers, and immigrants to specific geographic areas. For some conditions, two complementary target populations (e.g., infants and regional immigrants for borrelia) were defined. For others, alternative vaccination strategies targeting different populations were considered, and each was examined as a separate case. For group B streptococcus, for example, one case is based on adolescent girls as the target population for immunization and a second case considers immunization of pregnant women. The target population influences factors such as the number of doses of vaccine used per year and the time interval between average age at the time of vaccination and average age at the time of onset of a condition.

93

IMPLEMENTING THE ANALYSIS

Basic Model

The essential components used to calculate the cost-effectiveness ratio for each candidate vaccine are the costs of vaccine development, the costs of administering the vaccine to the target population, the reduction in the cost of care expected with the use of the vaccine, and the expected gain in health benefits. The basic calculation can be represented by the following equation:

$$CE_V = (C_D + C_I - C_C) / Q, \tag{1}$$

where CE_V is the cost-effectiveness ratio for case V, which is the analysis for a specific combination of health condition or pathogen, vaccine type, and target population; C_D is the cost of vaccine development; C_I is the annual cost of immunizing the target population; C_C is the annualized costs of care averted by use of the vaccine; and Q is the annualized health benefit from use of the vaccine.

Each of the components of this basic equation must be discounted to account for the time lag between the present and when the cost or health benefit will be realized. The anticipated health benefits and changes in the cost of care must also be reduced to reflect the estimated limits to the efficacy and use of the vaccine. The costs of immunization are also reduced to reflect less than universal use of the vaccine. This more complete characterization of the model can be represented as follows:

$$CE_V = [[\, rC_D + \{[C_I / (1+r)^{T(use)}] \bullet U \} - \{[C_C / (1+r)^{T(use) + T(lag)}] \bullet Eff \bullet U \} \,]] /$$

$$\{[Q / (1+r)^{T(use) + T(lag)}] \bullet Eff \bullet U \}, \tag{2}$$

where r is the discount rate; $T(use)$ is the time until steady-state vaccine use, which includes the time until licensure plus the time to adoption at the assumed rate of use; U is the assumed rate at which the target population will use the vaccine; $T(lag)$ is the time between the use of the vaccine and the realization of health benefits; and Eff is the assumed efficacy of the vaccine. CE_V, C_D, C_I, C_C, and Q are as defined above for Equation 1. Each of the components of the analysis is reviewed in more detail in subsequent sections of this chapter.

Performing the Analysis

The elements of Equation 2 were operationalized through a multipage spreadsheet template developed with the Excel spreadsheet package, version 5

(Microsoft Corporation, 1984–1994), operating on a personal computer. Using the basic template, a separate file was created for each case. The following data were entered: age-specific incidence and death rates, average age at immunization, morbidity scenarios and associated quality-adjustment weights, typical health care provided for the condition and its associated costs, size of the target population, number of vaccine doses required, cost per dose, estimated vaccine efficacy, anticipated steady-state vaccine utilization rates among the target population, remaining development costs, expected time until licensure, and time from licensure until anticipated utilization rates are reached. The basic template was modified to accommodate variations among the cases in the patterns of illness (e.g., distinctive characteristics by age or sex), in the features of the morbidity scenarios (e.g., numbers of health states included and mix of acute and chronic health states), and in the types of care required. Detailed descriptions of the data and calculations used for each case are provided in the Appendixes.

CALCULATION OF HEALTH BENEFITS

Health benefits were measured using quality-adjusted life years (QALYs). Described below is the multistep process followed by the committee to estimate vaccine-related health benefits and calculate QALYs.

Quality-Adjusted Life Years

QALYs reflect the combined impact of morbidity and mortality on the health-related quality of years of life lived. To calculate QALYs, a quality-adjustment weight is applied to each period of time during which a person experiences a changed health state due to a particular condition. These quality-adjusted periods can be summed over a person's expected lifetime (or some other specified period of time). This can be illustrated in a simplified form as

$$Q = W_1 t_1 + W_2 t_2 + W_3 t_3, \tag{3}$$

where Q is the total QALYs experienced by the individual, W_1 is the quality-adjustment weight associated with health state 1, and t_1 is the amount of time spent in that health state. Thus, the lifetime QALYs for an individual who lives for 70 years in perfect health, experiences six months of impaired health from condition 1, and dies five years sooner than the average life expectancy can be represented as

$$Q = (1.0 \bullet 70) + (W_1 \bullet 0.5) + (0.0 \bullet 5.0) .$$

Quality-Adjustment Weights Based on the
Health Utilities Index

The committee considered two basic options for determining the quality-adjustment weights used to represent the impact of morbidity associated with the conditions under study. One option was for the committee, on the basis of its judgment and that of other experts, to assign quality-adjustment weights to each health state in each morbidity scenario associated with each condition. The other option was to use an existing generic health status assessment tool to characterize each health state. The committee chose to use a standard assessment tool to promote the comparability of the assessments for each condition. This approach also allows others who use the committee's work to use the same instrument to make their own assessments of these or other conditions.

The committee selected the Health Utilities Index (HUI) Mark II (Feeny et al., 1995: Torrance et al., 1995). The HUI Mark II characterizes morbidity by using seven health attributes (sensation, mobility, emotion, cognition, self-care, pain, and fertility), each of which is divided into three, four, or five levels. Each level has a fixed quantitative score between 0 and 1.0 representing the strength of the "preference" for that level of morbidity relative to full health (1.0) or death (0).

A health state is described by assigning to it a specific level from each attribute. The HUI quality-adjustment weight for the health state is then derived from the following formula:

$$U = 1.06 \ (b_1 \bullet b_2 \bullet b_3 \bullet b_4 \bullet b_5 \bullet b_6 \bullet b_7) - 0.06 \ , \qquad (4)$$

where U is the utility of the health state (i.e., the quality weight), and b_x is the score for the level assigned for attribute x (Torrance et al., 1995). U corresponds to W_i in Equation 3.

Although HUI Mark II was originally developed for a study of childhood cancer survivors, it has been adapted for use with adult populations. It has also been used with the Ontario Health Survey (Berthelot et al., 1992; Roberge et al., 1995) and the Canadian National Population Health Survey (NPHS) (Catlin and Will, 1992; Wolfson, 1996) to develop provisional estimates of age-specific health status at the population level.[*]

---

[*]Final estimates for the NPHS will be based on the scoring system under development for the HUI Mark III, a revised HUI with eight component attributes (Torrance et al., 1992; Boyle et al., 1995).

Steps in the Calculation of Anticipated Health Benefits from Vaccine Use

The calculation of health benefits from vaccine use for each condition under study is a multistep process. The steps are listed in Box 5-1 and are described in the sections that follow.

Develop Morbidity Scenarios

For each condition studied, the committee, with the advice of outside experts, developed morbidity scenarios to describe the characteristic sequences of acute or chronic health states, the duration of each health state, and the proportion of persons with the condition who experience each scenario. The scenarios also capture the premature mortality associated with a condition but which is delayed 1 or more years beyond the onset of the condition. For most of the conditions included in the committee's analysis, several scenarios were required to depict the associated morbidity.

Some pathogens or conditions affect specific subpopulations in distinctive ways. For example, the consequences of infection with chlamydia, a sexually transmitted disease, are very different in men and women. For those conditions, separate morbidity scenarios were defined for each appropriate subpopulation. The subpopulation analyses were combined in the final stages of the calculation of the cost-effectiveness ratio.

Calculate Quality-Adjustment Weights

Once the morbidity scenarios were developed, the committee reviewed each health state and assigned a level in each of the seven attributes of HUI Mark II. To better reflect the range of morbidity represented by some health states, the committee estimated the proportion of cases of illness that should be assigned to each level of a specific health utility attribute. The preference score for the attribute was calculated as a weighted average of the scores for each level. The quality-adjustment weight for the health state was obtained by combining the scores for each attribute according to Equation 4. The calculations were performed using an Excel spreadsheet template.

Calculate Discounted Quality-Adjusted Life Expectancies

The quality-adjustment weights for each condition's morbidity scenarios (described above) were used to measure QALYs without the vaccine intervention. Quality-adjustment weights reflecting the average health status of the

---

BOX 5-1 Steps Used in Calculation of Vaccine-Related Health Benefits for a Specific Condition

- Develop morbidity scenarios, including estimate of percentage of cases represented by each scenario.
- Calculate quality-adjustment weights for each health state in each scenario.
- Calculate discounted quality-adjusted life expectancies.
- Establish age-specific incidence and death rates for the condition.
- Calculate average age at onset and average age at death.
- Calculate average interval between vaccination and onset of illness.
- Calculate average interval between age at onset of illness and age at condition-related death.
- Calculate life expectancy at average age at onset and average age at death.
- Calculate a baseline quality-adjustment weight for the population.
- Adjust the health state weights to reflect the population baseline.
- Calculate discounted QALYs for each health state with and without the impact of condition-related morbidity.
- For each morbidity scenario, sum the QALYs for the component health states.
- For each morbidity scenario, subtract QALYs with the condition from QALYs without the condition (i.e., calculate the condition-related QALYs lost).
- Weight the condition-related QALYs lost in each scenario by the percentage of cases represented by that scenario and sum across all scenarios.
- Multiply the sum of QALYs lost by the total number of cases for the condition.

---

population were used to measure QALYs with the intervention. To measure the impact of mortality and lifetime impairment, standard life table values were "quality adjusted" for the average health status of the population and discounted to their present value. Described here are the population-level quality adjustments used in the committee's analysis and the calculation of the discounted quality-adjusted life table values.

Population-Based Quality-Adjustment Weights   The analysis takes into account the underlying average health status of the population, independent of a specific condition or use of a candidate vaccine. Although an individual might be considered to experience periods of perfect health, represented by a quality-adjustment weight of 1.0, the health status of a population will reflect a range of individual levels of health status and should not be represented by a quality-adjustment weight set at 1.0. This average health status in the population is assumed to be the maximum health status level that can be achieved by use of any of the vaccines considered in the committee's analysis. To represent the average health status of the U.S. population, the committee adopted quality-adjustment weights representing the HUI Mark II-based age- and sex-specific health status results from the Canadian NPHS (Wolfson, 1996). These weights reflect population-based values calculated from self-reported features of health status. They range from .93 for men aged 15–24 to .64 for women aged 85 and older. The separate NPHS health status estimates for men and women were combined as a weighted average based on the age-specific proportions of men and women in the U.S. population. Since NPHS did not produce health status estimates for the population younger than 15 years of age, the committee chose, in the absence of other data, to apply the value for ages 15–24 to the younger age groups. See Table 5-1 for the quality adjustment weights for health status of the general population.

Life Expectancies The discounted quality-adjusted life expectancies used in the committee's analysis are based on the 1993 abridged U.S. life tables for the total population and for males and females separately (National Center for Health Statistics, 1993). These adjustments were incorporated through calculations that use the life table stationary population in each age interval (the $_nL_x$ values, in life table notation), which can also be interpreted as the number of person-years lived from ages x to $x+n$. The quality adjustment was incorporated by multiplying the number of person-years by the corresponding age- and sex-specific quality-adjustment weight for the population (Sullivan, 1971; Erickson et al., 1995):

$$_nL_x^* = w_x \bullet {_nL_x}.$$ (5)

The quality-adjusted person-years in each age interval were then discounted for the period between age at the onset of a condition and the midpoint of the age interval. Because the average age at onset for the conditions under study varies from infancy to older than 70 years, a series of life expectancy calculations were made for selected ages at onset (0, 1, 5, 10, 20, 30, 40, 50, 60, 70, 80, and 85 years of age). The discounting period was defined as the difference between the midpoint of the age interval and the age at onset. For example, the discounting period for person-years lived in the age interval 60–65 with disease onset at age 20 was 42.5 years (62.5 – 20 = 42.5).

Once the discounted person-year values were obtained, standard life table calculations were used to calculate discounted quality-adjusted life expectancies at the selected ages of onset,[*] with life expectancy at age x designated as e_x^*.

---

[*]To calculate life expectancies, the person-years lived are summed from the oldest to the youngest ages. For each age interval, a cumulative total of all person-years lived in that interval and at all older ages is obtained. Dividing the cumulative total for age interval x (designated T_x) by the number of persons in the life table population alive at the beginning of that age interval (l_x) gives the life expectancy (e_x) at age x. See Erickson et al. (1995) for additional discussion and illustration of life table calculations incorporating quality adjustments.

TABLE 5-1 Population-Based Age-Specific Health Status (quality adjustment weights)

Age Group	Males	Females	Combined
<1			0.92
1–4			0.92
5–14			0.92
15–24	0.93	0.92	0.92
25–34	0.93	0.92	0.92
35–44	0.92	0.91	0.92
45–54	0.89	0.87	0.88
55–64	0.87	0.86	0.86
65–74	0.85	0.83	0.84
75–84	0.81	0.76	0.78
≥85	0.71	0.64	0.66

NOTE: Values are based on the overall population (both household and institutionalized); combined values calculated as weighted average of male and female values (weights from distribution of U.S. population); no direct estimates were made for population younger than age 15, values for ages 15–24 were assumed to apply.

SOURCE: Wolfson, 1996.

Establish Age-Specific Incidence and Death Rates

Estimates of current age-specific incidence and mortality for each condition were assembled. Rates and numbers of cases and deaths were estimated for the following age groups: under 1 year, 1–4, 5–14, 15–24, 25–34, 35–44, 45–54, 55–64, 65–74, 75–84, and ≥85.

Although some of the conditions included in the analysis (e.g., Lyme disease [caused by *Borrelia burgdorferi*], gonorrhea, shigellosis, and tuberculosis) are designated as "reportable" and numbers of reported cases are published by the CDC (1994), the completeness of reporting varies by condition, reflecting both undiagnosed cases and incomplete reporting of diagnosed cases. Separate surveillance programs by CDC and others for conditions such as tuberculosis are the basis for some estimates of incidence. In the absence of surveillance programs, some estimates have been based on data from state- or community-level studies. Others rest largely on expert judgment. The specific sources of data for each condition are described in the Appendixes.

It is important to emphasize that the analysis uses incidence data, that is, the number (or rate) of new cases that would be expected during 1 year. For chronic illnesses such as multiple sclerosis, these data will differ from the prevalence estimates that are often reported.

Calculate Time Intervals for Discounting Future Health Benefits

As noted above, the timing of the health benefits expected from the use of the potential new vaccines included in the committee's analysis will vary depending on the intervals between the typical age at immunization and the age at onset of an illness or the age at death. The intervals calculated for the analysis are the following: T_o, the time from vaccination to the average age at onset of illness, and T_d, the difference between the average age at onset of illness and average age at the time of illness-related death. T_d is of interest for those acute conditions for which the age at death from a condition differs markedly from the overall age of patients with that condition. The time interval related to premature death following a period of chronic illness is accounted for separately.

The distribution of cases and deaths by age was used to estimate the average age at the time of onset of the condition and the average age at the time of death. Specifically, the midpoint of each age group was weighted by the proportion of cases or deaths occurring in that age group:

$$A = \Sigma(a_g \bullet P_g), \tag{6}$$

where A is the average age of onset (A_o) or death (A_d), a is the midpoint of age group g, and P is the proportion of cases or deaths in age group g.

Age at vaccination, A_v, was determined by the vaccination strategy and the target population specified by the committee. Most cases fall into one of the following categories:

Target Population	**Age at Vaccination**
Infants	6 months
Adolescents	12 years
Pregnant women	Average age of mothers at first births, minus 2 months (24.7 years)
New cases (therapeutic vaccines)	Age at diagnosis (assumed to equal average age at onset)

See the Appendixes for detailed information on the age at vaccination used for each case.

Thus, the interval from vaccination to onset of illness is calculated as $T_o = A_o - A_v$, and the difference between age at onset of illness and illness-related death is calculated as $T_d = A_d - A_o$.

Calculate Condition-Related Life Expectancies

The discounted quality-adjusted life expectancies for selected ages were used to calculate the life expectancy in the population at the average age at onset of a condition and at the average age of condition-related death. Specifically, the discounted and adjusted life expectancies were weighted by the proportion of cases or deaths occurring in the appropriate age group:

$$e^* = \sum (e_g^* \bullet P_g) \, , \qquad\qquad (7)$$

where e^* is the discounted quality-adjusted life expectancy in the population at the average age at onset (e_o^*) or at the average age at condition-related death (e_d^*); P_g is the proportion of cases or deaths in age group g. For example, the life expectancy at age 20 years was weighted by the proportion of cases (or deaths) in the age group 15–24.

Adjust for the Underlying Health Status of the Population

HUI Mark II-based quality-adjustment weights for health states were calculated from attribute scores assigned by the committee without reference to the underlying health status of the general population. Because that underlying health status declines with age, the committee made an adjustment to reflect the differences in the age patterns of the conditions that it considered. First, a population "baseline" quality-adjustment weight (w') for a condition was calculated as the weighted average of the age-specific quality-adjustment weights for the general population. The age-specific values were weighted by the proportion of cases at each age and were summed to produce the baseline weight for that condition. In general, one population baseline weight was calculated for each condition under study. If separate analyses were performed for specific subpopulations, a baseline weight was calculated for each subpopulation.

Then, the original quality-adjustment weight for each health state was multiplied by the baseline weight for the condition to produce a baseline-adjusted quality weight:

$$w_i = h_i \bullet w' \, , \qquad\qquad (8)$$

where w_i is the baseline-adjusted quality weight for health state i, h_i is the quality adjustment weight for health state i calculated from the committee's HUI Mark II scores; and w' is the population baseline quality-adjustment weight.

Calculate Discounted QALYs for Each Health State

Morbidity   For each health state, two sets of QALYs—QALYs with the condition under study and QALYs without the condition under study—were calculated. QALYs with the condition were derived by multiplying the baseline-adjusted quality weight for the health state by the duration of the health state. A parallel calculation in which the population baseline quality-adjustment weight was multiplied by the duration of the health state determined the QALYs that the general population would experience without the condition under study. Both sets of QALYs were then discounted to adjust for the time from average age at vaccination to average age at onset. Calculation of QALYs when the condition under study is present can be represented as

$$q_i = (w_i \bullet t_i) / (1 + r)^{(T_o + t_m)},$$

where q_i is the QALY value for health state i, w_i is the baseline-adjusted quality weight for the health state, t_i is the duration of the health state, r is the discount rate, T_o is the time from average age at vaccination to average age at onset, and t_m is the duration of health states that intervene between the onset of the condition and health state i. If related health states that persist for at least 1 year intervene between the onset of the condition and health state i, the discount period must be increased by t_m. To calculate q'_i, the corresponding QALY value for the general population, w_i is replaced by w', the population baseline quality-adjustment weight.

Calculation of QALYs for two kinds of health states required alternative approaches. First, for states that persist for a specified multiyear period rather than a period of days or weeks, allowance must be made for discounting the stream of QALYs associated with the health state. In these health states, QALYs discounted to the beginning of the health state were calculated by using the Excel present-value function. This value is then further discounted for the period $T_o + t_m$.

Second, for health states that persist for the normal remaining lifetime, the discounted quality-adjusted life expectancy at onset (e_o^*) was used as the value of the QALYs that the general population would experience without the condition under study. To estimate QALYs with the condition, e_o^* was multiplied by the committee's quality-adjustment weight for the health state h_i. (Adjustment for the baseline health status of the population is already reflected in the quality-adjusted life expectancy.) Additional discounting for the period from vaccination to onset $(T_o + t_m)$ is performed.

Mortality The impact of mortality on QALYs was estimated as described above for morbidity associated with lifetime health states. The death rates obtained for each condition reflect deaths that occur within a short time following onset of the condition. The discounted quality-adjusted life expectancy at the average age at death (e_d^*) provides the estimate of QALYs lost due to deaths, which must be discounted for the period $T_o + T_d$, where T_o is the time from average age at vaccination to average age at onset and T_d is the difference between average age at onset of illness and average age at illness-related death. If the age pattern of deaths is similar to the age pattern of illness, $T_d = 0$. If deaths are more common among younger or older patients, $T_d \neq 0$.

For some conditions, deaths occur following a period of chronic impairment. These have been assumed to be additional condition-related deaths beyond those reflected in the age-specific death rates. The age at death is calculated as the average age at onset of the condition plus the duration of health states experienced between onset and death. The discounted quality-adjusted life expectancy at the age at death is used to calculate the QALYs lost due to these deaths. Additional discounting for the period T_o plus the interval between onset and death must be included. Life expectancy at the time of these deaths was estimated by interpolation from the values calculated for specific ages of onset of illness (see above).

Calculate Total QALYs Gained with Vaccine Use

The QALYs associated with each health state were combined. For each morbidity scenario, the state-specific QALYs were summed, and the QALYs lived with the condition under study were subtracted from the QALYs for the general population without the condition. This provides an estimate of the QALYs that could be gained in each scenario with vaccine use.

The scenario-specific QALYs to be gained were multiplied by the proportion of cases of illness experiencing that scenario and were summed across all scenarios. This total was multiplied by the number of cases, or by the number of deaths for the QALYs associated with mortality, to calculate the overall benefit that the use of a vaccine for the condition under study would be expected to have in the population. If subpopulations were used in the analysis, the results were calculated for each subpopulation and the subpopulation results were summed to produce an estimate of the total health benefit.

$$Q_{;s} = [\Sigma_j (q_j \bullet P_j)] \bullet N_s , \qquad (10)$$

where $Q_{;s}$ is the total QALYs to be gained with vaccine use across all subpopulations, q_j is the individual QALY gain in scenario j; P_j is the proportion of cases of illness experiencing scenario j, and N_s is the total number of cases of illness in subpopulations.

COST FACTORS

As shown in Equation 1, the cost components of the numerator of the cost-effectiveness ratio include the costs of vaccine development (C_D), the cost of vaccine use (C_I), and the reduction in health care and related costs (C_C) that would be expected with vaccine use. All cost estimates are presented in constant dollars.

Vaccine Development

The costs of future research and clinical trials that would be needed to complete development of a vaccine and have it licensed, designated C_D, are a mix of public- and private-sector expenditures. They were assumed to fall at one of six levels: $120 million, $240 million, $300 million, $360 million, $390 million, or $400 million. A development cost was assigned to each vaccine on the basis of the committee's assessment of the current stage of the vaccine's development. In terms of the analysis, the cost of vaccine development is treated as an amortized fixed cost. The committee also assigned each candidate vaccine to one of three development intervals: 3, 7, or 15 years. Discounting incorporated this development interval to adjust for the differences in the times when the associated costs and benefits of the vaccines will be realized.

Vaccine Use

The cost of vaccine use is a function of the cost per dose of the vaccine, the cost to administer the vaccine, the number of doses each person must receive to be fully immunized, and the size of the population targeted to receive the vaccine:

$$C_I = (d + a) \bullet Dose \bullet Pop , \qquad (11)$$

where C_I is the annual cost of immunizing the target population, d is the cost per dose of the vaccine, a is the cost of administering a dose of vaccine, *Dose* is the number of doses each person must receive, and *Pop* is the size of the target population.

A vaccine's cost per dose is represented by the purchase price rather than the marginal cost to manufacturers of producing a single dose. The cost of prophylactic vaccines was assumed to be either $50 or $100. The cost of therapeutic vaccines was set at $500. The marginal cost of administering a dose of vaccine was set at $10. For most vaccines, it was assumed that three doses would be needed to achieve full immunization. In specific cases (e.g., influenza vaccine), the number of doses required was altered to match the available evidence.

The committee defined a target population for each vaccine considered, and the size of that target population was determined by using current estimates of the U.S. population by age. For vaccines intended for use in infants or adolescents, the target population was assumed to equal the birth cohort or the population at age 12, respectively. For vaccines intended for use in special subpopulations (e.g., travelers, residents in a specific geographic region, persons with chronic illness) the basis for the estimate of the size of the target population is described in detail in the Appendixes.

It was assumed that 5 years would be required following licensing to achieve stable, maximum levels of use of preventive vaccines. For therapeutic vaccines, this interval was assumed to be 2 years. The appropriate interval was incorporated into the discounting calculations.

Cost of Care

To estimate the cost of health care associated with each condition, the committee developed a set of "clinical scenarios" that specified the health services required, including hospitalizations, procedures, medications, office visits, rehabilitation services, and long-term institutional care. An appropriate unit of service (e.g., hospital days, doses of medication) was specified, and the amount of care received was defined in terms of those units. Costs, represented by charges for specific services, also were specified in terms of units of service.

For inpatient hospitalizations, hospital costs were estimated by using diagnosis-related group average national payments by the Health Care Financing Administration (HCFA) (St. Anthony's Publishing, Inc., 1995). Outpatient costs and inpatient physician visits were estimated from HCFA data as well (HCFA, 1995). For these costs, the committee estimated general categories of costs (outpatient physician visit with and without tests, etc.) and applied these to the morbidity scenarios. See Table 5-2 for examples of unit costs.

In addition, for each form of care, the committee specified the proportion of patients within the scenario that received that form of care. It was assumed that all costs of care associated with the condition under study would be averted with vaccine use.

The total cost of each form of care was calculated as

$$c_c = (u_c \bullet n_c) \bullet p_c \bullet p_s \bullet N, \tag{12}$$

where c_c is the total cost of type of care c for health state i, u_c is the unit cost of this form of care, n_c is the number of units of care received, p_c is the percentage of patients within the scenario that received this form of care, p_s is the percentage of all patients that experience this scenario, and N is the total number of patients with the condition under study.

The cost c_c was then discounted to adjust for T_o, the time from average age at vaccination to average age at onset of the condition, plus t_m, the duration of intervening health states that persist for at least 1 year. For continuing care required for a specified multiyear period rather than a period of days or weeks, it was necessary to allow for discounting of the stream of future costs. As in the QALY calculations, these costs were discounted to the beginning of the health state by using the Excel present-value function. For some health states, care continues for the remaining lifetime. The length of the remaining lifetime was estimated from the unadjusted 1993 life table life expectancy value (NCHS, 1993) at the average age at onset of the health state.

TABLE 5-2 Examples of Health Care Cost Estimates Used

Outpatient Costs	
Physician A	$50
Physician B (specialist)	$100
Physician C (in hospital)	$150
Medication A (nonprescription)	$10
Medication B (inexpensive prescription)	$50
Medication C (expensive prescription)	$150
Diagnostic A	$50
Diagnostic B	$100
Diagnostic C	$500
Hospitalization Costs (per admission; based on hospitalization)	
Multiple Sclerosis	$3,000
Pneumonia	$3,000
Viral Meningitis	$3,000
Tuberculosis	$6,000
Cellulitis	$3,000
Amputation	$7,000
Cirrhosis	$5,000
Ectopic Pregnancies	$3,000
Ulcer	$3,000
Digestive	$4,000
Gastroenteritis	$2,000
Complicated delivery (additional cost)	$2,000
Infectious myocarditis	$3,000
Diabetic complications	$3,000
Melanoma	$4,000

The total discounted cost of care that would be averted with vaccine use, C_C in Equation 1, was obtained by summing the costs across all health states. As was done for health benefits, calculations for separate subpopulations were summed to produce an estimate of total costs.

VACCINE EFFICACY AND UTILIZATION

The analysis includes adjustments for incomplete efficacy and use of the candidate vaccines, either of which will reduce the expected health benefits and savings in the cost of care. A lower utilization rate will also reduce the costs ssociated with vaccinating the target population. These adjustments were made by multiplying the QALY and cost measures by the assumed efficacy (*Eff*) and utilization rates (*U*) (see Equation 2).

It was assumed that preventive vaccines would achieve an efficacy level of 75%. The efficacy of therapeutic vaccines was assumed to be 40%. A utilization rate of 10%, 30%, 50%, 60%, or 90% was assigned to each vaccine.

COST-EFFECTIVENESS RATIOS

For each condition, cost-effectiveness ratios were calculated at three stages in the analysis. The first ratio examines the potential impact of the vaccine on morbidity and costs under the assumption that the vaccines are available immediately without any additional cost or time for development and that they are fully efficacious and are used by the entire target population. This comparison focuses attention on what might be considered an ideal vaccine benefit. The second cost-effectiveness ratio factors in the adjustments for incomplete efficacy and use, which tend to increase the cost of achieving the anticipated health benefit. The final ratio, which corresponds to Equation 2, shows the impact of the time and money needed to develop these vaccines. Some vaccines that promise substantial benefit require longer and more expensive periods of development, whereas others that offer smaller benefits are expected to be available more quickly and cheaply. In general, the committee found that the adjustments for efficacy and utilization had a more substantial impact on a vaccine's cost-effectiveness than the additional time and cost needed for development.

6

Ethical Considerations and Caveats

The recommendations in this report regarding priorities in the development of vaccines over the next 10 and 20 years relies directly on the measurement of the burden of disease in recipient populations for each vaccine. The model employed by the committee allows comparisons of vaccines in quantitative terms for their relative cost-effectiveness in reducing the burden of disease. There are ethical or value judgments and assumptions built into this model, and it would be imprudent for policymakers to assume that the model alone constitutes a completely ethically appropriate and uncontroversial standard for priorities in resource allocation for vaccine development. This chapter will first discuss those ethical and value judgments implicit in the model and, secondly, those that present unresolved complexities. These unresolved matters tend, for the most part, to center on issues of fairness and justice. It is especially important for policymakers to be explicitly aware of these unresolved issues since it would often be inappropriate to move directly from the relative ranking of vaccine priorities yielded by the model to final priorities for policy without talking them into account.

Since resources for vaccine development, as for any publicly supported health intervention, are inevitably scarce, it may seem to be a virtual truism that these limited resources should be directed to those vaccines that would achieve the greatest reduction in the burden of disease. But the allocation of public resources by policymakers, for vaccine development as elsewhere, must be just or fair to the public that will be affected by the prioritization.

There are two main reasons the committee has not attempted to build ethical or value judgments about justice or fairness in allocation into the quantitative model. First, although much effort in health policy has been devoted to the development and validation of measures of the burden of disease, very little work has been done to integrate these considerations of fairness into cost-benefit or cost-effectiveness measures. To the extent that cost-effectiveness measures sometimes conflict with fairness, such integration of considerations of fairness into the measures could amount to partial abandonment of the cost-effectiveness standard. Second, these issues of fairness remain controversial, and there is no clear consensus with which the committee could have justified building specific positions into our model.

For these reasons, it is common in studies like the committee's to employ a cost-effectiveness analysis to develop a priority list, and then to remind policy-makers who will make use of the list that they must, of course, also consider distributive issues of fairness or justice concerning the distribution of benefits and burdens in the ultimate priorities that they adopt. While the committee was unable, for the two reasons cited above, to integrate these issues of fairness or justice into the formal model, the committee does attempt to advance attention to these issues beyond what they typically receive by discussing briefly the nature of some of the more important considerations and illustrating where they arise in determining priorities for vaccine development.

Before discussing ethical issues in the development and use of the model for prioritization of new vaccine development, the committee wants to underscore one important ethical limitation that was imposed from the outset by the scope of work: the committee was asked to consider only the U.S. health needs of the population. In some cases this resulted in diseases with a very high burden of disease worldwide, such as malaria, cholera, and shistosomiasis, not even appearing on the final list of candidates that the committee included in the analysis. In other cases, vaccines for diseases that were considered might have received a very different ranking if our study had not been restricted to the U.S. population. It would have been a challenge beyond our resources and mandate to include an assessment of international disease burden as an additional quantitative factor in this model, and the committee did not undertake this.

Clearly, U.S. government agencies like National Institute of Allergy and Infectious Diseases and the other components of the National Institutes of Health are justified in giving priority to the needs of U.S. citizens whose tax dollars support their work. However, a wide variety of government-supported programs and activities, from direct foreign aid and overseas disaster relief programs to support for international peacekeeping, human rights, and third-world development efforts, are concerned with the well-being of the population beyond our borders and reflect our recognition of international responsibilities even if they sometimes serve U.S. interests as well. Especially in an area like medical research in general and vaccine development in particular, in which the United States has long been a world leader, the committee believes that ethically justified priorities for new vaccine development cannot ignore health needs beyond our own borders. Both governmental agencies and private organizations that make use of this report are urged not to ignore worldwide needs and opportunities for disease prevention from new vaccine development.

ETHICAL AND VALUE JUDGMENTS
BUILT INTO THE MODEL

These comments begin with the main ethical or value judgments built into the quantitative model that the committee developed and employed.

All QALYs Count Equally

The quality-adjusted life year (QALY) has been widely used in health care and other contexts in recent years to compare the outcomes of different health or other interventions. The calculation of QALYs is described in Chapters 4 and 5. The QALY measures the impact an illness or a health intervention on an individuals' expected years of life and their quality of life. The QALY measure assumes that an additional year of life has the same value regardless of the age of the person who receives it, assuming the life years are of comparable quality; for example, assuming no difference in quality, an additional life year secured for an infant, a 30-year-old, and a 75-year-old all have equal value. In this respect, all QALYs have equal value no matter who receives them or how old individuals are when they receive them.

Recently, a measure of the burden of illness in terms of disability-adjusted life years (DALYs) was developed for the World Bank and World Health Organization (Murray and Lopez, 1996). In contrast to QALYs, DALYs assign different values to years of life depending on age, and independent of differences in health-related quality of life. Roughly, DALYs assign relatively low value to a year of life in infancy and childhood, significantly greater value in the economically productive young adult years, and less value again at older ages. The principal rationale offered for this difference in the social value of life extension based on age was that it is common in many countries for persons to fill different social roles at different ages. In particular, because both the young and the old tend to depend on adults in their productive years for their well-being, the social value of life extension during adult life, as opposed to childhood and old age, was deemed greater.

The committee chose QALYs rather than DALYs because it believes the proper societal perspective on the value of extending its members' lives focuses on the value to those individuals of extending their lives, not the value of those lives to others. Using the latter perspective would bring in other differentiations between individuals in their social and economic value to others that the committee believes should not be given ethical significance in health care resource allocation in general, or vaccine development priorities in particular.

Years of Life at Different Ages Are Weighted by Quality

There is one important respect in which the committee's model does not assign equal value to year of life no matter the age at which a person receives it. The model does not assume that population-averaged levels of health status are the same at all ages, since that assumption is clearly false. The model therefore does use population-based age-related adjustments for average health status of populations at different ages; for example, because the health status of the average 45-year-old is higher than that of the average 80-year-old, the model adjusts the value of life extension to reflect this difference and thereby assigns higher quality-adjustment value to a year of life at age 45 than at age 80. This does not give different value to a year of life at different ages simply because of the difference in age, but is only a way of adjusting for differences in average health status of populations at different ages. It also should not be confused with the age-weighting of the DALY which assigns different value to a year of life based simply on age itself and independent of the health-related quality of that life-year for the person who receives it.

The Value of Life Extension with and without Disabilities

There is a further respect in which adjustments for differences in the health-related quality of life of added life years is ethically controversial. Some vaccines are developed for a disease to which specific populations may be vulnerable because of predisposing conditions that also reduce their health-related quality of life. The vaccine will not affect the underlying health condition, nor its impact on the person's quality of life. For example, people with untreated AIDS have a reduced health-related quality of life, as measured with the HUI, and are predisposed to other infectious diseases. Preventing those other infectious diseases by itself will not affect the quality of life decrement due to AIDS. On the other hand, the current influenza vaccine does not prevent all disease in elderly persons, but it does tend to avert life-threatening illness.

In each of these cases, the value of preventing death or illness, or alternatively of the years of life gained, will be reduced according to the effects that the preexisting condition or the resultant limitation have on the health-related quality of life of survivors. This means, to use the example of a vaccine to be given to prevent opportunistic infections in patients with AIDS (who have an already compromised quality of life), that a year of life extension for the patients with AIDS will have less value than a year of life extension produced by a different vaccine given to healthy persons or which leaves survivors with their initial healthy quality of life. In the context of disabilities, of which AIDS is an example covered by the Americans with Disabilities Act, it has been charged that this method of valuing health benefits discriminates against persons with disabilities by holding that their lives, and preserving their lives, are of less value than the lives of persons without disabilities.

This is a deep and troubling difficulty for any prioritization method that adjusts the value of preventing death or life extension by the health-related quality of the additional life years produced. It is not one that the committee can fully explore here, much less resolve. In support of valuing life extension in this way is the uncontroversial point that any individual will value a treatment that extends his or her life with full quality of life over an alternative treatment that will provide an equal period of life extension, but with a seriously compromised quality of life.

The committee's model extends this difference in the value of alternative life-extending interventions, based on differences in the quality of those life years, from the case of a single person choosing alternative treatments or interventions for herself, to the case of the social judgments of the value of life-extending interventions for different persons. Here, the person with the compromised quality of life might reasonably argue that a year of life extension is of no less value to her, despite its compromised quality, than a year of life extension is to a person who has no limitation in quality of life. The alternative for each person without the life-extending intervention is the same, namely death; each loses everything if he or she loses his or her life. It might therefore be argued, for example, that so long as the life extension provides a quality of life acceptable to the person who receives it, it should be given a value or importance equal to that of extending another person's life at a higher level of quality.

Our analytic model does not take this last position, however, but instead adjusts the value of all life-extending interventions both for the length and quality of the years of life-extension. Members of the committee disagreed about the correct resolution of this difficulty. Consequently, the committee has followed the standard procedure of adjusting the value of life extension according to the health-related quality of the life extended, not just in *intrapersonal* choices and evaluations of alternative health care interventions, but in the *interpersonal* choices and evaluations required by our prioritization process as well. Our analytic model can also potentially discriminate against the disabled who receive vaccines that prevent morbidity, not just mortality. This can occur when the disability acts as a co-morbid condition reducing the benefits from disease treatment or prevention, and when the presence of the disability makes disease treatment or prevention more costly. Here, as at a number of points, the committee explicitly notes the ethical issue and the position the methodology used in the analysis takes regarding it, but does not purport to have established conclusively that this position is the correct position.

Discount Rates for Costs and Benefits

The committee's analytic model uses a discount rate of 3% per year for the costs and benefits of vaccine programs. This might seem to be simply an economic or accounting matter, unrelated to any ethical or value judgments, but it is not. Use of a discount rate for economic resources that represent the costs of producing a benefit is not ethically controversial. If an investment of resources produces an economic benefit or return—for example, in money—it is more valuable if that benefit is produced immediately than if the same economic benefit is produced 10 years hence. In the first case, the economic return can be invested over the subsequent 10 years and so will yield a substantially greater sum at the end of that period than in the second case, where the same initial return is not produced until the end of 10 years. Likewise, if a benefit—either an economic benefit or a direct improvement in people's health status—will be produced at some fixed time in the future, say again 10 years hence, it is better to be able to pay the costs of producing the benefit as late as possible—for example in 10 years instead of immediately—because the funds can then be invested to earn a return in the meantime until they must be expended; fewer current dollars are necessary to produce a given sum of money to pay the costs of the benefit if they are not needed until some time in the future.

The ethically controversial issue is whether a given degree and period of improvement in well-being is of greater value the sooner it occurs, and of less value the longer its occurrence is delayed. If two vaccines are typically given at the same age, but the first prevents a disease with a given burden within the first year after being given, while the second prevents a disease with the same burden in the 10th year after being given, is the health benefit of the second vaccine of less value than that of the first? Haemophilus influenzae b (Hib) vaccine, which is given to infants to prevent meningitis in the first year or two after vaccine administration, is an example of the first sort. Hepatitis B vaccine given to infants to reduce risk of liver cancer in adulthood is an example of the second sort. Applying a discount rate directly to benefits of health interventions measured as changes in well-being leads to the conclusion that the first vaccine provides a greater health benefit.

It is important to be clear about the nature of this issue, and not to confuse it with two other issues. First, the later improvement in well-being may be worth less than the immediate improvement if there is more uncertainty about realizing the benefit because of its later occurrence. Future benefits and costs should be discounted for their uncertainty. However, later effects on well-being are not necessarily less certain than immediate effects.

Second, sometimes a near-term improvement in well-being, such as restoring or preventing a person's loss of a particular function now as opposed to 10 years hence, will be of greater value because the improvement will have a positive impact on the person's level of function and well-being over the intervening 10 years. This difference in well-being because of the time at which the restoration or prevention of loss of function occurs will be captured directly by applying a QALY measure to the person's life over those 10 years. No discount rate need be applied to changes in well-being to reflect this difference.

Applying a discount rate directly to well-being assumes a pure time preference for well-being, a preference for achieving gains sooner rather than later and incurring losses later rather than sooner. The ethically controversial nature of this assumption can be seen with a simple example. It will be more valuable to prevent pain or suffering of a given duration and magnitude today than to prevent pain or suffering of a greater magnitude and duration in the future, so long as applying the discount rate to the future pain brings down its present disvalue to less than the disvalue of the current pain. But that appears to say that the life with more pain or suffering is better than the life with less, simply because of when the pain occurs in the person's life. Despite these complexities, it is common to apply a discount rate in studies such as this to both costs and health benefits, and there are technical problems and apparent paradoxes that arise if only costs but not health benefits are discounted (Gold et al., 1996). The committee has therefore chosen to follow common practice and to use a discount rate for economic costs as well as health benefits. We have shown in Chapter 4 (the previous chapter on methods) in the discussion of the hypothetical Vaccine X the difference doing so makes in comparison with not discounting well-being.

Which Benefits and Costs Should Be Counted in the Prioritization Process?

The committee's analytic model for prioritizing different potential vaccines attempts to measure the direct health benefits to the potential vaccine recipients from diseases prevented by those vaccines. This excludes two kinds of indirect benefits from consideration. First, sometimes there are nonhealth benefits to vaccine recipients, such as prevention of lost wages when the diseases prevented typically result in significant periods of time away from work.

Second, sometimes there are indirect benefits to others besides the direct recipients of a vaccine. For example, some childhood diseases, such as varicella typically require a parent to stay home from work to care for the child, resulting in lost wages to the parent and economic costs to the parent's employer. Many other diseases affecting adults during parenting years can result in the need for child care because of the parent's illness or death.

The committee believes that counting these indirect and nonhealth benefits can result in ethically unacceptable discrimination. For example, counting the prevention of lost wages among the benefits of a particular vaccination program will result in lower priority being given to the prevention of diseases typically acquired during the nonworking years of a person's life, specifically childhood and old age. It would also discriminate against diseases that affect lower-income individuals disproportionately, whose lost wages will be less on average than those of higher income groups. (In the development of vaccines for international use, this discriminatory impact would be far greater and would disproportionately favor vaccines used in developed countries.) We recognize that these non-health and indirect benefits to others are real benefits. Indeed, especially from a public health perspective for making resource allocation and investment decisions, it may appear incompatible with a cost-effectiveness prioritization to selectively ignore some benefits. But this is only one place among others that the committee cites in this chapter at which ethical concerns place some constraint on the single-minded maximization of benefits that an unconstrained cost-effectiveness standard would yield.

In the calculation of costs too, there are (potentially ethically) problematic implications of giving weight to the indirect costs of vaccination programs, as well as to their direct costs and the direct health care costs avoided for treatment of the disease prevented by the vaccination program. For example, if the indirect effects of smoking are considered, it may not be cost-effective to prevent smoking, although doing so would prevent the health care costs associated with treatment of smoking-related disease. Individuals who would have died earlier from those diseases will now live longer and incur other health care and non-health care costs, including the costs of treating whatever diseases they eventually die of, as well as the costs of public welfare and retirement benefits like Social Security. Yet any possible increase in overall social costs from a smoking prevention program is typically rejected as a reason for not pursuing, or downgrading the importance of, smoking prevention.

The same kinds of issues would arise concerning the prioritization of different vaccines if weight were given to the indirect costs of the different vaccine programs. For example, vaccines for life-threatening diseases that typically affect adults around normal retirement ages will have the additional indirect social cost of extending Social Security payments to those who otherwise would have died of those diseases. This would be a factor not only for traditional vaccines for diseases like pneumococcal pneumonia or influenza, but also for cancer vaccines likely to become available in coming years. Here again, however, the complexity of the ethical issue arises from the fact that such cost savings are real savings, even if the committee decides not to give them weight in prioritizing potential vaccination programs, and there may be broader public policy perspectives from which their consideration would be ethically defensible.

CONSIDERATIONS OF JUSTICE

Small Benefits to Many Versus Large Benefits to a Few

The analytic model the committee has developed compares vaccines on the basis of the total direct health benefits they would produce in reducing the burdens of disease. Leaving differences in costs aside, the model is sensitive only to the total burden imposed by different diseases, not to differences in how overall disease burdens are distributed to individuals. This is consonant with typical public health perspectives that look to the overall health benefits of different disease prevention programs targeted to a given population, but it overlooks a factor that is ethically important in many people's judgments about health care priorities.

For many people, preventing (or treating) a disease that has an extremely large disease burden for each affected individual has higher ethical priority than preventing a widespread disease that has a much smaller disease burden for each individual, even if the much higher incidence of the latter disease makes its aggregate burden equal to or even greater than that of the former disease. Many people think that the relative priority for treating different diseases should be determined by their relative severity for the individuals who contract them.

From this perspective, the relative priority of treating different diseases is determined by a one-to-one comparison of those diseases—the relative severity of one case of disease A versus one case of disease B. But this way of thinking about priorities ignores differences in incidence and in turn in the overall or aggregate level of disease burden from diseases A and B. In the context of vaccines, diseases like chicken pox, mononucleosis, or diarrhea in infancy have a high incidence but a relatively low disease burden for individuals in typical cases (see our HUI calculations). On the other hand, a disease like tetanus or meningitis has a much lower incidence but a much greater disease burden for the individuals who contract it. Because of the difference in overall disease burden, our model has the potential to yield the result that a higher priority should be given to preventing the high-incidence/low-individual-burden disease than to preventing the low-incidence/high-individual-burden disease.

This result might be defended by distinguishing between the clinical context, in which a physician treats individual patients, and the public health context in which health care resource allocation decisions are made that will affect different groups in the population. In the clinical context, a physician forced to prioritize between individual patients typically will treat first the patient who will suffer the more serious consequences without treatment or will benefit the most from treatment, even if that will prevent him or her treating a larger number of less seriously ill patients. The sickest patient, if he or she can be effectively treated, has the greatest, or first, claim on the physician's efforts. But from a public health or social perspective, arguably the appropriate perspective for the committee's task regarding public priorities for development of vaccines that will be available to the public at large, the potential overall or aggregate effects of alternative vaccines on the public health may seem the appropriate perspective.

Even from a public health perspective, however, there is controversy as to whether the ethically correct stance is a maximizing perspective that gives priority to producing the maximum aggregate benefits, whether by large benefits to a few or by small benefits to many. A recent prominent example in which that perspective was rejected for setting public health care treatment priorities may be helpful. In an early stage of reforming its Medicaid program, the state of Oregon ranked all treatment-patient condition pairs by what was essentially a cost-effectiveness standard, from the treatment providing the highest health benefit per dollar spent to the one providing the least benefit for its costs. The intent was to then use limited resources to cover treatments that would produce the greatest health benefits with the money available. One result of this ranking was that capping teeth for exposed pulp was ranked just above appendectomies for acute appendicitis, despite the fact that the latter is a life-saving intervention in most cases.

There were technical controversies about Oregon's methodology, but the fundamental reason for this result was that capping a tooth is vastly less expensive than doing an appendectomy—Oregon estimated that it could pay for tooth capping for 150 patients for the cost of each appendectomy. The Oregon Health Services Commission, the body responsible for developing the proposed revision of the state's Medicaid plan, found this result unacceptable, as did the public; from a one-by-one comparison of treatments, it was clearly a higher priority to fund appendectomies than tooth capping. To avoid results such as this, Oregon essentially abandoned its cost-effectiveness ranking in favor of a relative-benefit ranking that disregarded the cost differences that lead to aggregating small benefits to many patients against large benefits to a few. Oregon did this from a social or public perspective of deciding how to allocate limited public resources, which is also the committee's perspective, not just from a clinical perspective where physicians confront individual patients one-by-one.

Moreover, unacceptable or unintuitive results because of aggregation can arise not only from large differences in costs of health interventions, but from large differences in the incidence of different diseases. This latter version of the aggregation problem is the form it will typically take in the context of vaccine development, where very serious but relatively uncommon diseases like meningitis must be compared with much less serious but much more common diseases like mononucleosis (caused by Epstein-Barr virus) or diarrhea (caused by rotavirus and other infectious agents). Even from a public health perspective, it is ethically controversial when, and for what reasons, small benefits to many patients may be aggregated so as to have higher priority than large benefits to a few. We did not attempt to resolve this issue, but have used a methodology that places no restrictions on such aggregation. Policymakers using our report should be attentive to this issue and must decide whether vaccine programs that provide small benefits to many should receive higher priority than other programs that provide large benefits to a few, so long as the former produce larger aggregate benefits.

What Priority Should Be Given to the Worst-Off or Sickest?

It is easy to confuse the question of priority to the sickest with the aggregation problem just discussed, since both our vaccine and nonvaccine examples of aggregation put a few of the sickest up against many less sick, but the issues are distinct. An initial abstract example applied to treatment instead of prevention will make the point most clearly. Suppose group A patients have a serious disease that leaves them with a health utility level of .25 as measured by the HUI, and their HUI level would be raised only to .45 with the best available treatment because no treatment is very effective for their disease. A similar number of group B patients have a health utility level of .60 because they have a considerably less serious disease, but since treatment for their disease is more effective although no more costly than for Group A patients, it would raise their health utility to .90. Suppose we only have funds to treat one of these groups. Should we prefer to treat B because doing so would produce a 50% greater benefit than treating A (an increase in HUI of .3 for group B compared to an increase in HUI of .2 for group A) or should we give priority to treating group A who are sicker or worse-off?

There is some empirical evidence that when asked about choices like this, most persons, both in this country and elsewhere, would prefer to treat the sickest or worst-off in our example group A, even at the cost of a significant reduction in overall benefits, compared with treating the less sick or better off, that is group B. This may be because they view doing so as fairer or more just. Justice or fairness may favor preferring first to help group A who suffer from the worse or greater disadvantage; to treat group B instead would only widen the already undeserved difference in the levels of well-being between A and B. If group A is treated, their level of well-being after successful treatment (.45) will still be below that of B even if that group receives no treatment (.60). Some people would prefer to treat group A over group B because they believe that treatment would be subjectively more important for persons in group A, despite the greater measured benefit that could be produced for B.

Although setting priorities among potential vaccines does not involve choices about treatments of different diseases, but rather choices between different diseases that might be prevented, the committee believes essentially the same issue is at stake. The issue is what priority, if any, should be given to patients who would be the sickest if their disease is not prevented—for example, preventing opportunistic infections such as cryptosporidiosis in patients with AIDS whose health status will remain low because of their AIDS—compared to greater health benefits that could be produced by preventing generally less serious diseases like mumps or chicken pox in patients without AIDS or other serious predisposing conditions.

Part of the complexity of this issue is that virtually no one would prefer not to treat the sickest, no matter how costly their treatment and how small the benefit to them from doing so, and no matter how beneficial and how inexpensive the treatment for the less sick. If fairness or equity is what is at stake here, there is a limit to how much gain in the well-being of others we will sacrifice in order to treat all fairly or equitably by giving priority to those with the most serious diseases. However, there does not seem to be any objective, principled basis for determining how much gain in overall well-being should be sacrificed in order to treat the sickest or, more generally, to avoid different forms or instances of unfairness. Here again, there is no consensus among ordinary persons, bioethicists, or health policy analysts about whether, first, fairness or equity requires some priority be given to the sickest or worst-off and, second, if so, how much and in what circumstances. Although this controversy has prevented the committee from attempting to incorporate any such priority into our analytic model, it is no reason for policymakers to ignore the issue in setting priorities for vaccine development or, for that matter, for health care allocation and investment more generally. That is why the committee has flagged, briefly discussed, and given examples of the issues that arise specifically in the prioritization of potential vaccines.

Fair Chances Versus Best Outcomes

The final issue of justice or fairness in the distribution of health benefits to which the committee calls attention here has been characterized as the conflict between fair chances and best outcomes. The conflict is most pressing when the health care intervention is life-saving, and not all whose lives are threatened can be saved, although it arises when the threat is to health and function as well. The issue has received the most attention in the context of organ transplantation where there is a scarcity of life-saving organs such as hearts and lungs, resulting in many deaths each year of patients waiting for an organ for transplant. An abstract example in the area of transplantation illustrates the problem. Suppose two patients are each in need of a heart transplant to prevent imminent death, but only one heart is available for transplant. Patient A has a life expectancy with a transplant of 10 years and patient B has a life expectancy with a transplant of 9 years, with no difference in their expected quality of life. (Of course, precise estimates of this sort are typically not possible, but the point is that there is a small difference in the expected benefits to be gained depending on which patient gets the scarce organ).

Once again, if the we wish to use scarce resources to maximize health benefits or QALYs, then we should straightaway prefer patient A. But patient B might argue that it is unfair to give her no chance to receive the scarce heart. Just like A, she needs the heart for life itself and will lose everything—that is, her life—if she does not receive it. It is unfair, B charges, to give the organ to A because of the small difference in expected benefits from doing so; that difference is too small to justly determine who lives and who dies. Instead, each should receive a fair chance of getting the organ, which might in this case be either an equal chance through a random selection between A and B, or a weighted lottery that gives the patient who would benefit more some greater likelihood of being selected to receive the organ. Like the other two considerations of justice just discussed, this too is far more complex and controversial than the committee can pursue here, but it is another example of when society might reasonably choose to constrain resource allocation aimed at maximizing health benefits in order to be fair to the individuals who will be affected by the resource allocation.

Does this conflict arise in choices about priorities for vaccine development? Perhaps the closest parallel would be a choice between potential vaccines for two life-threatening diseases, A and B, where A has a slightly greater burden of disease than B because there is a slightly greater incidence of A than B. If A is given priority over B, and a successful vaccine to prevent A is developed and employed, but no effort is supported to develop a vaccine for B, then people who develop life-threatening disease B may complain that they did not have a fair chance to survive through the development of a vaccine to prevent their disease.

There are at least three considerations that mitigate this ethical conflict in the context of vaccine development as compared with organ transplantation. The first is that vaccine development need not be an all-or-nothing choice, as in the case of recipient selection for scarce heart transplants, but a matter of the relative priority for funding to be given to the development of vaccines for different diseases. If disease A is given a higher priority for vaccine development than disease B because of A's greater burden of disease, this need not and typically does not mean that no resources go to the development of a vaccine for B, but rather that a greater effort with more resources will go to A than to B. Suppose the effort to develop the vaccine for A succeeds, while the effort for B fails, at least in part because of the lesser effort and resources that went to B. Individuals who contract B cannot complain that the small difference in expected benefits from a vaccine for A instead of for B was an unfair basis for selecting who will live—those who would have contracted A—and who will die—those who contract B. The small difference in expected benefits from a vaccine for A as opposed to B resulted only in a comparable small difference in the effort and resources devoted to vaccine development for A and B. Even if that small difference results in the earlier development of a vaccine for A than for B, it is not obvious that that is unfair to those who contract B and even die from it.

The second consideration that mitigates some of the conflict between fair chances and best outcomes in the case of vaccine development is that the prioritization of different potential vaccines is not a choice between identified patients, as in organ transplantation, but a choice between potential vaccines for different diseases made for the most part before we know which individuals will contract the different diseases. In that respect, the prioritization of disease A over B is not a life-and-death choice between identified patients who have diseases A or B because it is made before we know who will get A or B, even if the choice will eventually have life-and-death consequences for identified individuals (in fact, with the disease for which a successful vaccine is developed and deployed, the individuals who would have died from that disease without the vaccine will typically never be identified or known). It could be argued that before one knows whether one will get disease A or B, one would give greater priority to preventing whichever has the greater disease burden. Thus, it is less clear that the vaccine development choice in favor of the disease with the greatest health burdens and potential benefits is unfair to those who contract the lower priority disease for which a vaccine was not developed, than is the choice of transplant recipients in our earlier example.

The third consideration that mitigates some of the fair chances and best outcomes conflict in the case of vaccine development is that the diseases for which vaccines are sought are frequently not, at least usually, life threatening to most people who experience them, but often instead only have some impact on individuals' health status, and often for only a limited period of time. In these cases, the difference in impact on individuals who avoid a disease because a vaccine was developed and individuals who contract a disease for which no vaccine was developed is much less, and so the possible concern about fairness is less compelling.

CONCLUSION

The committee emphasizes that the aim in this chapter has been to identify some of the principal ethical issues involved in developing and using the model presented in this report to help set priorities for vaccine development. The use of a quantitative analytic model for determining those priorities can help focus those ethical issues, just as it helps focus the various empirical considerations that bear on the recommendation for priorities. The committee has tried to say enough about these ethical issues to give readers a sense of the nature of the controversies. In some cases, the committee has given reasons for the ethical position our quantitative model and recommendations take on the issues, but in others the aim was only to focus the issue for policymakers who will make use of this report.

7

Observations

The committee's sole recommendation is that decisionmakers use, when possible, objective and quantitative tools, such as that developed for this report for assessment of vaccine development, to guide and inform their actions. This particular cost-effectiveness model can help the vaccine research and development (R&D) community think systematically about the investments it might make. The model can also be used by vaccine program policymakers to inform their decisions about investments in delivery programs. The model is not static and may be modified. As new data emerge, specific elements can be changed or new candidate vaccines can be assessed. Major components of the model can also be modified if the needs or interests of a user differ from those envisioned by this committee. Should individuals wish to modify the model, the committee urges them to study carefully the chapters on ethics (Chapter 6) and methods (Chapters 4 and 5) so that the model is not used for purposes for which it is unsuited and inappropriate.

In the course of developing and illustrating this model, the committee discussed general issues related to the funding of research, neglected opportunities for vaccine R&D, the qualitative judgments integral to this modeling exercise, and vaccine program concerns. The committee thus closes this report with a series of observations that it hopes are considered as seriously as the analytic model that was the focus of the project.

THE FUNDING OF RESEARCH

Vaccinology exemplifies the centuries-old experience that science moves ahead in ways that one cannot always predict. Since the publication of the 1985

Institute of Medicine (IOM) report on priorities for vaccine development, vaccines can now be envisioned for the treatment and prevention of diseases not previously considered to be potential vaccine targets: for example, therapeutic vaccines for noninfectious diseases such as multiple sclerosis and melanoma were absent from consideration in the 1985 exercise, and in the future, preventive vaccines for these diseases will also likely be studied. The role of hepatitis B virus in liver cancer was recognized in 1985, but the current report includes many more examples of vaccine-preventable infections as causes of chronic conditions; for example, hepatitis C virus infection and liver damage, including cancer; *Helicobacter pylori* infection and gastric ulcers and cancers; and human papillomavirus infection and cervical cancer. Furthermore, scientific studies are emerging indicating a role for infectious agents in the pathogenesis of coronary artery disease and in a predisposition to asthma.

Stable and sufficient funding of basic research by the federal government, the use of creative funding mechanisms, and the creation of alliances between the public and private sectors are crucial to ensuring that effective, safe, and needed vaccines will be carried through the development stage into licensure. Funding of basic research in fields such as immunology, virology, and microbiology can also lead young investigators into more applied research on vaccines. In addition to basic research in molecular and cellular biology, progress in vaccine development and program implementation depends on research in fields such as epidemiology, health services research, health economics, human behavior, and even ecology. The lack of data and research in these fields, information that would have been useful to the committee in assessing disease burden, was surprising. In some cases, no significant new data had been published since that referenced in the 1985 IOM report on vaccine priorities, particularly national data on disease characteristics such as morbidity states and patterns of care.

R&D is an expensive enterprise currently supported through a natural and fluid mix of public and private funding. The federal funds used to support intramural research within government laboratories or dispensed by the extramural programs to researchers, most of whom are in academic institutions, have traditionally supported the vast majority of basic science research. New knowledge resulting from basic research is the essential first step that allows applied R&D to move forward into the private sector. Chapter 3 discusses how the lack of fundamental understanding of immune responses to *Treponema pallidum*, for example, led the committee to not consider the development of a vaccine against this agent, which is the cause of a very important public health problem, syphilis. Although it is sometimes difficult to demonstrate the benefits of investment in basic research with a direct link to a health intervention, the reader is referred to a classic paper for examples (Comroe and Dripps, 1976).

The National Institute of Allergy and Infectious Diseases (NIAID) of the National Institutes of Health (NIH) provides the majority of the approximately $250 million of public money spent annually on vaccine research (Mercer Management Consulting, 1995). Much of this is investigator-initiated basic research.

Some research, however is very targeted, and funding mechanisms such as Cooperative Research and Development Awards, sponsorship of centers for clinical trials such as the Vaccine Treatment and Evaluation Units, or support for acellular pertussis vaccine trials are used. Other NIH institutes, such as the National Cancer Institute and the National Institute of Child Health and Development, and other federal agencies, such as the Centers for Disease Control and Prevention (CDC) and the U.S. Department of Defense, also fund research related to vaccine R&D. Private philanthropic organizations such as the Rockefeller Foundation, the Burroughs Wellcome Fund, and the Josiah Macy Foundation also support basic and applied R&D related to vaccines.

Although private industry supports basic research, the most important role it plays is to assume the costs of applied R&D. The impetus for a company to invest in the development phase of a vaccine begins with the establishment of proof in principle, which is evidence that the vaccine could protect against disease. Such proof in principle results from the basic research findings of researchers funded by either public or private money. Another impetus is the potential of a return on investment by a company, which depends on the likelihood of product licensure, the market for that product, and the predicted costs of development and production. Manufacturer's profits from the sales of existing vaccines contribute approximately twice the amount of money to R&D as the federal investment in R&D. Another important source of funding is risk capital invested in small biotechnology firms. Once private industries invest significant amounts of money in the development of a product, they stand to make or lose money on the basis of the quality of the product, the size of the market, the purchase price of the product, and the profit associated with the sale of the licensed product.

However, R&D opportunities frequently come to fruition only if the government or other nonprofit organizations leverage their resources in partnership with private, for-profit organizations to develop products or gather data in phase III clinical trials to support efficacy and safety claims sufficient for approval of the products by the Food and Drug Administration (FDA). Program staff at NIAID, for example, work to stimulate creative and targeted research and collaborations at critical periods in the natural life cycle of some products to keep the R&D cycle moving until private sponsors are prepared to take on the project.

Many of the challenges to commercial interests in vaccine R&D are fairly well documented (IOM, 1995; Mercer Management Consulting, 1995). It is widely believed that vaccines do not generate large profits—either as a percentage of revenue from the sales of an individual product or as a percentage of the total profit of the parent pharmaceutical firm. In contrast to many pharmaceuticals, which are sometimes taken several times a day for years, most vaccines are used only a few times in each person's lifetime. Because of these market forces, the committee has heard compelling arguments that federal investment in vaccine R&D—as well as in fields such as health services research and health communication, which are necessary to understand how to stimulate the appropriate use of vaccines once they are developed—is all the more necessary.

The cooperation and synergistic activities of the public and private sectors have led to remarkable successes. The development of the acellular pertussis vaccines is one such example. NIAID invested significant funds to support clinical trials of acellular pertussis vaccines, which are now licensed and recommended for use. Tensions, however, are inevitable and probably healthy. For example, the committee is aware of tensions between the needs of FDA for mechanisms that it believes are necessary for ensuring the safety and efficacy of the vaccines and the effect that some of these mechanisms have on the financial requirements for licensure. Examples of these discussed by the committee include the financial burdens of pilot production and the high costs of the complex clinical trials required by FDA to demonstrate efficacy as well as safety. Although the committee did not study in detail the relationship between public and private research on vaccines, it is clear that improvements can be made to foster collaboration when market forces cannot guarantee that a for-profit vaccine manufacturer will risk an investment in the development and manufacture of a particular vaccine or a particular type of vaccines.

The private companies involved in vaccine research, development, and manufacturing expect and are entitled to a reasonable return on their investments. In fact, market forces have led to the development of many vaccines, such as the *Haemophilus influenzae* type b (Hib) vaccine. The burden of disease caused by Hib infection was significant, the target population (the annual birth cohort of approximately 4 million infants) had regular contact with the medical community, vaccinations were already an integral part of health care for this population, and a guaranteed market was confidently predicted. The Hib vaccine was, in fact, recommended for routine use by major advisory bodies such as the Advisory Committee on Immunization Practices of CDC and the Red Book Committee of the American Academy of Pediatrics, and immunization with the Hib vaccine was required for entrance into most day-care centers.

NEGLECTED OPPORTUNITIES FOR VACCINE R&D

In an ideal world, every vaccine of medical or public health importance would be developed. It is not clear that 20 years prior to licensure of polio vaccines either the disease burden or the basic science knowledge required for vaccine development would have been sufficient for inclusion in a modeling exercise such as the one undertaken for this report. However, it most certainly would have been a compelling candidate for analysis by 3 to 7 years prior to licensure, owing to the increase in paralytic disease and to advances in tissue culture and virology. This underscores the need for a dynamic research program that is not limited to the candidate vaccines discussed in this report and for the dynamic use of a model for ongoing evaluation of R&D priorities.

Sometimes this development is impeded by other than scientific or technical obstacles. Development can be abandoned if a return on investment seems unlikely because the vaccine would not be used optimally due to a lack of resources available to purchase and administer the vaccine, or to low acceptance of a vaccine. Candidate vaccines intended primarily for use in less-developed countries often are not pursued due to concerns that they will be unaffordable. Additional impediments to a return on investment include a very small target population or financial risks for litigation to a manufacturer. Three specific examples are discussed: candidate vaccines to be used primarily in less-developed countries, in pregnant women, or in very small target populations.

International Considerations

The committee focused on the burden of disease in the United States. There are many diseases of great importance to other countries that do not currently pose a significant burden on domestic health. However, policymakers in this country should factor these diseases and the international burden to health into their decisionmaking for both parochial considerations related to the potential threat to the United States from new and emerging infections, as well as the altruistic considerations involved in aiding other countries.

The experiences of recent years regarding new and emerging infections can only serve as a stern reminder that the United States cannot afford to be complacent about the potential threat to the health of its population from infections currently of importance mostly to other countries. Infectious agents know no boundaries, and a threat to another country's population today could be a threat to the U.S. population tomorrow. An example considered by the committee, but ultimately not included in the full analysis, is the threat in the United States of dengue hemorraghic fever. In addition, throughout the world the increasing levels of resistance of a variety of bacterial diseases to antibiotics make the need for disease prevention, including the use of vaccines, more compelling than ever. It is thus to the benefit of the United States to help protect the population of other countries from infectious diseases that could someday become a threat to its population.

In addition to the threat that emerging diseases could pose to the United States, it is incumbent upon the United States to assist in R&D for vaccines against these diseases, because without U.S. help, the products will not come to market. Developed countries frequently directly or indirectly assume the burden of financing advances that can benefit people in less-developed countries. The basic R&D for all vaccines used in the Expanded Programme on Immunization and the Children's Vaccine Initiative was supported by the United States and other developed countries, and mechanisms are in place to use these vaccines to the benefit of less-developed countries in Africa and Asia. When the development of vaccines against diseases in the United States is compelling, as evidenced by the results obtained with the model whose development has been described in this report, it would be prudent to at least qualitatively consider the nature of the international burden of disease potentially averted by use of the vaccine outside the United States.

Small Target Populations

Some infections threaten the health of only a small group of people, but that threat is nevertheless quite serious for that population. Chapter 6 discusses ethical considerations and provides some insight into how this situation can be considered. These groups can be identified by geography, age, or chronic health conditions. The committee felt that a *Pseudomonas aeruginosa* vaccine was not necessarily compelling for the general population, but that the threat to the health of people with cystic fibrosis was severe. Although the committee did not analyze the cost-effectiveness of a candidate vaccine for *P. aeruginosa*, it recognizes the benefit to be gained from a vaccine for that targeted group of people. The committee did analyze the cost-effectiveness of a candidate vaccine against two conditions of relatively low incidence but serious morbidity. These are the geographically-confined infections of *Histoplasma capsulatum* and *Coccidioides immitis*. As the results demonstrate (Chapter 4), these candidate vaccines fall into Level IV, despite the very serious morbidity associated with these infections. One significant difference in the consideration of a candidate vaccine for *P. aeruginosa* compared to one for *H. capsulatum* or *C. immitis* is that the health status of the target populations is very different. The impaired baseline health status of the *P. aeruginosa* target population would affect the cost-effectiveness ratio in ways that are unfavorable. Equity considerations, such as those discussed in Chapter 6, might have an important qualitative influence on policy-making regarding development or use of a *P. aeruginosa* vaccine.

Liability Concerns

As described in other sections of the report, concerns about liability have influenced vaccine R&D over the past two decades. The creation of the Vaccine Injury Compensation Program (VICP) successfully stabilized and encouraged the development of vaccines primarily intended for use in children. However, many existing vaccines are not covered by that program. The lack of compensation or indemnity against liability is perceived as a serious impediment to the development of some new vaccines; in particular, vaccines that would be beneficial if given to pregnant women. Vaccine manufacturers and other researchers interested in the use of vaccines directed against group B streptococcus and other infectious agents believe that some form of legal protection from lawsuits is imperative before these vaccines can be developed and licensed. The rationale for the immunization of pregnant women as a crucial strategy for reducing the rates of morbidity and mortality from group B streptococcus in both mothers and infants is presented in other sections of the report. The committee notes here, however, that the analysis described in this report identifies many infectious agents whose disease burden could be prevented most effectively with a strategy of immunization of pregnant women, and it hopes that serious consideration will be given to addressing the significant impediment to all vaccine development brought on by liability concerns. The committee did not believe it was the appropriate group, however, to recommend a specific policy solution.

QUALITATIVE JUDGMENTS

Models put a framework around previously incomparable data, and imperfect as the data can be, the committee nonetheless encourages the use of such evidence-based tools as *aids*, not *mandates*, for decisionmaking. If the results—the relative ranking of vaccine candidates—make intuitive sense (that is, if they conform to the informed judgment of the health care community) the model is probably correct. If the results are surprising (that is, a vaccine candidate ranks much higher or much lower relative to others than one would have predicted), a decisionmaker might ask if either the model or the data inputs are suspect. If not, then the model has been particularly useful. The experience in prioritizing reimbursement for health care interventions described in Chapter 6 is instructive. At times relative rankings run counter to the community's beliefs, and thus, this model, like any model, should be viewed as malleable. There is always a role for informed judgment when deciding to what degree the results of a modeling tool drive policies, particularly when the limitations of the model have been made explicit. The 1985 IOM committee on vaccine priorities, in fact, included an acellular pertussis vaccine mostly because of the pivotal role that its development would play in increasing confidence in vaccine safety and ensuring a supply of vaccine. This was a qualitative consideration that the committee valued but that it could not enter directly into the model.

Ethical concerns are another such consideration. Health status measurements are discussed in detail in Chapters 4, 5, and 6. The committee used quality-adjusted life years (QALYs) in this exercise. The disability-adjusted life year is used by some researchers in these kinds of analyses, but for reasons explained in the chapters on methods (Chapter 4) and ethical considerations (Chapter 6), QALYs are a respectable and valid choice preferred by the committee. Although QALYs are a quantitative measure, they embody ethical considerations that cannot be directly quantified or weighted. The committee struggled with applying the health utility index in its QALY calculations, but in the end, it noticed remarkable inter- and intraperson consistency in the values obtained for similar health states. The committee expects and encourages continued research on this and other measures of health status.

VACCINE PROGRAM CONCERNS

The committee discussed barriers in addition to those identified above in the section on R&D. Vaccine delivery poses significant barriers to the effective prevention and control of infectious disease. Children in the United States can receive up to 16 injections and three oral doses of vaccine delivered against 8 infectious diseases before the age of 2 years. The rate of compliance with the recommended immunizations at 2 years of age is below that achieved for children a few years older due to compliance with vaccination requirements for school entry. Combination vaccines promise to reduce the number of vaccine doses that must be administered separately, but these will not be a panacea. The combinations will help to increase the level of acceptance and the rates of utilization of vaccines, but clinical trial design issues are not trivial. The committee hopes that the Federal government and state governments, the medical community, the public, and vaccine manufacturers carefully think about rational approaches to combination vaccines and vaccination schedules. Furthermore, noninjection routes of delivery (for example, oral, intranasal, or cutaneous routes of delivery) should receive serious consideration. At the same time, the committee knows that market forces and corporate alliances will influence the availability of combination products.

Despite the impediments of delivering so many immunizations during infancy, mandatory childhood immunization is a fundamental part of health care for children in the United States. Adolescents and adults have received less information about the importance of vaccines to protect their health and are less accessible than children to health care providers, especially for preventive health care services. Patient and provider education about the benefits of new vaccines will be crucial.

Vaccines are one of the few preventive measures that save money. It is not clear that people are willing to accept, use, and pay for vaccines that do not save money. For example, it is the opportunity cost savings for a parent who does not need to take time off from work to care for a sick child that has helped make the varicella-zoster virus vaccine a marketable preventive health intervention. Saving a child from illness and the very rare cases of death due to chicken pox was not enough to convince some in the medical establishment and some parents that the varicella-zoster virus vaccine was important.

The model described in this report demonstrates that not all vaccines will save money. Some new vaccines might be very expensive. However, the health benefits might still be compelling. Use of these vaccines will require a shift in thinking from an expectation that vaccines always save money to an acknowledgment that the health benefits of some vaccines might be worth the cost.

Many vaccines are not covered by health insurance, under either indemnity plans or managed care plans. Financial incentives might be crucial for encouraging the use of vaccines. The Vaccines for Children Program and other public health initiatives have helped provide childhood vaccines to those who can not afford them. Federal and state governments need to prepare now to work with insurers, providers, and communities to ensure that all who need the many vaccines that will be developed in the next two decades can receive them.

However, the cost of vaccines to the individual and to insurers is not the only impediment to vaccine use. Vaccines, like other public health successes, such as clean water, fluoridation for the prevention of caries, and food safety measures are victims of their own success: people forget how dangerous vaccine-preventable diseases can be and become complacent. This false sense of security strikes individuals, communities, health care providers, and policymakers. It is not until the medical and public health systems fail and illness from infectious disease surges (for example, as a result of antibiotic resistance, nosocomial infections, measles outbreaks in the late 1980s, or food-borne illness) that society pays the price for interventions, such as vaccines, not yet developed, maintained, or implemented.

The committee urges careful consideration but not rigidity in the use of evidence-based approaches, such as the qualitative framework and quantitative model developed for this report, for prioritization of research, development, and use of vaccines, as well as other preventive and therapeutic interventions. The committee, while acknowledging the limitations of modeling exercises in general and of the one it developed and used in particular, does believe that modeling is useful and important when attempting to compare widely divergent vaccine-preventable conditions. It hopes that the inferences derived from the model will be useful to the vaccine science community, the vaccine manufacturers, and research and program policymakers.

References

Abraham R, Minor P, Dunn G, et al. Shedding of virulent poliovirus revertants during immunization with oral polio vaccine after prior immunization with inactivated polio vaccine. *Journal of Infectious Diseases* 1993; 168:1105–1109.

ACP (American College of Physicians). *Guide for Adult Immunization,* 2nd ed. Philadelphia: American College of Physicians, 1990.

Allan CH, Mendrick DL, Trier JS. Rat intestinal M cells contain acidic endosomal-lysosomal compartments and express class 11 major histocompatibility complex determinants. *Gastroenterology* 1993; 104:698–708.

Baker CJ, Rench MA, Edwards MS, et al. Immunization of pregnant women with a polysaccharide vaccine of group B streptococcus. *New England Journal of Medicine* 1988; 319:917–921.

Bart K, Foulds J, Patricia P. The global eradication of poliomyelitis: benefit-cost analysis. *Bulletin of the World Health Organization* 1996; 74:1.

Bennett NM, Lewis B, Doninger AS et al. A coordinated, community-wide program in Monroe County, New York, to increase influenza immunization rates in the elderly. *Archives of Internal Medicine* 1994; 154:1741–1745.

Bergner M, Bobbit RA, Carter WB, et al. The sickness impact profile: development and final revision of a health status measure. *Medical Care* 1981; 19:787–805.

Berthelot JM, Roberge R, Wolfson MC. The calculation of health-adjusted life expectancy for a Canadian province using a multi-attribute utility function: a first attempt. *In 6th Working-Group Meeting REVES, International Research Network for Interpretation of Observed Values of Health Life Expectancy,* Montpelier, Vermont, October 1992.

Bodian D. Differentiation of types of poliomyelitis viruses. 1. Reinfection experiments in monkeys (second attacks). *American Journal of Hygiene* 1949; 49: 200–224.

Bodian D. Poliomyelitis immunization. Mass use of oral vaccine in the United States might prevent definitive evaluation of either vaccine. *Science* 1961; 134:819.

Boyle MH, Furlong W, Feeny GW, et al. Reliability of the Health Utilities Index— Mark III used in the 1991 cycle 6 Canadian General Social Survey Health Questionnaire. *Quality of Life Research* 1995; 4:249–257.

Brodie M, Park WH. Active immunization against poliomyelitis. *American Journal of Public Health* 1936; 26:119–125.

Buffington J, Bell KM, LaForce FM. The Genesee Hospital Medical Staff. A target-based model for increasing influenza immunizations in private practice. *Journal of General Internal Medicine* 1991; 6:204–209.

Catlin G, Will P. The national population health survey: highlights of initial developments. *Health Reports* 1992; 4(3):313–319.

CDC (Centers for Disease Control and Prevention). Certification of poliomyelitis eradication in the Americas. *Morbidity and Mortality Weekly Report* 1994a; 54: 720–722.

CDC. General recommendations on immunization. Recommendations of the advisory committee on immunization practices (ACIP). *Morbidity and Mortality Weekly Report* 1994b; 43(No. RR-1-4).

CDC. Summary of notifiable diseases, United States, 1994. *Morbidity and Mortality Weekly Report* 1994c; 43(53).

CDC. Influenza and pneumococcal vaccination coverage levels among persons aged greater than or equal to 65 years 1973–1993—United States 1995. *Morbidity and Mortality Weekly Report* 1995a; 44:506–507, 513–515.

CDC. Mass vaccination with oral poliovirus vaccine—Asia and Europe. *Morbidity and Mortality Weekly Report* 1995b; 44:234–236.

CDC. Progress towards global poliomyelitis eradication 1985–1994. Morbidity and Mortality Weekly Report 1995c; 44:273–275, 281.

CDC. Recommended childhood immunization schedule. *Morbidity and Mortality Weekly Report* 1995d:44:1–9.

CDC. National, state, and urban area vaccination coverage levels among children aged 19–35 months—United States, July 1996–June 1997. *Morbidity and Mortality Weekly Report* 1998; 47:108–116.

CDC. Recommended childhood immunization schedule—United States, 1999. *Morbidity and Mortality Weekly Report* 1999; 48:12–16.

Chatfield SN, Fairweather N, Charles I, et al. Construction of a genetically defined Salmonella typhi Ty2 aroa, aroc mutant for the engineering of candidate oral typhoid-tetanus vaccine. *Vaccine* 1992; 10:53–60.

Chen ST, Edsall G, Pell MM, et al. Timing of antenatal tetanus immunization for effective protection of the neonate. *Bulletin of the World Health Organization* 1983; 61:159–165.

Claassen I, Osterhaus A. The ISCOM structure as an immune-enhancing moiety: experience with viral systems. *Research Immunology* 1992; 143:531–541.

Coffman RL, Varkila K, Scott P, et al. Role of cytokines in the differentiation of $CD4^+$ T-cell subsets in vivo. *Immunology Review* 1991; 123:189–207.

Commission on the Cost of Medical Care. *The Economic Significance of the Prevention of Paralytic Poliomyelitis 1955–1961.* Report of the Commission on the Cost of Medical Care 1964; 4:29–46.

Comroe JH, Dripps RD. Scientific basis for the support of biomedical science. *Science* 1976; 192:105–111.

Conley ME, Delacroix DL. Intravascular and mucosal immunoglobulin A: two separate but related systems of immune defense. *Annals of Internal Medicine* 1987; 106:892–899.

Czinn SJ, Cai A, Nedrud JG. Protection of germ-free mice from infection by *Helicobacter felis* after active oral or passive IgA immunization. *Vaccine* 1993; 11:637–642.

Davies MDJ, Parrott DMW. Cytotoxic T cells in small intestine epithelial, lamina propria and lung lymphocytes. *Immunology* 1981; 44:367–371.

Drummond MF, Stoddart GL, Torrance GW. *Methods for the Economic Evaluation of Health Care Programmes.* New York: Oxford University Press, 1987.

Eddy, DM. Oregon's methods: did cost-effectiveness analysis fail? *Journal of the American Medical Association* 1991; 266:2135–2141.

Eldridge JH, Hammond CJ, Meulbroek JA, et al. Controlled vaccine release in the gut-associated lymphoid tissue. Orally administered biodegradable microspheres target the Peyer's patches. Controlled Release 1990; 11:205–214.

Enders JF. General preface to studies on the cultivation of poliomyelitis viruses in tissue culture. *Journal of Immunology* 1952; 69:639.

Enders JF, Weller TH, Robinson FC. Cultivation of the Lansing strain of poliomyelitis virus in cultures of various human embryonic tissues. *Science* 1949; 109: 85–87.

Erickson P, Wilson R, Shannon I. Years of Healthy Life. *Healthy People 2000 Statistical Notes.* No. 7:95–1237. Hyattsville, Md.: National Center for Health Statistics, 1995.

Ermak TH, Dougherty EP, Bhagat HR, et al. Uptake and transport of copolymer biodegradable microspheres by rabbit Peyer's patch M cells. *Cell and Tissue Research* 1995; 279:433–436.

Ernst PB, Befus AD, Bienenstock J. Leukocytes in the intestinal epithelium: an unusual immunological compartment. *Immunology Today* 1985; 6:50–55.

Farstad IN, Halstensen TS, Fausa O, et al. Heterogeneity of M-cell-associated B and T cells in human Peyer's patches. *Immunology* 1994; 83:457–464.

Fedson DS. Influenza and pneumococcal immunization strategies for physicians. *Chest* 1987; 91:436–443.

Fedson DS. Influenza and pneumococcal vaccination in Canada and the United States, 1980–1993: what can the two countries learn from each other? *Clinical Infectious Diseases* 1995; 20:1371–1376.

Feeny D, Furlong W, Boyle M, et al. Multi-attribute health status classification systems: health utilities index. *PharmacoEconomics* 1995; 7:490–502.

Fynan EF, Webster RG, Fuller DH, et al. DNA vaccines: protective immunization by parenteral, mucosal and gene-gun inoculations. *Proceedings of the National Academy of Sciences* 1993; 90:11478–11482.

General Accounting Office. Immunization: Health and Human Services Could Do More to Increase Vaccination Among Older Adults. A report to congressional requesters. GAO/PEMD-95-14. Washington, D.C.: General Accounting Office; 1995.

Gold MR, Siegel JE, Russell LB, et al. *Cost-Effectiveness in Health and Medicine.* New York: Oxford University Press, 1996.

Gregoriadis G. Immunological adjuvants: a role for liposomes. *Immunology Today* 1990; 11:89–97.

Guyer B, Hughart N, Holt E, et al. Immunization coverage and its relationship to preventive health care visits among inner-city children in Baltimore. *Pediatrics* 1994; 94:53–58.

Halsey N, Klein D. Report of a workshop: immunization of pregnant women. *Pediatric Infectious Disease Journal* 1990; 9:574–581.

Haq TA, Mason HS, Clements JD, et al. Oral immunization with a recombinant bacteria antigen produced in transgenic plants. *Science* 1995; 268:714–716.

Harrington H. Review of literature in International Committee for the Study of Infantile Paralysis. Poliomyelitis: A survey made possible by a grant from the International Committee for the Study of Infantile Paralysis. Baltimore, Md.: Williams & Wilkins Co.; 1932:130–144.

HCFA (Health Care Financing Administration). *Health Care Financing Review: Medicare and Medicaid Statistical Supplement.* HCFA Pub. No. 03348. Baltimore, Md.: U.S. Department of Health and Human Services, 1995.

Health Information Foundation. The changing status of polio. *Progress in Health Services.* 1959; 8:1–6.

Hinman AR, Koplan JP, Orenstein WA, et al. Live or inactivated poliomyelitis vaccine: an analysis of benefits and risks. *American Journal of Public Health* 1987; 77:1–5.

Hone DM, Harris AM, Chatfield S, et al. Construction of genetically defined double aro mutants of Salmonella typhi. *Vaccine* 1991; 9:810–816.

Hsieh CS, Macatonia SE, Tripp CS, et al. Development of Th1 CD4[+] T cells through IL-12 produced by Listeria-induced macrophages. *Science* 1993; 260:547–549.

Insel RA, Amstey M, Woodin K, et al. Immunization of pregnant women to prevent infectious diseases in the neonate or infant. *International Journal of Technical Assessment of Health Care* 1994; 10:143–153.

IOM (Institute of Medicine). *New Vaccines Development: Establishing Priorities, Vol. 1. Diseases of Importance in the United States.* Washington, D.C.: National Academy Press, 1985a.

IOM. *New Vaccines Development: Establishing Priorities, Vol. 2. Diseases of Importance in Developing Countries.* Washington, D.C.: National Academy Press, 1985b.

IOM. *Adverse Effects of Pertussis and Rubella Vaccines.* Washington, D.C.: National Academy Press, 1991.

IOM. *Setting Priorities for Health Technology Assessment: A Model Process.* Washington, D.C.: National Academy Press, 1992.

IOM. *Adverse Events Associated with Childhood Vaccines: Evidence Bearing on Causality.* Washington, D.C.: National Academy Press, 1994a.

IOM. *DPT Vaccine and Chronic Nervous System Dysfunction: A New Analysis.* Washington, D.C.: National Academy Press; 1994b.

IOM. *The Children's Vaccine Initiative: Continuing Activities. A Summary of Two Workshops.* Washington, D.C.: National Academy Press, 1995.

IOM. *Options for Poliomyelitis Vaccination in the United States: Workshop Summary.* Howe CJ, Johnston RB (eds.). Washington, D.C.: National Academy Press, 1996a.

IOM. *Vaccines Against Malaria: Hope in a Gathering Storm.* Washington, D.C.: National Academy Press, 1996b.

IOM. *America's Vital Interest in Global Health: Protecting Our People, Enhancing Our Economy, and Advancing Our International Interests.* Washington, D.C.: National Academy Press, 1997a.

IOM. *Risk Communication and Vaccination: Summary of a Workshop.* Washington, D.C.: National Academy Press, 1997b.

IOM. *Summarizing Population Health: Directions for the Development and Application of Population Metrics.* Washington, D.C.: National Academy Press, 1998.

Jones BD, Ghori N, Falkow S. *Salmonella typhimurium* initiates murine infection by penetrating and destroying the specialized epithelial M cells of the Peyer's patches. *Experimental Medicine* 1994; 180:15–23.

Kaetzel CS, Robinson JK, Chintalacharuvu KR, et al. The polymeric immunoglobulin receptor (secretory component) mediates transport of immune complexes across epithelial cells: a local defense function for IgA. *Proceedings of the National Academy of Sciences* 1991; 88:8796–8800.

Kaetzel CS, Robinson JK, Lamm ME. Epithelial transcytosis of monomeric IgA and IgG cross-linked through antigen to polymeric IgA. A role for monomeric antibodies in the mucosal immune system. *Immunology* 1994; 152:72–76.

Kaplan RM, Anderson JP. A general health policy model: update and applications. *Health Services Research* 1988; 23:203–235.

Kind P, Gudex CM. Measuring health status in the community: a comparison of methods. *Journal of Epidemiology and Community Health* 1994;486:86–91.

Kolmer JA, Klugh Jr. G, Rule AM. A successful method for vaccination against acute anterior poliomyelitis. *Journal of the American Medical Association* 1935; 104:456–460.

Koprowski H, Jervis GA, Norton TW. Immune responses in human volunteers upon oral administration of a rodent-adapted strain of poliomyelitis virus. *American Journal of Hygiene* 1952; 55:108–126.

Kraehenbuhl JP, Neutra MR. Molecular and cellular basis of immune protection of mucosal surfaces. *Physiological Reviews* 1992; 72:853–879.

Landauer KS, Stickle G. An analysis of residual disabilities (paralysis and crippling) among 100,000 poliomyelitis patients with special reference to the rehabilitation of past poliomyelitis patients. *Archives of Physical Medical Rehabilitation* 1958; 39:141–151.

Lieu TA, Cochi SL, Black SB, et al. Cost-effectiveness of a routine varicella vaccination program for U.S. children. *Journal of the American Medical Association* 1994; 271: 375–381.

Linder N, Ohel G. In utero vaccination. *Clinical Perinatology* 1994; 21:663–674.

Ma JCK, Hiatt A, Hein M, et al. Generation and assembly of secretory antibodies in plants. *Science* 1995; 268:716–719.

Mazanec MB, Nedrud JG, Kaetzel CS, et al. Intracellular neutralization of virus by immunoglobulin A antibodies. Proceedings of the National Academy of Sciences 1992; 89:6901–6905.

Mazanec MB, Nedrud JG, Kaetzel CS, et al. A three-tiered view of the role of IgA in mucosal defense. Immunology Today 1993; 14:430–435.

McCormick J, Gusmao, H, Nakamura S, et al. Antibody response to serogroup A and C meningococcal polysaccharide vaccine in infants born of mothers vaccinated during pregnancy. Journal of Clinical Investigation 1980; 65:1141–1144.

McDonald CJ, Hui SL, Tierney WM. Computing—effects of computer reminders for influenza vaccination on morbidity during influenza epidemics. *MD Computing* 1992; 9:304–312.

McDowell I, Newell C. *Measuring Health: A Guide to Rating Scales and Questionnaires.* Second edition. New York: Oxford University Press, 1996.

Mercer Management Consulting. *Report on the United States Vaccine Industry.* New York: Mercer Management Consulting, 1995.

Merkel PA, Caputo GC. Evaluation of a simple office-based strategy for increasing influenza vaccine administration and the effect of differing reimbursement plans on the patient acceptance rate. *Journal of General Internal Medicine* 1994; 9:679–683.

Mestecky J, McGhee JR. Immunoglobulin A (IgA): Molecular and cellular interactions involved in IgA biosynthesis and immune response. *Advances in Immunology* 1987; 40:153–245.

Michetti P, Mahan MJ, Slauch JM, Mekalanos JJ, Neutra MR. Monoclonal secretory immunoglobulin A protects mice against oral challenge with the invasive pathogen S*almonella typhimurium. Infection and Immunity* 1992; 60:1786–1792.

Moldoveanu Z, Porter DC, Lu A, et al. Immune responses induced by administration of encapsidated poliovirus replicons which express HIV-1 gag and envelope proteins. *Vaccine* 1995; 13:1013–1022.

Morein B, Sundquist B, Hoglund S, et al. ISCOM, a novel structure for antigenic presentation of membrane proteins from enveloped viruses. *Nature* 1984; 308:457–460.

Morgan IM. Immunization of monkeys with formalin-inactivated poliomyelitis viruses. *American Journal of Hygiene* 1948; 48:394–406.

Mosmann TR, Coffman, RL. Thl and Th2 cells: different patterns of lymphokine secretion lead to different functional properties. *Annual Review of Immunology* 1989; 7:145–173.

Mulholland K, Suara RO, Siber G, et al. Immunization of pregnant women with *Haemophilus influenzae* type b polysaccharide-tetanus protein conjugate vaccine in The Gambia. *Journal of the American Medical Association* 1996; 275:1182–1188.

Murray, CJL, Lopez, AD, eds. *The Global Burden of Disease: A Comprehensive Assessment of Mortality and Disability from Diseases, Injuries, and Risk Factors in 1990 and Projected to 2020.* Cambridge, Mass.: Harvard School of Public Health on behalf of the World Health Organization and the World Bank, 1996.

NCHS (National Center for Health Statistics). 1993. Abridged Life Table, United States [WWW document]. URL: http://www.cdc.gov/nchswww/datawh/statab/unpubd/ mortabs/lewk1.htm (accessed April 24, 1997).

Nichol KL, Korn JE; Margolis KL, et al. Achieving the national health objective for influenza immunization: success of an institution-wide vaccine program. *American Journal of Medicine* 1990; 89:156–160.

O'Dempsey TJ, McArdle T, Ceesay SJ, et al. Meningococcal antibody titres in infants of women immunized with meningococcal polysaccharide vaccine during pregnancy. *Archives of Diseases of Children* 1996; 74:F43–F46.

O'Hagan DT, McGee JP, Holmgren J, et al. Biodegradable microparticles for oral immunization. *Vaccine* 1993; 11:149–154.

Ogra P, Faden H. Poliovirus vaccines: Live or dead. *The Journal of Pediatrics* 1986; 108: 1031–1033.

Ogra P, Karzon D. Formation and function of poliovirus antibody in different tissues. *Progress in Medical Virology* 1971; 13:156–193.

Owen RL, Jones AL. Epithelial cell specialization within human Peyer's patches: an ultrastructural study of intestinal lymphoid follicles. *Gastroenterology* 1974; 66: 189–203.

Patrick D, Erickson P. Health Status and Health Policy: *Quality of Life in Health Care Evaluation and Resource Allocation*. New York: Oxford University Press, 1993.

Paul JR. *Clinical Epidemiology*. Chicago: University of Chicago Press; 1958:204–220.

Pearson DC, Thompson RS. Evaluation of Group Health Cooperative of Puget Sound's senior influenza immunization program. *Public Health Reports* 1994; 109:571–578.

Phillips-Quagliata JM, Lamm ME. Lymphocyte homing to mucosal effector sites. In Ogra R, Mestecky J, Lamm M, et al. (eds.), *Handbook of Mucosal Immunology*. Orlando, Fla.: Academic Press; 1994:225–239.

Plotkin SA. Inactivated polio vaccine for the United States: a missed vaccination opportunity. *Pediatric Infectious Disease Journal* 1995; 14:835–839.

Porter DC, Ansardi DC, Choi WS, et al. Encapsidation of genetically engineered poliovirus minireplicons which express HIV type 1 gag and pol proteins upon infection. *Virology* 1993; 67:3712–3719.

Porter DC, Ansard DC, Morrow CD. Encapsidation of poliovirus replicons encoding the complete human immunodeficiency type virus type 1 gag gene by using a complementation system which provides the Pl capsid proteins in trans. *Virology* 1995; 69:1548–1555.

Renegar KB, Small Jr. PA. Passive transfer of local immunity to influenza virus infection by IgA antibody. *Immunology* 1991; 146:1972–1978.

Rivers TM, Ward SM, Baird RD. Amount and duration of immunity induced by intradermal inoculation of cultured vaccine virus. *Journal of Experimental Medicine* 1939; 69:857.

Roberge R, Berthelot JM, Wolfson M. The health utility index: measuring health differences in Ontario by socioeconomic status. *Health Reports* 1995; 7:25–32.

Roberts M, Chatfield SN, Dougan G. Salmonella as carriers of heterologous antigens. In: O'Hagan DT (ed.), *Novel Delivery Systems for Oral Vaccines*. Boca Raton, Fla.: CRC Press; 1994:27–58.

Rodriguez RM, Baroff LJ. Emergency department immunization of the elderly with pneumococcal and influenza vaccines. *Annals of Emergency Medicine* 1993; 22: 1729–1732.

Rosser RM. A health index and output measure. In: Walker SR, Roser RM (eds.), *Quality of Life: Assessment and Application.* Lancaster, England: MTP Press, 1987; 133–160.

Rosser R, Cotte M, Rabin R, et al. Index of health-related quality of life. In: Hopkins A (ed.), *Measure of the Quality of Life and the Uses to Which Such Measures May Be Put.* London: Royal College of Physicians of London, 1992;81–89, 147–153.

Russell LB, Gold MR, Siegel JE, et al. The role of cost-effectiveness analysis in health and medicine. *Journal of the American Medical Association* 1996; 276: 1172–1177.

Sabin AB. Characteristics and genetic potentialities of experimentally produced and naturally occurring variants of poliomyelitis virus. *Annals of the New York Academy of Science* 1955; 61:924–938.

Sadoway DT, Loucraft JR, Johnston BA. Maximizing influenza immunization in Edmonton: a collaborative model. *Canadian Journal of Public Health* 1994; 85:47–50.

Salk JE. Principles of immunization as applied to poliomyelitis and influenza. American *Journal of Public Health* 1953; 43:1384–2398.

Schofield F. Selective primary health care: strategies for control of disease in the developing world. XXII. Tetanus: a preventable problem. *Review of Infectious Diseases* 1986; 8:144–156.

Seder RA, Paul WE. Acquisition of lymphokine-producing phenotype by CD4[+] T cells. *Allergy and Clinical Immunology* 1994; 94:1195–1202.

Siegel B, Mahan C, Witte J, et al. Influenza and pneumococcal pneumonia immunization. *Journal of Florida Medical Association* 1990; 77:593–595.

Smith JS. *Patenting the Sun: Polio and Salk Vaccine.* New York: Doubleday; 1991.

St. Anthony's Publishing, Inc. *St. Anthony's DRG Guidebook: 1996.* Reston, Va.: St. Anthony's Publishing, 1995.

Sullivan DF. A single index of morbidity and mortality. *HSMHA Health Reports* 1971; 86(4):347–355.

Tackett CO, Hone DM, Curtiss R, III, Kelly SM, Losonsky G, Guers L, Harris AM, Edelman R, Levin MM. Comparison of the safety and immunogenicity of • aroC • aroD and • cya • crp *Salmonella typhi* strains in adult volunteers. *Infection and Immunity* 1992; 60:536–541.

Taylor PM, Askonas BA. Influenza nucleoprotein specific cytotoxic T cell clones are protective in vivo. *Immunology* 1986; 58:417–420.

Thanavala Y, Yang YF, Lyons P, et al. Immunogenicity of transgenic plant-derived hepatitis B surface antigen. *Proceedings of the National Academy of Sciences* 1995; 92:3358–3361.

The National Foundation. *Poliomyelitis: Annual Statistical Review.* New York: The National Foundation; 1961.

The National Foundation. *What You Should Know about Polio Vaccine?* Publication 19. New York: The National Foundation; 1962.

Torrance GW and Feeny D. Utilities and quality-adjusted life years. *International Journal of Technology Assessment in Health Care* 1989; 5:559–575.

Torrance GW, Furlong W, Feeny D, et al. Provisional Health Status Index for the Ontario Health Survey. Final Report Submitted to Statistics Canada (Contract

44400900187). Hamilton, Ontario: Centre for Health Economics and Policy Analysis, McMaster University, 1992.

Torrance GW, Furlong W, Feeny D, et al. Multi-attribute health preference functions: health utilities index. *PharmacoEconomics* 1995; 34:503–520.

Waksman BH. Adjuvants and immune regulation by lymphoid cells. Springer Seminar. *Immunopathology* 1979; 2:5–33.

Ware JE, Sherbourne DC. The MOS 36-item short-form health survey. *Medical Care* 1992; 30:473–483.

Williams WW, Hickson MA, Kane MA, et al. Immunization policies and vaccine coverage among adults: the risk for missed opportunities. *Annals of Internal Medicine* 1988; 108:616–625. (Erratum, *Annals of Internal Medicine* 1988; 109:348.)

Winner III, L, Mack J, Weltzin R, Mekalanos JJ, Kraehenhbuhl JP, Neutra MR. New model for analysis of mucosal immunity: intestinal secretion of specific monoclonal immunoglobulin A from hybridoma tumors protects against *Vibrio cholerae* infection. *Infection and Immunity* 1991; 59:977–982.

Wolf JL, Bye WA. The membranous epithelial (M) cell and the mucosal immune system. *Annual Review of Medicine* 1984; 35:95–112.

Wolf JL, Rubin DH, Finberg R, et al. Intestinal M cells: a pathway for entry of reovirus into the host. *Science* 1981; 212:471–472.

Wolfson MC. Health-adjusted life expectancy. *Health Reports* 1996; 8:41–46.

Wrenn K, Zeldin M, Miller O. Influenza and pneumococcal vaccination in the emergency department: Is it feasible? *Journal of General Internal Medicine* 1994; 9: 425–429.

Yang Y, Nunes FA, Berencs K, et al. Cellular immunity to viral antigens limits El-deleted adenoviruses for gene therapy. *Proceedings of the National Academy of Sciences* 1994; 91:4407–4411.

Yap KL, Ada GL, McKenzie IFC. Transfer on specific cytotoxic T lymphocytes protects mice inoculated with influenzae virus. *Nature* 1978; 273:238–239.

Zinkernagel RM, Doherty PC. MHC-restricted cytotoxic T cells: studies on the biological role of polymorphic major transplantation antigens determining T-cell restriction-specificity, function, and responsiveness. *Advances in Immunology* 1979; 27:51–177.

Zweerink HJ, Courtneidge SA, Skehel JJ, et al. Cytotoxic T cells kill influenzae virus-infected cells but do not distinguish between serologically distinct type A viruses. *Nature* 1977; 267:354–356.

APPENDIX 1

Borrelia burgdorferi

DISEASE BURDEN

Epidemiology

For the purposes of the calculations in this report, the committee estimated that there are 12,000 new cases of infection each year in the United States. The risk of borrelia infection is highest in certain regions of the United States, such as, New England, the Mid-Atlantic states, and certain areas in the Midwest. The committee assumed that within epidemic regions new infections occur equally in males and females and that there are no deaths. The incidence rate is 4.56 per 100,000, but varies slightly by age group. The highest incidence is estimated to occur in the age groups that spend the most amount of time out of doors, that is, those up to 14 years of age. Table A1-1 illustrates the age distribution of new cases of borrelia infection used in the model. Approximately half of all new infections are assumed to occur in people born in the region and half in migrants into the area.

Disease Scenarios

For the purposes of the calculations in this report, the committee assumed that 90% of people newly infected with borrelia experience acute manifestations and seek treatment. The morbidity results in 3 weeks of minor illness associated with a health utility index (HUI) of .89. Another 2% of the new infections experience the same acute illness but do not seek treatment. The committee estimated that 8% of all new infections lead to chronic morbidity expressed as recurrences over a long period of time. The committee estimated that such people experience approximately 2 months per year of illness associated with a HUI of .79 and that

143

Table A1-1 Incidence Rates—*Borrelia burgdorferi*

5-Year Age Groups	Total Population	Incidence Rates (per 100,000) (5-yr age groups)	Cases	Age Groups	Population	Incidence Rates (per 100,00)
0-4	20,182,000	4.95	998	<1	3,963,000	4.95
5-9	19,117,000	4.95	945	1-4	16,219,000	4.95
10-14	18,939,000	4.95	937	5-14	38,056,000	4.95
15-19	17,790,000	4.27	759	15-24	36,263,000	4.27
20-24	18,473,000	4.27	789	25-34	41,670,000	4.27
25-29	19,294,000	4.27	824	35-44	42,149,000	4.88
30-34	22,376,000	4.27	955	45-54	30,224,000	4.61
35-39	22,215,000	4.88	1,084	55-64	21,241,000	4.27
40-44	19,934,000	4.88	973	65-74	18,964,000	4.27
45-49	16,873,000	4.88	823	75-84	11,088,000	4.27
50-54	13,351,000	4.27	570	• 85	3,598,000	4.27
55-59	11,050,000	4.27	472			
60-64	10,191,000	4.27	435	**Total**	263,435,000	4.56
65-69	10,099,000	4.27	431			
70-74	8,865,000	4.27	378			
75-79	6,669,000	4.27	285			
80-84	4,419,000	4.27	189			
• 85	3,598,000	4.27	154			
Total	263,435,000		12,000			

these recurrences occur for 10 years. Table A1-2 summarizes the disease scenarios associated with borrelia infections.

COST INCURRED BY DISEASE

Health care costs are incurred through diagnostic evaluation, physician visits, and antibiotics. Table A1-3 summarizes the health care costs incurred by borrelia infections. For the purposes of the calculations, it was assumed that all people with acute manifestations incur two physician visits and a prescription antibiotic, and that half receive diagnostic tests. It was assumed that each recurrence is associated with two physician visits and a prescription medication, and that the recurrences occur for 10 years.

VACCINE DEVELOPMENT

The committee assumed that the development of a Borrelia burgdorferi vaccine is feasible and that licensure is imminent (a Borrelia vaccine for use in persons 15 years of age and older was licensed prior to the completion of this report). The estimates for this report are that it will take 3 years until licensure is completed and that $120 million needs to be invested. Table 4-1 summarizes vaccine development assumptions for all vaccines considered in this report.

VACCINE PROGRAM CONSIDERATIONS

Target Population

The committee's analysis assumes that immunization with this vaccine will occur only in those geographic regions discussed under the epidemiology section. Immunization will occur during infancy or within 1 year of migration to the area. It is estimated that 90% of infants will receive the immunization. The committee estimates that only 10% of migrants into an area will receive the immunization.

Vaccine Schedule, Efficacy, and Costs

The committee estimated that this vaccine would cost $100 per dose. Vaccine administration would cost an additional $10. The committee has accepted default assumptions for this vaccine that estimate it will require a series of 3 doses and that efficacy will be 75%. Table 4-1 summarizes vaccine program assumptions for all vaccines considered in this report.

Table A1-2 *Borrelia burgdorferi*

	No. of Cases	% of Cases	Committee HUI Values	Duration (years)
MORBIDITY SCENARIOS				
Total Deaths	0			
Total Cases	12,000			
I. **Patients who receive treatment**				
Acute manifestations		90%	0.89	0.0575 (3 weeks)
II. **Untreated patients—no recurrence**				
Acute manifestations		2%	0.89	0.0575 (3 weeks)
III. **Complications in untreated patients—recurrences**		8%		
Acute manifestations			0.89	0.0575 (3 weeks)
Recurrences (over 10 years)			0.79	0.1667 (2 months/year over 10 years)

Table A1-3 Health Care Costs—*Borrelia burgdorferi*

	Duration (years)	% with Care	Cost per Case	Cost per Unit	Units per Case (or per year)	Form of Treatment
I. **Patients who receive treatment**						
Acute manifestations	0.0575	100%	$100	$50	2.0	Physician A
	0.0575	100%	$50	$50	1.0	Medication B
	0.0575	50%	$100	$100	1.0	Diagnostic B
II. **Complications in untreated patients—recurrences**						
(2 months per year over 10 years)	10,000	100%	$100	$50	2.0	Physician A
		100%	$50	$50	1.0	Medication B per recurrence

RESULTS

If a vaccine program for *B. burgdorferi* were implemented today and the vaccine was 100% efficacious and utilized by 100% of the target population, the annualized present value of the QALYs gained would be 200. Using committee assumptions of less-than-ideal efficacy and utilization and including time and monetary costs until a vaccine program is implemented, the annualized present value of the QALYs gained would be 39.

If a vaccine program for *B. burgdorferi* were implemented today and the vaccine was 100% efficacious and utilized by 100% of the target population, the annualized present value of the health care costs saved would be $2 million. Using committee assumptions of less-than-ideal efficacy and utilization and including time and monetary costs until a vaccine program is implemented, the annualized present value of the health care costs saved would be $410,000.

If a vaccine program for *B. burgdorferi* were implemented today and the vaccine was 100% efficacious and utilized by 100% of the target population, the annualized present value of the program cost would be $690 million. Using committee assumptions of less-than-ideal efficacy and utilization and including time and monetary costs until a vaccine program is implemented, the annualized present value of the program cost would be $280 million.

Using committee assumptions of time and costs until licensure, the fixed cost of vaccine development has been amortized and is $3.6 million for a *B. burgdorferi* vaccine.

If a vaccine program were implemented today and the vaccine were 100% efficacious and utilized by 100% of the target population, the annualized present value of the cost per QALY gained is $3.5 million. Using committee assumptions of less-than-ideal utilization and including time and monetary costs until a vaccine program is implemented, the annualized present value of the cost per QALY gained is $7.3 million.

See Chapters 4 and 5 for details on the methods and assumptions used by the committee for the results reported.

READING LIST

Byerly E, Deardorff K. National and State Population Estimates: 1990 to 1994, U.S. Bureau of the Census, Current Population Reports, pp. 25–1127, U.S. Government Printing Office, Washington, DC, 1995.

CDC. Summary of Notifiable Diseases, United States 1994. Morbidity and Mortality Weekly Report 1994; 43:1–80.

Hansen KA. Geographical Mobility: March 1993 to March 1994, U.S. Bureau of the Census, Current Population Reports, pp. 20–485, U.S. Government Printing Office, Washington, DC, 1995.

Stechenberg BW. Borrelia: Lyme Disease. In: Textbook of Pediatric Infectious Diseases. RD Feigin and JD Cherry eds. Philadelphia, PA: WB Saunder Company, 1992, pp. 1062–1067.

Steere AC. Borrelia burgdorferi (Lyme Disease, Lyme Borreliosis). In: Principles and Practice of Infectious Diseases. GL Mandell, JE Bennett, Dolin R eds. New York: Churchill Livingstone, 1995, pp. 2143–2155.

Ventura SJ, Martin JA, Mathews TJ, et al. Advance Report of Final Natality Statistics, 1994. Monthly Vital Statistics Report 1996; 44.

Wormser GP. Prospects for a Vaccine to Prevent Lyme Disease in Humans. Clinical Infectious Diseases 1995; 21:1267–1274.

APPENDIX 2

Chlamydia

DISEASE BURDEN

Epidemiology

For the purposes of the calculations in this report, the committee has estimated that there are 4 million new cases of chlamydia infections in noninfants in the United States each year. These cases are split equally between men and women. The committee estimated that there are 130,000 cases annually of chlamydia infections in infants. There is very minimal mortality associated with this infection; the committee has indicated a nominal number of 5 deaths in women annually for purposes of modeling. The morbidity is extensive and manifests in many different ways.

The committee estimated that the age distribution of new chlamydia infections is the same for men and women. The vast majority (90%) of new cases in noninfants occur in people between the ages of 15 and 34 years of age. Table A2-1 illustrates the age distribution of new annual chlamydia infections in women and men used in the model.

Disease Scenarios: Women

The committee estimated that 70% of infections in women are asymptomatic and that 55% of those go untreated. 15% of asymptomatic cases are detected through screening. 30% of new infections in women are symptomatic.

See Appendix 28 for more information.

149

TABLE A2-1 Incidence of Chlamydia in Men and Women

Age Groups	Male Population	Incidence Rates (per 100,000)	Cases
<1	2,030,000	0.00	0
1–4	8,314,000	120.28	10,000
5–14	19,502,000	461.49	90,000
15–24	18,516,000	6,480.88	1,200,000
25–34	20,835,000	2,879.77	600,000
35–44	20,911,000	334.75	70,000
45–54	14,777,000	135.35	20,000
55–64	10,101,000	99.00	10,000
65–74	8,420,000	0.00	0
75–84	4,274,000	0.00	0
≥85	1,005,000	0.00	0
Total	128,685,000	1,554.18	2,000,000

Age Groups	Female Population	Incidence Rates (per 100,000)	Cases
<1	1,933,000	0.00	0
1–4	7,905,000	126.50	10,000
5–14	18,554,000	485.07	90,000
15–24	17,747,000	6,761.71	1,200,000
25–34	20,835,000	2,879.77	600,000
35–44	21,238,000	329.60	70,000
45–54	15,447,000	129.47	20,000
55–64	11,140,000	89.77	10,000
65–74	10,544,000	0.00	0
75–84	6,814,000	0.00	0
85+	2,593,000	0.00	0
Total	134,750,000	1,484.23	2,000,000

Health consequences of chlamydia infection in women accounted for in the model include acute urethral syndrome, mild cervicitis, pelvic inflammatory disease (PID) and its sequelae (ectopic pregnancy, chronic pelvic pain, and infertility, assumed for calculation purposes to incur costs and decreased health states with a 5-year lag from infection), Reiter's syndrome, and arthritis. Table A2-2 illustrates the estimated number of cases in each state, the duration of time that state is experienced, and the health utility index (HUI) associated with each state. These vary greatly. At one end of the spectrum are a large number of relatively minor conditions such as acute urethral syndrome (100,000 cases experiencing three days of an HUI of .75). At the other end are many fewer

Table A2-2 Morbidity Scenarios for Chlamydia Infection in Women, Men and Infants

	No. of Cases	% of Cases	Committee HUI Values	Duration
WOMEN				
Asymptomatic	1,400,000	70.0%	1.00	
untreated		55.0%		
treated (detected in screening, etc)		15.0%		
Acute Urethral Syndrome	100,000	5.0%	0.75	0.0082 (3 days)
Mild (cervicitis, bartholinitis)	500,000	25.0%	0.90	0.0767 (4 weeks)
PID	280,500	14.0%		
outpatient treatment only			0.63	0.0274 (10 days)
PID	33,000	1.7%		
inpatient treatment—no surgery			0.57	0.0055 (2 days)
PID	16,500	0.8%		
inpatient treatment with surgery			0.46	0.0055 2 days)
PID	49,500	2.5%		
outpatient treatment after inpatient treatment			0.83	0.0274 (10 days)
Ectopic Pregnancy— Outpatient Treatment	14,850	0.7%		
PID sequelae: 5-year lag			0.58	0.0767 (4 weeks)
Ectopic Pregnancy—Inpatient Treatment	14,850	0.7%		
PID sequelae: 5-year lag inpatient			0.23	0.0082 (3 days)
outpatient treatment after inpatient treatment			0.66	0.0767 (4 weeks)
Chronic pelvic pain	59,400	3.0%		
PID sequelae: 5-year lag			0.60	22.7313 (duration remaining lifetime)
Infertility	66,000	3.3%		
PID sequelae: 5-year lag			0.82	22.7313 (duration remaining lifetime)
Reiter's Syndrome	2,000	0.1%	0.63	0.0384 (2 weeks)
Arthritis	10,000	0.5%	0.69	0.1151 (6 weeks)
MEN				
Asymptomatic untreated	500,000	25.0%	1.00	0
Urethritis	1,500,000	75.0%	0.84	0.0192 (7 days)
Epididymitis outpatient	36,000	1.8%	0.46	0.0192 (7 days)
Epididymitis inpatient	3,600	0.2%	0.30	0.0082 (3 days)
Reiter's Syndrome	2,000	0.1%	0.63	0.0384 (2 weeks)

Continued

Table A2-2 *Continued*

	No. of Cases	% of Cases	Committee HUI Values	Duration (years)
Arthritis	10,000	0.5%	0.69	0.1151 (6 weeks)
INFANTS				
Conjunctivitis neonatal infection	100,000	76.9%	0.97	0.5000 (6 months)
Pneumonia outpatient	40,000	30.8%	0.79	0.1667 (onset: 6 weeks; duration: 2 months)
Pneumonia w/ sequelae inpatient	10,000	7.7%	0.55	0.0137 (onset: 6 weeks; duration: 5 days)

cases with a much more serious decrement in health status for longer periods of time. Examples include ectopic pregnancy (14,850 cases treated as an inpatient for 3 days and 4 weeks recuperation as an outpatient at an HUI of .66) and chronic pelvic pain (59,400 cases of an HUI state of .60 for the duration of lifetime).

Disease Scenarios: Men

The committee estimated that 25% of infections in men are asymptomatic. The symptomatic cases all involve urethritis. A small percentage of these symptomatic infections also involve more serious manifestations, such as epididymitis, Reiter's syndrome, and arthritis. Table A2-2 illustrates the estimated number of cases in each state, the duration of time that state is experienced, and the health utility index (HUI) associated with each state in men. These vary greatly. At one end of the spectrum are a large number of cases of urethritis (1,500,000 cases lasting 7 days with an HUI of .84). At the other end are many fewer cases with a more serious decrement in health status for longer periods of time, such as epidymitis and arthritis.

Disease Scenarios: Infants

The committee estimated that there are 130,00 new infections in infants each year. Most of these are neonatal conjunctivitis, but there are some cases of pneumonia. Table A2-2 illustrates the estimated number of cases in each state, the duration of time that state is experienced, and the health utility index (HUI) associated with each state in infants.

COSTS INCURRED BY DISEASE

Table A2-3 summarizes the health care costs incurred by chlamydia infections. For the purposes of the calculations used in the report, it was assumed that women with asymptomatic infections (e.g. identified through screening) and with mild manifestations (acute urethral syndrome, cervicitis, bartholinitis) treated as an outpatient incur costs associated with a limited physician visit, an inexpensive diagnostic, and an inexpensive prescription medication. Women with pelvic inflammatory disease (PID) treated as an outpatient only incur costs associated with a limited physician visit, a specialist physician visit, a mid-level diagnostic, and an inexpensive prescription medication. More severe cases of PID requiring hospitalization are associated with hospitalization costs, specialist in-patient physician visits, and a mid-level diagnostic. Those requiring surgery incurs additional costs (e.g., surgeons, anesthesiologists, anesthetists). Outpatient costs following hospitalization include a specialist visit.

Ectopic pregnancy was assumed to be associated with both outpatient and inpatient costs. The outpatient costs include a specialist visit for diagnosis for all women and, for half the women with ectopic pregnancy, lab tests and multiple follow-up visits. Inpatient costs include the hospitalization charges, physician costs, mid-level diagnostics, and costs for surgeons and anesthesiologists. Follow-up visits are also included.

Chronic pelvic pain was assumed to be associated with multiple general physician visits (general and specialist), analgesics, and intermediate diagnostics. It was assumed that 75% of women with chronic pelvic pain would receive outpatient laparoscopy and associated physician charges and that 30% would require inpatient surgery with associated charges.

For the purposes of the calculation, it was assumed that half of women infertile due to chlamydia infection receive treatment for infertility. Costs incurred were assumed to include multiple specialist visits and expensive diagnostics. Slightly fewer would receive outpatient laparoscopy and other surgeries. It was assumed that a small fraction would undergo in vitro fertilization.

Costs incurred due to both Reiter's syndrome and arthritis for both men and women were assumed to include two visits to a specialist and inexpensive prescription medications.

Costs incurred for urethritis in men infected with chlamydia were assumed to include a limited physician visit, an inexpensive diagnostic, and an inexpensive prescription medication. Outpatient costs incurred by men with epididymitis include a limited and a specialist physician visit, and an inexpensive diagnostic and prescription medication. Inpatient costs associated with those few patients hospitalized for epididymitis include hospital costs, comprehensive in patient physician visits, medications, and surgeons and anesthesiologists for a minority who require surgery.

Table A2-3 Treatment Scenarios for Chlamayida Infection in Women, Men and Infants

	% with Care	Cost per Unit	Units per Case	Form of Treatment
WOMEN				
Asymptomatic	100%	$50	1	physician a
	100%	$50	1	diagnostic a
	100%	$50	1	prescription b
Acute Urethral Syndrome: outpatient	100%	$50	1	physician a
	100%	$50	1	diagnostic a
	100%	$50	1	prescription b
Mild conditions (cervicitis, bartholinitis): outpatient	100%	$50	1	physician a
	100%	$50	1	diagnostic a
	100%	$50	1	prescription b
PID: outpatient only	100%	$50	1	physician a
	100%	$100	1	physician b
	100%	$100	1	diagnostic b
	100%	$50	1	prescription b
PID: inpatient—no surgery	100%	$4,000	1	hospitalization
	100%	$150	3	physician c
	100%	$100	1	diagnostic b
PID: inpatient with surgery	100%	$4,000	1	hospitalization
	100%	$150	3	physician c
	100%	$500	4	surgical staff
PID: outpatient after inpatient	100%	$100	1	physician b
Ectopic Pregnancy : outpatient	100%	$100	1	physician b
	50%	$50	1	physician a
	50%	$100	6	follow-up physician b
	10%	$50	1	diagnostic a
	10%	$130	1	follow-up visits and tests (2 visits) outpatient laparoscopy
	50%	$1,250	1	laparoscopy
	50%	$300	2	surgeon
	50%	$500	2	anesthesiologist
	50%	$100	1	diagnostics b
	50%	$100	1	physician b
Ectopic Pregnancy—Inpatient PID sequelae: 5-year lag inpatient	100%	$3,000	1	hospitalization
	100%	$150	1	physician c
	100%	$100	1	diagnostics b
	100%	$500	1	surgeon
	100%	$500	1	anesthesiology
outpatient after inpatient	100%	$100	2	physician b

Table A2-3 *Continued*

	% with Care	Cost per Unit	Units per Case	Form of Treatment
Chronic pelvic pain				
PID sequelae: 5 year lag				
treatment assumed to occur	100%	$100	1	physician b
5 years after onset of				
infection				
	100%	$50	4	physician a
	100%	$100	1	analgesics (6 months)
	100%	$100	1	diagnostic b
				outpatient laparascopy
	75%	$1,000	1	hospital charges
	75%	$500	2	surgeon/anesthesiologist
	75%	$150	1	physician c
				lower abdominal
				surgery
	30%	$4,000	1	hospitalization
	30%	$500	1	surgeon
	30%	$500	1	anesthesiologist
	30%	$150	1	physician c
	30%	$50	1	post-discharge visit
				(physician a)
Infertility				
PID sequelae: 5-year lag	50%	$150	6	physician c
treatment assumed to occur	50%	$500	1	diagnostic c
5 years after onset of				
infection				
				outpatient laparoscopy
	38%	$1,000	1	hospitalization
	38%	$500	2	surgeon/anesthesiologist
	38%	$150	1	physician c
				tubal surgery
	15%	$1,000	1	outpatient surgery
	15%	$500	2	surgeon/
				anesthesiologist
	15%	$150	1	physician c
Reiter's Syndrome	100%	$100	2.0	physician b
	100%	$50	1.0	medication b
Arthritis	100%	$100	2.0	physician b
	100%	$50	1.0	medication b
MEN				
Urethritis	100%	$50	1	physician a
	100%	$50	1	diagnostics a
	100%	$50.00	1	medication b
Epididymitis: outpatient	100%	$100	1	physician b
	100%	$50	1	physician a
	100%	$50	1	diagnostics a
	100%	$50	1	medication b

Continued

Table A2-3 *Continued*

	% with Care	Cost per Unit	Units per Case	Form of Treatment
Epididymitis: inpatient	100%	$3,000	1	hospitalization
	100%	$150	3	physician c
	100%	$50	1	medication b
	0.03	$500	2	surgical staff
Reiter's Syndrome	100%	$100	2.0	physician b
	100%	$50	1.0	medication b
Arthritis	100%	$100	2.0	physician b
	100%	$50	1.0	medication b
INFANTS				
Conjunctivitis: neonatal infection	100%	$50	1	limited visit
	100%	$50	1	diagnostics a
	100%	$50	1	medication b
Pneumonia: outpatient	100%	$100	2	physician b
	100%	$100	1	diagnostic b
	100%	*$50	1	medication b
Pneumonia w/ sequelae: inpatient	100%	$4,000	1	hospital (3 days)
	100%	$150	1	comprehensive
	100%	$100	1	intermediate
	100%	$50	2	brief
	100%	$50	1	diagnostic
	100%	$50	1	medication b

and prescription medications. Inpatient costs for the smaller number of infants with pneumonia requiring hospitalization include hospitalization costs, physician visits (specialists and general), diagnostics, and medications.

VACCINE DEVELOPMENT

The committee assumed that the development of a chlamydia vaccine is feasible and that licensure can occur within the time frame of its charge, but is not imminent. The estimates for the model are that it will take 15 years until licensure and that $360 million needs to be invested. Table 4–1 summarizes vaccine development assumptions for all vaccines considered in this report.

VACCINE PROGRAM CONSIDERATIONS

Target Population

The committee's model assumes that chlamydia immunization will occur during puberty. As described in the body of the report, for these purposes, that is set at 12 years of age. Both males and females would receive the immunization. It is estimated that only 50% of the target population will accept the immunization.

Vaccine Schedule, Efficacy, and Costs

The committee estimated that this would be a relatively low-cost vaccine, costing $50 per dose. Vaccine administration would cost an additional $10. The committee has accepted default assumptions for this vaccine that it will require a series of 3 doses and that efficacy will be 75%. Table 4–1 summarizes vaccine program assumptions for all vaccines considered in this report.

RESULTS

If a vaccine program for *Chlamydia* were implemented today and the vaccine was 100% efficacious and utilized by 100% of the target population, the annualized present value of the QALYs gained would be 525,000. Using committee assumptions of less-than-ideal efficacy and utilization and including time and monetary costs until a vaccine program is implemented, the annualized present value of the QALYs gained would be 110,000. Although the number of new chlamydia infections in men equal those in women in this model, the number of QALYs lost due to disease in men is much less due to the decreased severity of the disease experienced in men.

If a vaccine program for *Chlamydia* were implemented today and the vaccine was 100% efficacious and utilized by 100% of the target population, the annualized present value of the health care costs saved would be $850 million. Using committee assumptions of less-than-ideal efficacy and utilization and including time and monetary costs until a vaccine program is implemented, the annualized present value of the health care costs saved would be $175 million.

If a vaccine program for *Chlamydia* were implemented today and the vaccine was 100% efficacious and utilized by 100% of the target population, the annualized present value of the program cost would be $680 million. Using committee assumptions of less-than-ideal efficacy and utilization and including time and monetary costs until a vaccine program is implemented, the annualized present value of the program cost would be $190 million.

Using committee assumptions of time and costs until licensure, the fixed cost of vaccine development has been amortized and is $11 million for a *Chlamydia* vaccine.

If a vaccine program were implemented today and the vaccine were 100% efficacious and utilized by 100% of the target population, the annualized present value of the cost per QALY gained is -$350. A negative value represents a saving in costs in addition to a saving in QALYs. Using committee assumptions of less-than-ideal utilization and including time and monetary costs until a vaccine program is implemented, the annualized present value of the cost per QALY gained is $200.

See Chapters 4 and 5 for details on the methods and assumptions used by the committee for the results reported.

READING LIST

Alexander LL, Treiman K, Clarke P. A National Survey of Nurse Practitioner Chlamydia Knowledge and Treatment Practices of Female Patients. Nurse Practitioner 1996; 21:48, 51–4.

CDC. Ectopic Pregnancy—United States, 1990–1992. Morbidity and Mortality Weekly Report 1995; 44:46–48.

CDC. Evaluation of Surveillance for *Chlamydia trachomatis* Infections in the United States, 1987 to 1991. Morbidity and Mortality Weekly Report 1993; 42:21–27.

CDC. Recommendations for the Prevention and Management of *Chlamydia trachomatis* Infections. Morbidity and Mortality Weekly Report 1993; 42:1–4.

Institute of Medicine. The Hidden Epidemic: Confronting Sexually Transmitted Diseases. Eng TR, Butler WT (eds.). Washington, DC: National Academy Press, 1997.

Jones RB. Chlamydia trachomatis (trachoma perinatal infections, lymphogranuloma vernereum, and other genital infections). In: Principles and Practice of Infectious Diseases. GL Mandell,, JE Bennett, Dolin R eds. New York, NY: Churchill Livingstone, 1995, pp. 1679–1693.

Magid D, Douglas JM, Schwartz JS. Doxycycline Compared with Azithromycin for Treating Women with Genital Chlamydia trachomatis Infections: An Incremental Cost-Effectiveness Analysis. Annals of Internal Medicine 1996; 124:389–99.

U.S. Bureau of the Census. Statistical Abstract of the U.S.: 1995 (115th edition). Washington, DC, 1995.

Ventura SJ, Martin JA, Mathews TJ, et al. Advance Report of Final Natality Statistics, 1994. Monthly Vital Statistics Report 1996; 44.

APPENDIX 3

Coccidioides immitis

DISEASE BURDEN

Epidemiology

For the purposes of the calculations in this report, the committee estimated that there are 100,000 new cases of *C. immitis* infection each year in the United States. *C. immitis* infections are most prominent in several geographic locations in the United States, primarily California, Texas, New Mexico, Arizona, Nevada. The committee estimated that half of new infections occur to people born in those regions and half occur to people who have migrated into those regions. This distinction has significant implications in other portions of the modeling exercise. The highest incidence was estimated to occur in people between the ages of 15 and 44 years of age. Table A3-1 shows the age distribution of incidence and mortality associated with *C. immitis*. The committee estimated that males and females are equally vulnerable to coccidioides infection. The committee estimated there are 117 deaths per year associated with the infection.

The treatment of HIV infection and AIDS and the effect of those changes on the health status and costs of care experienced by those with HIV has changed rapidly in recent years and is expected to continue to do so. Therefore, the committee has chosen not to include a scenario specific to infection in those

---

See Appendix 28 for more information.

Table A3-1 Incidence and Mortality Rates for Coccidioides

5-year Age Groups	Total Population	Incidence Rates (per 100,000) (5-year age groups)	Cases
0-4	20,182,000	0.00	0
5-9	19,117,000	0.00	0
10-14	18,939,000	57.73	10,934
15-19	17,790,000	57.73	10,270
20-24	18,473,000	57.73	10,665
25-29	19,294,000	57.73	11,139
30-34	22,376,000	57.73	12,918
35-39	22,215,000	57.73	12,825
40-44	19,934,000	57.73	11,508
45-49	16,873,000	57.73	9,741
50-54	13,351,000	14.65	1,956
55-59	11,050,000	14.65	1,619
60-64	10,191,000	14.65	1,493
65-69	10,099,000	14.65	1,480
70-74	8,865,000	14.65	1,299
75-79	6,669,000	14.65	977
80-84	4,419,000	14.65	648
85+	3,598,000	14.65	527
Total	263,435,000		100,000

Age Groups	Population	Mortality Rates (per 100,000)	% Distribution of Deaths
<1	3,963,000	0.000	0.000
1-4	16,219,000	0.000	0.000
5-14	38,056,000	0.003	0.009
15-24	36,263,000	0.019	0.058
25-34	41,670,000	0.039	0.139
35-44	42,149,000	0.030	0.109
45-54	30,224,000	0.054	0.139
55-64	21,241,000	0.064	0.115
65-74	18,964,000	0.148	0.239
75-84	11,088,000	0.147	0.139
85+	3,598,000	0.181	0.055
Total	263,435,000	0.045	1.0000

with HIV/AIDS. Consideration of this population would result in differences in the calculations achieved with this model, but the uncertainties associated with doing so were thought to be quite extreme.

Disease Scenarios

For the purposes of the calculations in this report, the committee estimated that 40% of all *C. immitis* infections were asymptomatic. Symptomatic infections manifested as mild respiratory illness with and without complications of erethyma nodosum, pneumonia, and as a persistent, disseminated infection. The health utility indices associated with *C. immitis* infection vary from .65 for hospitalization with disseminated infection to .90 for the prolonged outpatient phase of a persistent, disseminated infection. Table A3-2 illustrates the estimated number of cases in each health state, the duration of time that state is experienced, and the health utility index (HUI) associated with each state.

COST INCURRED BY DISEASE

Table A3-3 summarizes the health care costs incurred by *C. immitis* infections. For the purposes of the calculations used in this report, it was assumed that the mild respiratory illness associated with *C. immitis* infection leads to the costs of a limited physician visit and that only half of those with this illness would seek medical attention. It is assumed that 100% of people with more severe complications seek medical attention. Those people with complications of erythema incur costs associated with the respiratory illness (limited physician visit, diagnostic, medication) and several specialist visits for assessment and treatment of the complications.

Outpatient pneumonia is assumed to be associated with physician visits, diagnostics, and medications. Inpatient hospital costs were included for the few patients who were assumed to require it. Persistent/disseminated infection was associated with several hospitalizations as well as numerous outpatient visits, diagnostics, and medications over a 3-year period.

Although the health care scenarios are the same for those who would be immunized in infancy and as migrants (at older ages), the costs are calculated separately to allow for the effects of discounting, which will be different in infants (who might have a lag of many years until disease manifestations) and in migrants (some of whom will have much less of a lag between immunization and prevention of disease and the associated health care costs).

VACCINE DEVELOPMENT

The committee estimated that development is feasible but is not imminent. The estimates are that it will take 15 years until licensing and that $360 million needs to be invested.

Table A3-2 Morbidity Scenarios for *Coccidioides* Infection

	No. of Cases	% of Cases	Committee HUI Values	Duration
Total Deaths	117			
Total Cases (new symptomatic and asymptomatic infections)	100,000			
No Symptoms		40%	1.00	
Mild respiratory illness		17%	0.81	0.0192 (1 week)
Mild respiratory illness with erythema complications		3%		
mild respiratory illness			0.81	0.0192 (1 week)
erythema nodosum / toxic erythema / arthritis			0.75	0.0575 (3 weeks)
Pneumonia: outpatient only		30%	0.75	0.0575 (3 weeks)
Pneumonia		5%		
self-limiting: inpatient			0.73	0.0192 (1 week)
self-limiting: outpatient			0.75	0.0575 (3 weeks)
Persistent/disseminated		5%		
P/D: inpatient			0.65	0.0384 (2 weeks)
P/D: outpatient: 3-year period			0.90	3.0000 (3 years)

Table A3-3 Health Care Costs Associated with *Coccidioides* Infection

	% with Care	Cost per Unit	Units per Case	Form of Treatment
Mild respiratory illness	50%	$50	1.0	physician a
Mild respiratory illness with erythema complications				
mild respiratory illness	100%	$50	3.0	physician a, diagnostic a, medication b
erythema nodosum / toxic erythema / arthritis	100%	$100	2.0	physician b
Pneumonia: outpatient only	100%	$250	1.0	outpatient treatment (physician a and b, diagnostic a, medication b)
Pneumonia				
self-limiting: inpatient	100%	$4,000	1.0	inpatient treatment
self-limiting: outpatient	100%	$250	1.0	outpatient treatment (e.g., physician a and b, medication b, diagnostic a)
Persistent/disseminated				
P/D: Inpatient	100%	$4,000	2.0	inpatient treatment
P/D: outpatient : 3-year period	100%	$50	7.0	outpatient treatment (physician a, diagnostic a, medication b)

VACCINE PROGRAM CONSIDERATIONS

Target Population

The target population for this vaccine is approximately 1,035,300 people: all infants born in the geographic regions identified above and migrants into the area. The model assumes that half of immigrants into the area from the western part of the United States would not have had the vaccine already. For the purposes of the model, the average age for migrants into the area is estimated to be 27.9 years, and immunization is estimated to occur within 1 year of migration. The committee estimated that 90% of infants would receive the vaccine, compared with only 10% of migrants.

Vaccine Schedule, Efficacy, and Costs

The committee estimated that this would be a relatively low-cost vaccine, costing $50 per dose. Vaccine administration would cost an additional $10. The committee has accepted default assumptions for this vaccine that it will require a series of 3 doses and that efficacy will be 75%. Table 4-1 summarizes vaccine program assumptions for all vaccines considered in this report.

RESULTS

If a vaccine program for *c. immitis* were implemented today and the vaccine was 100% efficacious and utilized by 100% of the target population, the annualized present value of the QALYs gained would be 1,700. Using committee assumptions of less-than-ideal efficacy and utilization and including time and monetary costs until a vaccine program is implemented, the annualized present value of the QALYs gained would be 240.

If a vaccine program for *c. immitis* were implemented today and the vaccine was 100% efficacious and utilized by 100% of the target population, the annualized present value of the health care costs saved would be $44.8 million. Using committee assumptions of less-than-ideal efficacy and utilization and including time and monetary costs until a vaccine program is implemented, the annualized present value of the health care costs saved would be $6.3 million.

If a vaccine program for *c. immitis* were implemented today and the vaccine was 100% efficacious and utilized by 100% of the target population, the annualized present value of the program cost would be $190 million. Using committee assumptions of less-than-ideal efficacy and utilization and including time and monetary costs until a vaccine program is implemented, the annualized present value of the program cost would be $53.4 million.

164   *VACCINES FOR THE 21ST CENTURY*

Using committee assumptions of time and costs until licensure, the fixed cost of vaccine development has been amortized and is $10.8 million for a *C. immitis* vaccine.

If a vaccine program were implemented today and the vaccine were 100% efficacious and utilized by 100% of the target population, the annualized present value of the cost per QALY gained is $85,000. Using committee assumptions of less-than-ideal utilization and including time and monetary costs until a vaccine program is implemented, the annualized present value of the cost per QALY gained is $240,000.

See Chapters 4 and 5 for details on the methods and assumptions used by the committee for the results reported.

READING LIST

Byerly E, Deardorff K. National and State Population Estimates: 1990 to 1994, U.S. Bureau of the Census, Current Population Reports, pp. 25–1127, U.S. Government Printing Office, Washington, DC, 1995.

California Department of Finance. Population of California Counties and the State and Components of Change [WWW document]. URL http://library.ca.gov/california/4e2tab1.html (accessed January 24, 1997).

CDC. Compressed Mortality Database. WONDER (wonder.cdc.gov). 1997. ICD–9, Number 114.

Dugger KO, Villareal KM, et al. Cloning and Sequence Analysis of the cDNA for a Protein from *C. immitis* with Immunogenic Potential. Biochemical and Biophysical Research Communications 1996; 218:485.

Galgiani JN, Catanzaro A, Cloud GA, et al. Fluconazole Therapy for Coccidioidal meningitis—The NIAID–Mycoses Study Group. Annals of Internal Medicine 1993; 19:28–35.

Hansen KA. Geographical Mobility: March 1993 to March 1994, U.S. Bureau of the Census, Current Population Reports, pp. 20–485, U.S. Government Printing Office, Washington, DC, 1995.

Kirkland TN, Fierer J. Coccidioidomycosis: a Reemerging Infectious Disease. Emerging Infectious Diseases 1996; 2:192–9.

Libke RD, Granoff DM. Coccidioidomycosis. In: Textbook of Pediatric Infectious Diseases. RD Feigin and JD Cherry eds. Philadelphia, PA: WB Saunder Company, 1992, pp. 1916–1928.

Pappagianis D. Evaluation of the Protective Efficacy of the Killed *C. immitis* Spherule Vaccine in Humans. American Review of Respiratory Disease 1993; 148:656–660.

Pappagianis D. Marked Increase in Cases of Coccidioidomycosis in California: 1991, 1992, and 1993. Clinical Infectious Diseases 1994; 19(Suppl 1):S14–8.

Stevens DA. *C. immitis*. In: Principles and Practice of Infectious Diseases. GL Mandell, JE Bennett, R Dolin, eds. New York, NY: Churchill Livingstone, 1995, pp. 2365–2374.

Texas Agricultural Experiment Station, Department of Rural Sociology. 1994 Total Population Estimates for Texas Counties [WWW document]. URL http://www-txsdc.tamu.edu/txpop94.html (accessed February 13, 1997).

Texas Department of Health. Bureau of Vital Statistics Annual Report 1994.

Cytomegalovirus

DISEASE BURDEN

Epidemiology

For the purposes of the calculations in this report, the committee estimated cases of cytomegalovirus infection in infants born to infected mothers and in organ-transplant patients in the United States. The committee estimated that there are 40,000 infants born every year with CMV infection and that 2,800 transplant patients acquire CMV infection. The committee assumed 400 deaths annually from the congenitally acquired CMV infection, and 160 deaths from CMV infection in organ transplant patients.

The treatment of HIV infection and AIDS and the effect of those changes in the health status and costs of care experienced by those with HIV has changed rapidly in recent years and is expected to continue to do so. Therefore, the committee has chosen not to include a scenario specific to infection in those with HIV/AIDS. Consideration of this population would result in differences in the calculations achieved with this model, but the uncertainties associated with doing so were thought to be quite extreme.

Disease Scenarios

For the purposes of the calculations in this report, the committee estimated that 90% of congenitally acquired CMV infections are asymptomatic at birth. Of these 36,000 new cases per year, 5,400 infants develop neurologic sequelae, such as deafness. These sequelae are estimated to lead to a health utility index (HUI) of .89 and persist for the duration of that infant's life. The committee estimated that 10% of the 4,000 congenitally acquired cases of CMV that are symptomatic at birth (400 cases annually) lead to death after a brief hospitalization following birth.

Of those 3,600 infants who live beyond the initial phase described above, the committee estimated that 90%, or 3,240 infants, experience severe sequelae, and 10%, or 360 infants, experience mild sequelae. These sequelae are life-long. The HUI associated with the mild and severe sequelae were estimated to be .89 and .48, respectively. Those experiencing severe sequelae were estimated to have a reduced lifespan to only 20 years. Table A4-1 illustrates the estimated number of cases in each health state, the duration of time that state is experienced, and the health utility index (HUI) associated with each state.

For the purposes of the calculations in this report, the committee estimated that there are 1,200 cases of moderate CMV disease (e.g., pneumonia and gastrointestinal disease) lasting 1 month, and 1,600 cases of severe CMV disease lasting 2 months in organ-transplant recipients each year. The HUI associated with moderate and severe CMV disease was estimated at .91 and .68 (further adjusted to reflect an altered baseline HUI for organ transplant patients compared to the general population). Further, the committee estimated that 10% of organ transplant patients with severe CMV disease die.

COST INCURRED BY DISEASE

Table A4-2 summarizes the health care costs incurred by cytomegalovirus infections. For the purposes of the calculations used in the report, it was assumed that costs for neurologic sequelae of CMV infection in newborns (whether symptomatic at birth or not) includes regular visits to a specialist for the lifetime of all infected individuals, and special schooling expenses. A small percentage of more severely affected newborns incur costs for hospitalization and long-term care. For infants who are symptomatic at birth, costs for hospitalization, diagnostics, and specialists are included in the calculations. Outpatient follow-up for these patients include several physician visits. For those infants who experience severe sequelae of the CMV infection, costs for 20 years of long-term care are included.

The other group of patients with CMV infections assessed in this report are organ transplant recipients. Patients who develop CMV infections incur costs associated with hospitalization, diagnostics, and multiple physician visits.

Table A4-1 Disease Scenarios for CMV Infection in Infants

	No. of Cases	% of Cases	Committee HUI Values	Duration (years)
Asymptomatic at birth	36,000	90.0%	1.00	
Asymptomatic at birth: neurologic sequelae	5,400	13.5%		
neurologic sequelae (especially deafness) (15% of asymptomatic): for normal lifespan			0.89	26.854 (discounted quality adjusted life expectancy at 6 months)
Symptomatic at birth	4,000	10.0%		
initial infection (hospitalization)			0.50	0.0384 (14 days)
death (10% of symptomatic)		1.0%	0.00	
Symptomatic at birth: mild sequelae	360	0.9%		
mild sequelae (deaf, blind, mild retardation) (10% of survivors): for normal lifespan			0.89	26.854 (discounted quality adjusted life expectancy at 6 months)
Symptomatic at birth: severe sequelae	3,240	8.1%		
severe sequelae (severe mental retardation) (90% of survivors): for 20-year period			0.48	20
death by age 20			0.00	23.955 (discounted quality adjusted life expectancy at age 20)

VACCINE DEVELOPMENT

The committee assumed that the development of a CMV vaccine is feasible and that licensure can occur within 7 years. The estimates for the model are that 360 million needs to be invested. Table 4-1 summarizes vaccine development assumptions for all vaccines considered in this report.

VACCINE PROGRAM CONSIDERATIONS

Target Population

The committee's model assumes that immunization with this vaccine will occur during puberty. As described in the body of the report, for these purposes that is 12 years of age. Both males and females would receive the immunization.

Table A4-2 Health Care Costs for CMV Infection in Infants and Transplant Patients

	Duration (years)	% with Care	Cost per Case	Units per Case (or per year)	Form of Treatment
INFANTS					
Asymptomatic at birth (no treatment)					
Asymptomatic at birth: neurologic sequelae					
Yearly costs	75.350	10%	$225	365	Long-term care (per year)
		90%	$100	6	Physician B (per year)
	10.000	90%	$2,000	1	Schooling for moderately deaf ($ per year)
Acute care	0.0384	10%	$2,500	14	Neonatal intensive care
Symptomatic at birth					
Initial infection (hospitalization)	0.0384	10%	$12,000	1	Hospitalization
		90%	$7,000	1	Hospitalization
		100%	$500	4	Diagnosis C
		100%	$150	14	Physician C
Outpatient follow-up		90%	$100	2	Physician B

Symptomatic at birth: mild sequelae					
Mild sequelae (deaf, blind, mild retardation) (10% of survivors): for normal lifespan	75.350				Care for neurologic sequelae
	75.350	100%	$100	4	Physician B or other (per year)
	10.000	10%	$8,000	1	Schooling (per year)
Symptomatic at birth: severe sequelae					
Severe sequelae (severe mental retardation) (90% of survivors): for 20-year period	20.000	100%	$225	365	Long-term care (per year)
	10.000	10%	$8,000	1	Schooling (per year)
TRANSPLANT PATIENTS					
Severe CMV disease					
(pneumonia, GI disease)	0.1667	100%	$14,000	1	Additional hospitalization
	0.1667	100%	$500	1	Diagnostic C
	0.1667	100%	$150	60	Physician C
Moderate CMV disease					
(pneumonia, GI disease)	0.0833	100%	$7,000	1	Additional hospitalization
	0.0833	100%	$500	1	Diagnostic C
	0.0833	100%	$150	30	Physician C

It is estimated that only 50% of the target population will accept the immunization.

Vaccine Schedule, Efficacy, and Costs

The committee estimated that this would be a relatively low-cost vaccine, costing $50 per dose. Vaccine administration would cost an additional $10. The committee has accepted default assumptions for this vaccine that it will require a series of 3 doses and that efficacy will be 75%. Table 4-1 summarizes vaccine program assumptions for all vaccines considered in this report.

RESULTS

If a vaccine program for CMV were implemented today and the vaccine was 100% efficacious and utilized by 100% of the target population, the annualized present value of the QALYs gained would be 70,000. Using committee assumptions of less-than-ideal efficacy and utilization and including time and monetary costs until a vaccine program is implemented, the annualized present value of the QALYs gained would be 18,000. The vast majority of these QALYs are attributable to the long-term sequelae experienced by infants who acquire congenital-CMV infections.

If a vaccine program for CMV were implemented today and the vaccine was 100% efficacious and utilized by 100% of the target population, the annualized present value of the health care costs saved would be $4 billion. Using committee assumptions of less-than-ideal efficacy and utilization and including time and monetary costs until a vaccine program is implemented, the annualized present value of the health care costs saved would be $1.1 billion.

If a vaccine program for CMV were implemented today and the vaccine was 100% efficacious and utilized by 100% of the target population, the annualized present value of the program cost would be $680 million. Using committee assumptions of less-than-ideal efficacy and utilization and including time and monetary costs until a vaccine program is implemented, the annualized present value of the program cost would be $240 million.

Using committee assumptions of time and costs until licensure, the fixed cost of vaccine development has been amortized and is $10.8 million for a CMV vaccine.

If a vaccine program were implemented today and the vaccine were 100% efficacious and utilized by 100% of the target population, the annualized present value of the cost per QALY gained is -$50,000. A negative value represents a saving in costs in addition to a saving in QALYs. Using committee assumptions of less-than-ideal utilization and including time and monetary costs until a vaccine program is implemented, the annualized present value of the cost per QALY gained is -$45,000.

See Chapters 4 and 5 for details on the methods and assumptions used by the committee for the results reported.

READING LIST

Demmler GJ. Acquired Cytomegalovirus Infections. In: Textbook of Pediatric Infectious Diseases. RD Feigin and JD Cherry eds. Philadelphia, PA: WB Saunder Company, 1992, pp. 1532–1547.

Demmler GJ. Congenital Cytomegalovirus Infection. Seminars in Pediatric Neurology 1994; 1:36–42.

Demmler GJ. Summary of a Workshop on Surveillance for Congenital Cytomegalovirus Disease. Reviews of Infectious Diseases 1991; 13:315–29.

Demmler GJ. Vaccines for Cytomegalovirus. Seminars in Pediatric Infectious Diseases 1991; 2:186–190.

Ho M. Cytomegalovirus. In: Principles and Practice of Infectious Diseases. GL Mandell, JE Bennett, Dolin R eds. New York, NY: Churchill Livingstone, 1995, pp. 1351–1363.

Institute of Medicine. New Vaccines Development: Establishing Priorities, Volume 1. Diseases of Importance in the United States. Washington, DC: National Academy Press, 1985a.

Istas AS, Demmler GJ, Dobbins JG, et al. Surveillance for Congenital Cytomegalovirus Disease: A Report from the National Congenital Cytomegalovirus Disease Registry. Clinical Infectious Diseases 1995; 20:665–70.

Pass RF. Immunization Strategy for Prevention of Congenital CMV Infection. Infectious Agents and Disease 1996; 5:240–4.

Porath A, McNutt RA, Smiley LM, et al. Effectiveness and Cost Benefit of a Proposed Live Cytomegalovirus Vaccine in the Prevention of Congenital Disease. Reviews of Infectious Diseases 1990; 12:31–40.

Starr SE. Cytomegalovirus Vaccines: Current Status. Infectious Agents and Disease 1992; 1:146–148.

U.S. Bureau of the Census. Statistical Abstract of the U.S.: 1995 (115th edition). Washington, DC, 1995.

Ventura SJ, Martin JA, Mathews TJ, et al. Advance Report of Final Natality statistics, 1994. Monthly Vital Statistics Report 1996; 44.

Yow MD, Demmler GJ. Congenital Megalovirus Disease—20 Years is Long Enough. New England Journal of Medicine 1992; 326:702–703.

APPENDIX 5

Enterotoxigenic *E. coli*

DISEASE BURDEN

Epidemiology

Enterotoxigenic *E. coli* (ETEC) is a common causes of "traveler's diarrhea" and a very important cause of diarrhea in infants in developing countries. ETEC can produce nausea, abdominal cramps, low fever, and a sudden-onset profuse watery diarrhea that is like a mild cause of cholera. Traveler's diarrhea can be severe but is rarely fatal. For the purposes of the calculations in this report, the committee estimated that there are 660,000 new cases of ETEC infection each year in the United States. The incidence rate is 250 per 100,000 within all age groups and in both males and females. It is assumed that 90% of the infections occur in travelers. There are no deaths associated with ETEC infection for the purposes of the modeling in this report.

Disease Scenarios

For the purposes of the calculation in this report, the committee assumed that the vast majority of infections manifest as mild to moderate diarrhea lasting 4 days and associated with a health utility index (HUI) of .75. For 10% of the patients, the diarrhea was estimated to last 8 days.

COST INCURRED BY DISEASE

Table A5-1 summarizes the health care costs incurred by ETEC infections. For the purposes of the calculations in this report, it was assumed that all people infected with ETEC use over-the-counter medications and that only a small fraction see a physician. Costs for additional diapers and oral rehydration are included for some of the infected individuals, whether travelers or not. It is these costs which are increased for those who experience a more prolonged diarrhea.

VACCINE DEVELOPMENT

The estimates for the model are that it will take 7 years until licensure and that $240 million needs to be invested. Table 4-1 summarizes vaccine development assumptions for all vaccines considered in this report.

VACCINE PROGRAM CONSIDERATIONS

Target Population

The target population was estimated to include the annual birth cohort and overseas travelers. For the purposes of this report, the number of targeted travelers is 2,500,000 annually. It is estimated that 90% of infants and 30% of travlers will receive the immunization.

Vaccine Schedule, Efficacy, and Costs

The committee estimated that this vaccine would cost $50 per dose and that vaccine administration would cost an additional $10. The committee has accepted default assumptions for this vaccine that it will require a series of 3 doses and that efficacy will be 75%. Table 4-1 summarizes vaccine program assumptions for all vaccines considered in this report.

RESULTS

If a vaccine program for ETEC were implemented today and the vaccine was 100% efficacious and utilized by 100% of the target population, the annualized present value of the QALYs gained would be 1,600. Using committee assumptions of less-than-ideal efficacy and utilization and including time and monetary costs until a vaccine program is implemented, the annualized present value of the QALYs gained would be 280.

Table A5-1 Health Care Costs Associated with ETEC Disease

	% of Cases	Duration (years)	% with Care	Cost per Case	Cost per Unit	Units per Case	Form of Treatment
Mile-moderate illness	90%						
Diarrhea		0.0110	100%	$10	$10	1.0	Medication A
		0.0110	15%	$50	$50	1.0	Physician A
		0.0110	15%	$10	$10	1.0	Other costs (diapers/oral rehydration therapy)
Prolonged illness	10%						
Acute manifestations		0.0219	100%	$10	$10	1.0	Medication A
		0.0219	15%	$50	$50	1.0	Physician A
		0.0219	15%	$20	$10	2.0	Other costs (diapers/oral rehydration therapy)

If a vaccine program for ETEC were implemented today and the vaccine was 100% efficacious and utilized by 100% of the target population, the annualized present value of the health care costs saved would be $11.7 million. Using committee assumptions of less-than-ideal efficacy and utilization and including time and monetary costs until a vaccine program is implemented, the annualized present value of the health care costs saved would be $2 million.

If a vaccine program for ETEC were implemented today and the vaccine was 100% efficacious and utilized by 100% of the target population, the annualized present value of the program cost would be $1.2 billion. Using committee assumptions of less-than-ideal efficacy and utilization and including time and monetary costs until a vaccine program is implemented, the annualized present value of the program cost would be $550 million.

Using committee assumptions of time and costs until licensure, the fixed cost of vaccine development has been amortized and is $7.2 million for a ETEC vaccine.

If a vaccine program were implemented today and the vaccine were 100% efficacious and utilized by 100% of the target population, the annualized present value of the cost per QALY gained is $700,000. Using committee assumptions of less-than-ideal utilization and including time and monetary costs until a vaccine program is implemented, the annualized present value of the cost per QALY gained is $2 million.

See Chapters 4 and 5 for details on the methods and assumptions used by the committee for the results reported.

READING LIST

Braden C, Keusch GT. Diarrhea and Dysentery-Causing *Escherichia Coli*. In: Textbook of Pediatric Infectious Diseases. RD Feigin and JD Cherry eds. Philadelphia, PA: WB Saunder Company, 1992, pp. 607–620.

APPENDIX 6

Epstein-Barr Virus

DISEASE BURDEN

Epidemiology

For the purposes of the calculations in this report, the committee estimated that there are 118,546 new infections with Epstein-Barr virus (EBV) each year in the United States. The infection occurs primarily in teenagers and young adults. 80% of the cases were estimated to occur in people between the ages of 15 and 24 years of age. It was assumed that males and females are affected equally. The committee assigned a case fatality rate of 0 to this infection.

Disease Scenarios

For the purposes of the calculation in this report, the committee estimated that 95% of infections manifest as uncomplicated mononucleosis (fever, lymphadenopathy, and pharyngitis). This state lasts three weeks and is associated with a health utility index (HUI) of .94. Approximately 5% of infections manifest in a more complicated manner (e.g. hepatitis). This state lasts 8 weeks and is associated with a much lower HUI, .47. Table A6-1 illustrates the estimated number of cases in each health state, the duration of time that state is experienced, and the health utility index (HUI) associated with each state.

See Appendix 28 for more information.

Table A6-1 Health Care Costs Associated with EBV Infection

	% of Cases	Duration (years)	Committee HUI Values	% with Care	Units per Case (or per year)	Form of Treatment
Uncomplicated infectious mononucleosis	95%					
Fever, lymphadenopathy, pharyngitis		0.0575	0.94	100%	1.0	Physician A
				100%	1.0	Diagnostic A
Complicated infectious mononucleosis	5%					
e.g., hepatitis		0.1534	0.47	50%	1.0	Medication B
				100%	2.0	Physician B
				100%	1.0	Diagnostic B
				50%	1.0	Medication B

COST INCURRED BY DISEASE

Table A6-1 summarizes the health care costs incurred by EBV infections. For the purposes of the calculations in this report, it was assumed that patients with uncomplicated mononucleosis incur costs associated with a physician visit, a diagnostic, and medications. Patients with complicated mononucleosis incur slightly more costs due to more physician visits (to a specialist) and more expensive diagnostics.

VACCINE DEVELOPMENT

The committee assumed that the development of an EBV vaccine is feasible and that licensure can occur within the time frame of its charge, but is not imminent. The estimates for the model are that it will take 15 years until licensure and that $390 million needs to be invested. Table 4-1 summarizes vaccine development assumptions for all vaccines considered in this report.

VACCINE PROGRAM CONSIDERATIONS

Target Population

The committee's model assumes that immunization with this vaccine will occur during puberty. As described in the body of the report, for these purposes, that is set at 12 years of age. Both males and females would receive the immunization. It is estimated that only 50% of the target population will accept the immunization.

Vaccine Schedule, Efficacy, and Costs

The committee estimated that this would be a relatively low-cost vaccine, costing $50 per dose. Vaccine administration would cost an additional $10. The committee has accepted default assumptions for this vaccine that it will require a series of 3 doses and that effectiveness will be 75%. Table 4-1 summarizes vaccine program assumptions for all vaccines considered in this report.

RESULTS

If a vaccine program for EBV were implemented today and the vaccine was 100% efficacious and utilized by 100% of the target population, the annualized present value of the QALYs gained would be 630. Using committee assumptions of less-than-ideal efficacy and utilization and including time and monetary costs until a vaccine program is implemented, the annualized present value of the QALYs gained would be 130. Although the number of people experiencing uncomplicated mononucleosis is far greater than those experiencing complications, slightly more than half of the QALYs lost are attributable to complicated mononucleosis due to the much lower HUI value and the longer duration.

If a vaccine program for EBV were implemented today and the vaccine was 100% efficacious and utilized by 100% of the target population, the annualized present value of the health care costs saved would be $12.6 million. Using committee assumptions of less-than-ideal efficacy and utilization and including time and monetary costs until a vaccine program is implemented, the annualized present value of the health care costs saved would be $2.6 million.

If a vaccine program for EBV were implemented today and the vaccine was 100% efficacious and utilized by 100% of the target population, the annualized present value of the program cost would be $680 million. Using committee assumptions of less-than-ideal efficacy and utilization and including time and monetary costs until a vaccine program is implemented, the annualized present value of the program cost would be $190 million.

Using committee assumptions of time and costs until licensure, the fixed cost of vaccine development has been amortized and is $11.7 million for a EBV vaccine.

If a vaccine program were implemented today and the vaccine were 100% efficacious and utilized by 100% of the target population, the annualized present value of the cost per QALY gained is $1.1 million. Using committee assumptions of less-than-ideal utilization and including time and monetary costs until a vaccine program is implemented, the annualized present value of the cost per QALY gained is $1.5 million.

See Chapters 4 and 5 for details on the methods and assumptions used by the committee for the results reported.

READING LIST

Sumaya CV. Epstein-Barr Virus. In: Textbook of Pediatric Infectious Diseases. RD Feigin and JD Cherry eds. Philadelphia, PA: WB Saunder Company, 1992, pp. 1547–1557.

Schooley RT. Epstein-Barr Virus (Infectious Mononucleosis). In: Principles and Practice of Infectious Diseases. GL Mandell, JE Bennett, Dolin R eds. New York, NY: Churchill Livingstone, 1995, pp. 1364–1376.

U.S. Bureau of the Census. Statistical Abstract of the U.S.: 1995 (115th edition). Washington, D.C. 1995.

APPENDIX 7

Helicobacter pylori

DISEASE BURDEN

Epidemiology

H. pylori is also believed to play a role in peptic ulcer disease. This speculation came about after the organism was found to be present more frequently in idiopathic peptic ulcer disease than in age-matched controls. Furthermore, *H. pylori* has been associated with duodenal ulcers. Chronic superficial gastritis may progress to chronic gastric atrophy with the possible risk of gastric adenocarcinoma. Therefore, *H. pylori* can be considered a risk factor for gastric cancer.

For the purposes of the calculations in this report, the committee estimated that there are approximately 1,240,000 new infections of Helicobacter pylori (*H. pylori*) each year in the United States. The incidence rate is highest in people between the ages of 1 and 24 years of age; it was assumed that there are no new infections after 44 years of age. It was assumed that there are approximately 14,500 deaths annually due to *H. pylori* infection. Most of these deaths occur in people 65 years of age or older. See Table A7-1.

See Appendix 28 for more information.

Table A7-1 Incidence and Mortality Rates of *H. pylori* Infection

Age Groups	Population	% Distribution of Cases	Cases
INCIDENCE			
<1	3,963,000	.0160	19,815
1-4	16,219,000	.1309	162,190
5-14	38,056,000	.3072	380,560
15-24	36,263,000	.2927	362,630
25-34	41,670,000	.1682	208,350
35-44	42,149,000	.0851	105,373
45-54	30,224,000	.0000	0
55-64	21,241,000	.0000	0
65-74	18,964,000	.0000	0
75-84	11,088,000	.0000	0
85+	3,598,000	.0000	0
Total	263,435,000	1,000	1,238,918

Age Groups	Population	% Distribution of Deaths	Cases
MORTALITY			
<1	3,963,000	0.0004	6
1-4	16,219,000	0.0002	3
5-14	38,056,000	0.0001	2
15-24	36,263,000	0.0016	23
25-34	41,670,000	0.0085	431
35-44	42,149,000	0.0296	943
45-54	30,224,000	0.0647	1,781
55-64	21,241,000	0.1223	3,572
65-74	18,964,000	0.2453	4,510
75-84	11,088,000	0.3096	3,169
85+	3,598,000	0.2176	
Total	263,435,000	1.0000	14,500

Disease Scenarios

For the purposes of the calculation in this report, the committee assumed that there are acute and chronic manifestations of *H. pylori* infection (see Table A7-2). Some of the chronic manifestations last for decades; others manifest for much shorter periods of time. It was assumed that 30% of people infected with *H. pylori* experience a week of acute gastritis. Half of those people go on to experience recurrent attacks of gastritis (approximately 2 days per month) for the lifetime of the person with no other complications. The health utility index (HUI) associated with gastritis was estimated to be .74. It was assumed that approximately 10% of infections are associated with approximately 30 years of recurrent gastritis, followed by peptic ulcer disease.

Table A7-2 Disease Scenarios for *H. pylori* Infection

	No. of Cases	% of Cases	Committee HUI Values	Duration (years)
GASTRITIS:				
Gastritis	371,675	30.0%		
acute gastritis at initial infection			0.74	0.0192 (1 week)
Gastritis—recurrent	185,838	15.0%		
chronic mild symptoms— **no** transition to PUD			0.74	1.5848 (2 days/month for life)
Gastritis to Peptic Ulcer Disease	123,892	10.0%		
chronic mild symptoms until PUD diagnosis made			0.74	2 days/month; continues for average of 30 years
PEPTIC ULCER DISEASE				
Peptic Ulcer Disease	123,892	10.0%		
acute PUD			0.61	0.0192 (1 week)
Peptic Ulcer Disease (untreated or recurrence)	61,946	5.0%	0.74	1.0832 (2 days/month for life)
Peptic Ulcer Disease (w/complications)	2,478	0.2%	0.4	0.0384 (2 weeks)
GASTRIC CANCERS				
Gastric Adenocarcinoma	12,389	1.0%	0.82	1.0000 (average life expectancy from diagnosis)
Lymphomas/MALTomas	6,195	0.5%	0.82	7.5000 (average life expectancy from diagnosis)

It was assumed that there is a 30-year latency between time of infection and acute peptic ulcer disease; half of the people with acute peptic ulcer disease experience chronic peptic ulcer disease for the duration of their lives.

It was further assumed that a small proportion (1.5%) of infected people develop cancer secondary to the *H. pylori* infection and that the cancers are diagnosed around age 70 and that these people die within a year. HUI states associated with these latent conditions range from .40 for acute complications of peptic ulcer disease to .74 for recurrences of chronic, mild peptic ulcer disease, to .82 for the average state during the year of life from diagnosis of cancers to death.

COST INCURRED BY DISEASE

Table A7-3 summarizes the health care costs incurred by *H. pylori* infections. For the purposes of the calculations in this report, it was assumed that

Table A7-3 Health Care Costs Associated with *H. pylori* Infections

	% with Care	Cost per Unit	Units per Case	Form of Treatment
GASTRITIS				
acute gastritis at initial infection	100%	$10	1.0	medication a
	80%	$50	1.0	physician a
	25%	$100	1.0	physician b
	50%	$50	1.0	diagnostic a
	50%	$100	1.0	diagnostic b
	10%	$1,000	1.0	outpatient surgery
	5%	$500	2.0	surgical staff
	25%	$150	1.0	medication c
Gastritis—recurrent				
chronic mild symptoms—no transition to PUD	100%	$10	1.0	medication a
2 days per month; continues for remaining lifetime	10%	$50	1.00	physician a
	5%	$100	1.00	physician b
Gastritis to PUD				
chronic mild symptoms until PUD diagnosis made	100%	$10	6.0	medication a
2 days per month; continues for 30 years	10%	$50	1.00	physician a
PEPTIC ULCER DISEASE: average 30-year lag from initial infection				
Peptic Ulcer Disease				
acute PUD	100%	$10	1.0	medication a
	100%	$50	1.0	physician a
	100%	$100	2.0	physician b
	50%	$500	1.0	diagnostic c
	25%	$1,000	1.0	outpatient surgery
	25%	$500	2.0	surgical staff
	25%	$500	1.0	diagnostic c
	75%	$150	1.0	medication c
Peptic Ulcer Disease (untreated)				
chronic mild symptoms	100%	$10	1.0	medication a
2 days per month; continues for remaining lifetime	100%	$50	1.00	physician a
	25%	$100	1.00	physician b
	50%	$50	1.00	diagnostic a
	50%	$150	1.00	medication c
Peptic Ulcer Disease (w/complications)				
	100%	$50	1.0	physician a
	100%	$100	2.0	physician b
	100%	$500	1.0	diagnostic c
	75%	$3,000	1.0	hospitalization w/o surgery

Continued

Table A7-3 *Continued*

	% with Care	Cost per Unit	Units per Case	Form of Treatment
Peptic Ulcer Disease (w/complications) *Continued*	25%	$6,000	1.0	hospitalization w/ surgery
	100%	$150	1.0	medication c
GASTRIC CANCERS:				
Gastric adenocarcinoma, lymphomas, MALTomas	100%	$50	6.0	physician a
	100%	$75	6.0	physician b
	100%	$500	1.0	diagnostic c
	100%	$4,000	1.0	hospitalization
	100%	$500	2.0	surgical staff
	100%	$500	1.0	diagnostic c

100% of people experiencing gastritis incur costs for inexpensive over-the-counter medication, but that only 10% incur costs for a limited visit to a physician. It was assumed that 5% of patients with gastritis visit a specialist. For recurrent disease, it was assumed that costs incurred include 1 visit to a physician per year and 6 purchases of over-the-counter medication per year for lifetime or until a diagnosis of peptic ulcer disease is made.

It was assumed that all patients with acute peptic ulcer disease (PUD) incur costs associated with over-the-counter medications, a limited visit to a physician, and two visits to a specialist. It was assumed that half these patients receive a relatively expensive diagnostic procedure. It was assumed that 25% of patients receive ambulatory surgery for these symptoms, and that 75% of acute PUD patients receive expensive prescription medications. Similar patterns and costs of care were assumed for the patients with chronic, mild peptic ulcer disease (each year for the remainder of life). The patients who experience serious complications of PUD incur costs for hospitalization and follow-up.

It was assumed that all patients with gastric adenocarcinomas and lymphomas receive extensive care during the year of life from diagnosis to death. Costs included in the analysis are multiple visits to a general physician and a specialist, expensive diagnostics, and one hospitalization.

The annualized present value of the cost of care averted by a vaccine strategy (with the program assumptions described below) is approximately $70,000,000.

VACCINE DEVELOPMENT

The committee assumed that will take 7 years until licensure and that $240 million needs to be invested. Table 4-1 summarized vaccine development estimates for all candidates considered in this report.

VACCINE PROGRAM CONSIDERATIONS

Target Population

For the purposes of the calculations in this report, it is assumed that the target population for this vaccine the annual birth cohort of the United States. It was assumed that 30% of the target population would utilize the vaccine.

Vaccine Schedule, Efficacy, and Costs

For the purposes of the calculations in this report, it was estimated that this vaccine would cost $50 per dose and that administration costs would be $10 per dose. Default assumptions of a 3-dose series and 75% efficacy were accepted. Table 4-1 summarizes vaccine program assumptions for all vaccines considered in this report.

RESULTS

If a vaccine program for *H. pylori* were implemented today and the vaccine was 100% efficacious and utilized by 100% of the target population, the annualized present value of the QALYs gained would be 90,000. Using committee assumptions of less-than-ideal efficacy and utilization and including time and monetary costs until a vaccine program is implemented, the annualized present value of the QALYs gained would be 14,000. The majority of these lost QALYs are associated with gastritis, because of the large number of cases.

If a vaccine program for *H. pylori* were implemented today and the vaccine was 100% efficacious and utilized by 100% of the target population, the annualized present value of the health care costs saved would be $430 million. Using committee assumptions of less-than-ideal efficacy and utilization and including time and monetary costs until a vaccine program is implemented, the annualized present value of the health care costs saved would be $67.3 million.

If a vaccine program for *H. pylori* were implemented today and the vaccine was 100% efficacious and utilized by 100% of the target population, the annualized present value of the program cost would be $720 million. Using committee assumptions of less-than-ideal efficacy and utilization and including time and monetary costs until a vaccine program is implemented, the annualized present value of the program cost would be $150 million.

Using committee assumptions of time and costs until licensure, the fixed cost of vaccine development has been amortized and is $7.2 million for a *H. pylori* vaccine.

If a vaccine program were implemented today and the vaccine were 100%

efficacious and utilized by 100% of the target population, the annualized present value of the cost per QALY gained is $3,300. Using committee assumptions of less-than-ideal utilization and including time and monetary costs until a vaccine program is implemented, the annualized present value of the cost per QALY gained is $6,500.

See Chapters 4 and 5 for details on the methods and assumptions used by the committee for the results reported.

READING LIST

Blaser MJ. *Helicobacter pylori* and Related Organisms. In: Principles and Practice of Infectious Diseases. GL Mandell, JE Bennett, Dolin R eds. New York, NY: Churchill Livingstone, 1995, pp. 1956–1964.

CDC. Compressed Mortality Database. WONDER (wonder.cdc.gov). 1997. ICD-9, Number 531–533.

Dubois A. Spiral Bacteria in the Human Stomach: The Gastric Helicobacters. Emerging Infectious Diseases 1995; (1)3: 79–83.

Fendrick AM, Chernew ME, Hirth RA, et al. Alternative Management Strategies for Patients with Suspected Peptic Ulcer Disease. Annals of Internal Medicine 1995; 123:260–268.

Hansson LE, Nyren O, Hsing HW, et al. The Risk of Stomach Cancer in Patients with Gastric or Duodenal Ulcer Disease. The New England Journal of Medicine 1996; 335:242–249.

Marshall BJ. *Helicobacter pylori*—The Etiologic Agent for Peptic Ulcer. JAMA 1995; 274:1064–1066.

Miller BA, Kolonel LN, Bernstein L, et al. (eds). Racial/Ethnic Patterns of Cancer in the United States 1988–1992, National Cancer Institute. NIH Pub. No. 96–4104. Bethesda, MD, 1996.

NIH. *Helicobacter pylori* in Peptic Ulcer Disease. JAMA 1994; 272:65–69.

Ofman JJ, Etchason J, Fullerton S, et al. Management Strategies for *Helicobacter pylori*-seropositive Patients with Dyspepsia: Clinical and Economic Consequences. Annals of Internal Medicine 1997; 126:280–291.

Parsonnet J. *Helicobacter pylori* in the Stomach—a Paradox Unmasked. The New England Journal of Medicine 1996; 335:278–280.

Ruiz-Palacios G, Pickering LK. *Campylobacter* and *Helicobacter* Infections. In: Textbook of Pediatric Infectious Diseases. RD Feigin and JD Cherry eds. Philadelphia, PA: WB Saunder Company, 1992, pp. 1062–1067.

Singh GK, Kochanek KD, MacDorman MF. Advance Report of Final Mortality Statistics, 1994. Monthly Vital Statistics Report 1996; 45.

Sonnenberg A, Everhart JE. The Prevalence of Self-Reported Peptic Ulcer in the United States. American Journal of Public Health 1996; 86:200–5.

Staat MA, McQuillan GM. A Population-Based Serologic Survey of *Helicobacter pylori* Infection in Children and Adolescents in the United States. The Journal of Infectious Diseases 1996; 174:1120–1123.

APPENDIX 8

Hepatitis C

The hepatitis C virus (HCV) is the major cause of parenteral non-A, non-B hepatitis. A chronic infection is usually asymptomatic even when liver damage is seen in biopsy. Eventually, the chronic infection can lead to cirrhosis and hepatocellular carcinoma. The prevalence of HCV is significantly greater in intravenous-drug users than in blood donors. At least half of the patients who have previously been diagnosed with posttransfusion non-A, non-B hepatitis have tested positive for HCV antibodies. Some countries, such as Japan, have a higher frequency of HCV infection, which is reflected in the high frequency of hepatocellular carcinoma.

DISEASE BURDEN

Epidemiology

For the purposes of the calculations in this report, the committee estimated that there are 150,000 new infections with HCV every year in the United States. It is assumed that all new infections occur in people between 15 and 54 years of age.

See Appendix 28 for more information.

189

Disease Scenarios

For the purposes of the calculation in this report, the committee assumed that 30% of people with HCV infection experience only an acute and mild disease lasting approximately 2 weeks. The health utility index (HUI) associated with this illness is .9. It was assumed that 50% of people with HCV infection experience lifelong but very mild intermittent illness (HUI of .97). It was assumed that 7% of HCV infections lead to chronic hepatitis associated with a rapid, progressive course leading to death within 7 years of infection. The remaining 13% of HCV infections were associated with the mortality from cirrhosis and liver failure 25 years after infection and cirrhosis and liver cancer 30 years after infection. See Table A8-1.

COST INCURRED BY DISEASE

Table A8-2 summarizes the health care costs incurred by HCV infections. For the purposes of the calculations in this report, it was assumed that a relatively small fraction of patients experiencing mild symptoms of acute hepatitis seek medical treatment. Hospitalization and related costs are included for a very few patients. For the 50% of patients with HCV who have lifelong, uncomplicated, mild hepatitis, it was assumed that, on average, 10% of these people see a physician for illness associated (but unrecognized in many cases) with the HCV infection.

HCV infections associated with a chronic course but leading to severe liver disease was associated with 20 and 30 years of treatment for low grade symptoms (diagnosed as HCV-related or not). 10% of patients visit a specialist every other year. The 4-year symptomatic phase was associated with quarterly specialist visits, 2 hospitalizations, and a biopsy (for 10% of the patients). The year spent in terminal cirrhosis, liver failure, or liver cancer was assumed to be associated with a hospitalization and monthly specialist visits.

The rapid, progressive course of HCV disease was assumed to be associated with antiviral medication, bimonthly specialist visits, 2 extensive diagnostics per year for 6 years, and 1 hospitalization during that time period. The final year of life was assumed to be associated with hospitalization and monthly visits to a specialist.

VACCINE DEVELOPMENT

The committee assumed that it will take 15 years until licensure of an HCV vaccine and that $360 million needs to be invested. Table 4-1 summarizes vaccine development assumptions for all vaccines considered in this report.

Table A8-1 Disease Scenarios for Hepatitis C Infection

	No. of Cases	% of Cases	Committee HUI Values	Duration (years)
Total Cases (new symptomatic and asymptomatic infections)	150,000			
Acute Hepatitis jaundice, malaise, etc.	45,000	30%	0.90	0.0384 (2 weeks)
Chronic Hepatitis: Slow course—No complications	75,600	50%		
low-grade symptoms			0.97	20.3164 (quality-adjusted life expectancy at onset). 43.3484 (unadjusted life expectancy at onset)
Chronic Hepatitis: Slow course—Cirrhosis to liver failure	3,780	3%		
low-grade symptoms			0.97	20.0000
symptomatic phase			0.90	4.0000
terminal cirrhosis; liver failure			0.59	1.0000
premature death			0.00	12.3902 (quality-adjusted life expectancy at onset + 25 years). 21.3870 (unadjusted life expectancy at onset +25 years)
Chronic Hepatitis: Slow course—Cirrhosis to carcinoma	15,120	10%		
low-grade symptoms			0.97	30.0000
symptomatic phase			0.90	4.0000
terminal carcinoma			0.59	1.0000
premature death			0.00	8.7664 (quality-adjusted life expectancy at onset + 35 years). 14.4048 (unadjusted life expectancy at onset +35 years)
Chronic Hepatitis: Rapid, progressive course	10,500	7%		
liver failure: symptomatic			0.90	6.0000
liver failure: terminal			0.59	1.0000
premature death			0.00	18.5549 (quality-adjusted life expectancy at onset + 7 years). 36.8422 (unadjusted life expectancy at onset + 7 years)

Table A8-2 Health Care Costs Associated with Hepatitis C Infection

	Duration (years)	% with Care	Cost per Unit	Units per Case	Form of Treatment (per year for chronic phases)
Acute Hepatitis					
	0.0384	20%	$50	2.0	physician a
	0.0384	5%	$2,000	1.0	hospitalization
	0.0384	5%	$100	2.0	physician b
	0.0384	5%	$100	2.0	diagnostics b
	0.0384	5%	$150	1.0	medication c
Chronic Hepatitis: Slow course—No complications					
low-grade symptoms	43.3484	10%	$50	1.0	physician a
Chronic Hepatitis: Slow course—Cirrhosis to liver failure					
low-grade symptoms	20.0000	10%	$100	0.5	physician visit
symptomatic phase	4.0000	100%	$100	4.0	physician b
	4.0000	10%	$12,000	0.25	biopsy (1 in 4 years)
	4.0000	100%	$5,000	0.5	hospitalization (1 in 2 years)
terminal cirrhosis; liver failure	1.0000	100%	$5,000	1.0	hospitalization
	1.0000	100%	$100	12.0	physician b
Chronic Hepatitis: Slow course—Cirrhosis to carcinoma					
low-grade symptoms	30.0000	10%	$100	0.5	physician a
symptomatic phase	4.0000	10%	$12,000	0.25	biopsy
	4.0000	100%	$100	4.0	physician b
	4.0000	100%	$5,000	0.5	hospitalization
terminal carcinoma	1.0000	100%	$5,000	1.0	hospitalization
	1.0000	100%	$100	12.0	physician b
Chronic Hepatitis: Rapid, progressive course					
liver failure: symptomatic	6.0000	100%	$150	12.0	medication c
	6.0000	100%	$100	6.0	physician b
	6.0000	100%	$1,000	2.0	diagnostics
	6.0000	100%	$12,000	0.2	hospitalization
liver failure: terminal	1.0000	100%	$5,000	1.0	hospitalization
	1.0000	100%	$100	12.0	physician b

VACCINE PROGRAM CONSIDERATIONS

Target Population

For the purposes of the calculations in this report, it is assumed that the target population for this vaccine is the annual birth cohort. It was assumed that 90% of the target population would utilize the vaccine.

Vaccine Schedule, Efficacy, and Costs

For the purposes of the calculations in this report, it was estimated that this vaccine would cost $50 per dose and that administration costs would be $10 per dose. Default assumptions of a 3-dose series and 75% efficacy were accepted. Table 4-1 summarizes vaccine program assumptions for all vaccines considered in this report.

RESULTS

If a vaccine program for HCV were implemented today and the vaccine was 100% efficacious and utilized by 100% of the target population, the annualized present value of the QALYs gained would be 110,000. Using committee assumptions of less-than-ideal efficacy and utilization and including time and monetary costs until a vaccine program is implemented, the annualized present value of the QALYs gained would be 41,000.

If a vaccine program for HCV were implemented today and the vaccine was 100% efficacious and utilized by 100% of the target population, the annualized present value of the health care costs saved would be $180 million. Using committee assumptions of less-than-ideal efficacy and utilization and including time and monetary costs until a vaccine program is implemented, the annualized present value of the health care costs saved would be $67.9 million.

If a vaccine program for HCV were implemented today and the vaccine was 100% efficacious and utilized by 100% of the target population, the annualized present value of the program cost would be $720 million. Using committee assumptions of less-than-ideal efficacy and utilization and including time and monetary costs until a vaccine program is implemented, the annualized present value of the program cost would be $360 million.

Using committee assumptions of time and costs until licensure, the fixed cost of vaccine development has been amortized and is $10.8 million for a HCV vaccine.

If a vaccine program were implemented today and the vaccine were 100% efficacious and utilized by 100% of the target population, the annualized present value of the cost per QALY gained is $5,000. If the target population was all 12-year-olds, the annualized present value of the cost per QALY gained is $3,000. Using committee assumptions of less-than-ideal utilization and including time and monetary costs until a vaccine program is implemented, the annualized present value of the cost per QALY gained is $7,400. If the target population was all 12-year-olds (assuming 50% utilization), the annualized present value of the cost per QALY gained is $4,000.

See Chapters 4 and 5 for details on the methods and assumptions used by the committee for the results reported.

READING LIST

Bhandari BN, Wright TL. Hepatitis C: An Overview. Annual Review of Medicine 1995; 46:309–317.

Lemon SM, Brown EA. Hepatitis C Virus. In: Principles and Practice of Infectious Diseases. GL Mandell, JE Bennett, Dolin R eds. New York, NY: Churchill Livingstone, 1995, pp. 1474–1486.

APPENDIX 9

Herpes Simplex Virus

The herpes simplex virus exists as two biologically distinct serotypes, HSV-1 and HSV-2, which differ mainly by their mode of transmission. Initially, the infection caused by either type is a mucocutaneous infection which is followed later by a latent infection of neuronal cells in the dorsal root ganglia.

The spread of HSV-1 generally occurs by direct contact, usually involving saliva. This strain of herpes typically presents itself in an infection known as herpes gingivostomatitis. Recurrences of this orolabial infection are commonly called fever blisters or cold sores. Other infections associated with HSV-1 include conjunctivitis, keratitis, and herpetic whitlow. A more serious infection, sporadic encephalitis, appears primarily in older children and adults. In some individuals with chronic skin diseases such as eczema, a severe primary HSV-1 infection known as Kaposi's varicelliform eruption may be encountered.

Acquisition of HSV-2 usually occurs by sexual contact or from a maternal genital infection to a newborn. The most common infection identified with HSV-2 is known as herpes genitalis. HSV-2 is responsible for approximately 85% of symptomatic primary genital HSV infections, most of which are recurrent infections. Some complications associated with genital herpetic infections include aseptic meningitis, extragenital lesions, and neonatal herpes (in the case of maternal transmission).

HSV infection can occur in patients who develop malignancy, an immunodeficiency (i.e., AIDS), or any disease which demands immunosuppressive therapy. The infection may become severe, causing extensive mucocuta-

---

See Appendix 28 for more information.

neous necrosis, viremia with dissemination to various organs causing meningo-encephalitis, pneumonitis, hepatitis, and coagulopathy.

DISEASE BURDEN

Epidemiology

For the purposes of the calculations in this report, the committee estimated that there are 500,000 new oral infections with HSV each year in the United States. These infections occur in people between 1 and 44 years of age. There are approximately 20,000 new ocular infections with HSV each year. These occur in people between 1 and 84 years of age. There are approximately 1,500 cases of central nervous system infection with HSV each year. The incidence was assumed to be highest in children between 5 and 14 years of age. It was also assumed that there are 300,000 new cases of genital HSV infections occurring primarily in people between 15 and 34 years of age. There are also 1,500 new cases of neonatal HSV infections each year. See Table A9-1.

Disease Scenarios

Oral Infections

For the purposes of the calculation in this report, the committee assumed that the vast majority of symptomatic primary oral infections with HSV last 1 week and are associated with an HUI of .9. 2% of the infections are associated with an HUI of .62. It is assumed that 30% of infections are associated with 10 years of minor recurrences (HUI of .9) lasting 1 week and 5% of infections are associated with 5 years of similar recurrences of a longer period per year.

Ocular Infections

For the purposes of the calculations in this report, it was assumed that all ocular infections are associated with 2 weeks of an acute conjunctivitis, keratitis, or blepharitis (HUI of .9). It is assumed that 30% of infections become chronic and result in an HUI of .9 for two weeks per year for 10 years.

Central Nervous System Infections

For the purposes of the calculations in this report, it was assumed that all CNS HSV infections are associated with a flu-like illness, and that chronic neurologic sequelae of HSV infection occurs in 20% of teenagers and 15% of

Table A9-1 Incidence and Mortality of HSV Infections

Age Groups	Populations	Incidence Rates (per 100,000)	% Distribution of Cases	Cases
INCIDENCE OF ORAL HSV INFECTIONS				
<1	3,963,000	0.00	0.0000	0
1-4	16,219,000	1,541.40	0.5000	250,000
5-14	38,056,000	394.16	0.3000	150,000
15-24	36,263,000	137.88	0.1000	50,000
25-34	41,670,000	60.00	0.0500	25,000
35-44	42,149,000	59.31	0.0500	25,000
45-54	30,224,000	0.00	0.0000	
55-64	21,241,000	0.00	0.0000	
65-74	18,964,000	0.00	0.0000	
75-84	11,088,000	0.00	0.0000	
85+	3,598,000	0.00	0.0000	
Total	263,435,000	189.80	1.0000	500,000
INCIDENCE OF OCULAR HSV INFECTIONS				
<1	3,963,000	0.00	0.0000	0
1-4	16,219,000	6.17	0.0500	1,000
5-14	38,056,000	7.88	0.1500	3,000
15-24	36,263,000	8.27	0.1500	3,000
25-34	41,670,000	7.20	0.1500	3,000
35-44	42,149,000	4.75	0.1000	2,000
45-54	30,224,000	6.62	0.1000	2,000
55-64	21,241,000	9.42	0.1000	2,000
65-74	18,964,000	10.55	0.1000	2,000
75-84	11,088,000	18.04	0.1000	2,000
85+	3,598,000	0.00	0.0000	0
Total	263,435,000	7.59	1.0000	20,000
INCIDENCE OF HSV CNS INFECTION				
<1	3,963,000	0.00	0.0000	
1-4	16,219,000	0.00	0.0000	
5-14	38,056,000	1.97	0.5000	750
15-24	36,263,000	0.00	0.0000	
25-34	41,670,000	0.00	0.0000	
35-44	42,149,000	0.00	0.0000	
45-54	30,224,000	0.62	0.1250	188
55-64	21,241,000	0.88	0.1250	188
65-74	18,964,000	0.99	0.1250	188
75-84	11,088,000	1.69	0.1250	188
85+	3,598,000	0.00	0.0000	
Total	263,435,000	0.57	1.0000	1,500

Continued

Table A9-1 *Continued*

Age Groups	Populations	Incidence Rates (per 100,000)	% Distribution of Cases	Cases
MORTALITY ASSOCIATED WITH HSV CNS INFECTION				
<1	3,963,000	0.00	0.0000	
1-4	16,219,000	0.00	0.0000	
5-14	38,056,000	0.39	0.2222	150
15-24	36,263,000	0.00	0.0000	
25-34	41,670,000	0.00	0.0000	
35-44	42,149,000	0.00	0.0000	
45-54	30,224,000	0.43	0.1944	131
55-64	21,241,000	0.62	0.1944	131
65-74	18,964,000	0.69	0.1944	131
75-84	11,088,000	1.18	0.1944	131
85+	3,598,000	0.00	0.0000	
Total	263,435,000	0.26	1.0000	675
INCIDENCE OF GENITAL HSV INFECTION				
<1	3,963,000	0.00	0.0000	
1-4	16,219,000	0.00	0.0000	
5-14	38,056,000	0.00	0.0000	
15-24	36,263,000	275.76	0.3333	100,000
25-34	41,670,000	479.96	0.6667	200,000
35-44	42,149,000	0.00	0.0000	
45-54	30,224,000	0.00	0.0000	
55-64	21,241,000	0.00	0.0000	
65-74	18,964,000	0.00	0.0000	
75-84	11,088,000	0.00	0.0000	
85+	3,598,000	0.00	0.0000	
Total	263,435,000	113.88	1.0000	300,000

adults who experience the acute CNS disease. This chronic condition is assumed to be associated with an HUI of .19 for the duration of the person's life.

Genital Infections

For the purposes of the calculations in this report, it was assumed that 100% of genital HSV infections are associated with a 2-week period at an HUI of .81 (genital lesions, fever, pain). It is assumed that 90% of infections lead to 10 years of minor recurrences; 10% of infections are associated with 5 years of more severe recurrences.

Neonatal Infections

For the purposes of the calculations in this report, it was assumed that 33% of neonatal HSV infections result in acute encephalitis and the other 67% result in serious non-CNS disease. It is assumed that 200 cases of neonatal HSV infection are associated with very severe, chronic neurologic sequelae (an HUI of .19 for approximately 20 years until premature death). See Tables A9-1 and A9-2.

COST INCURRED BY DISEASE

Table A9-3 summarizes the health care costs incurred by HSV infections.

Oral and Ocular Infections

For the purposes of the calculation in this report, it was assumed that oral and ocular infections with HSV are associated with costs for medication (over-the-counter and more expensive prescription medications, depending on severity), and physician visits (general or specialists, depending on the severity). A very few cases of severe infections are associated with brief hospitalization.

Central Nervous System Infections

For the purposes of the calculations in this report, it was assumed that all CNS infections are associated with hospitalization and multiple specialist examinations, plus diagnostic evaluation. Long-term-care costs are included for the few patients who experience lifelong, serious neurologic sequelae.

Genital Infections

For the purposes of the calculations in this report, it was assumed that genital HSV infections are associated with outpatient treatment consisting of physician visits, occasional diagnostic evaluation, and medication. The frequency of physician visits increases with the severity of the recurrences.

Table A9-2 Disease Scenarios for HSV Infection

	No. of Cases	% of Cases	Committee HUI Values	Duration (years)
ORAL				
asymptomatic primary infection		80%		
symptomatic primary infection	490,000	98.0%		
gingivostomatitis, pharyngitis, fever			0.90	0.0192 (1 week)
severe primary infection		2.0%		
gingivostomatitis, pharyngitis, fever	10,000		0.62	0.0192 (1 week)
minor recurrences	150,000	30.0%	0.90	0.0192 (1 week)
serious recurrences	25,000	5.0%	0.90	0.0384
OCULAR				
Primary infection	20,000	100.0%		
blepharitis, conjunctivitis, keratitis			0.90	0.0384 (2 weeks)
Recurrences	6,000	30.0%	0.90	0.0384 (2 weeks)
CNS (ENCEPHALITIS, MENINGITIS)				
Acute infection	1,500	100.0%		
flu-like symptoms, CNS disturbance			0.19	0.0833 (1 month)
Chronic neurologic sequelae—children/ teenagers	300	20.0%		
severe neurologic impairment for 20-year period			0.19	20.0000 (20 years)
death after 20 years impairment			0.00	21.7793 (discounted quality adjusted life expectancy at age 30)
Chronic neurologic sequelae— adults	225	15.0%		
severe neurologic impairment for 10-year period			0.19	10.0000 (10 years)
death after 10 years impairment			0.00	8.5536 (discounted quality adjusted life expectancy at age 70)

Table A9-2 *Continued*

	No. of Cases	% of Cases	Committee HUI Values	Duration (years)
GENITAL				
Acute symptomatic infection	300,000	100.0%		
genital lesions, pain, fever			0.81	0.0384 (2 weeks)
Minor recurrence	270,000	90.0%	0.95	0.0384 (2 weeks)
Serious recurrence	30,000	10.0%		
NEONATAL HSV				
Acute non-encephalitis	1,000	66.7%	0.24	0.0833 (1 month)
Acute encephalitis	500	33.3%	0.24	0.0833 (1 month)
Chronic neurologic sequelae	200	13.3%		
severe neurologic impairment for 20-year period			0.19	20.0000 (20 years)
death after 20 years impairment			0.00	47.0252 (discounted quality adjusted life expectancy at age 20)

Neonatal Infections

For the purposes of the calculations in this report, it was assumed that all neonates infected with HSV require hospitalization. It was assumed that hospitalization costs for encephalitis are higher than for the non-encephalitic manifestations. Additional costs related to labor and delivery of the neonate are included. Long-term-care costs are included for the few patients who experience lifelong serious neurologic sequelae from neonatal infections.

VACCINE DEVELOPMENT

The committee assumed that it will take 7 years until licensure of a HSV vaccine and that $240 million needs to be invested. Table 4-1 summarizes vaccine development assumptions for all vaccines considered in this report.

Table A9-3 Health Care Costs Associated with HSV Infection

	% of Cases	% with Care	Cost per Unit	Units per Case	Form of Treatment
ORAL					
Symptomatic primary infection	98.0%				
gingivostomatitis, pharyngitis, fever		100%	$10	1.0	medication a
		10%	$50	1.0	physician a
Severe primary infection	2.0%				
gingivostomatitis, pharyngitis, fever		10%	$3,000	1.0	hospitalization
		100%	$100	1.0	physician b
		100%	$50	1.0	medication b
		100%	$50	1.0	diagnostic a
Minor recurrences	30.0%				
		100%	$50	1.0	physician a
		100%	$50	1.0	medication b
Serious recurrences	5.0%				
		100%	$50	2.0	physician a
		100%	$50	2.0	medication b
OCULAR					
Primary infection	100.0%				
blepharitis, conjunctivitis, keratitis		100%	$50	1.0	medication a
		100%	$50	1.0	physician a
Recurrences	30.0%				
30% of primary cases 1 per year for 10 years		100%	$50	1.0	medication a
		25%	$50	1.0	physician a
CNS					
Acute infection	100.0%				
flu-like symptoms, CNS disturbance		100%	$6,000	1.0	hospitalization
		100%	$1,500	15.0	physician c
		100%	$500	2.0	diagnostics c
Chronic neurologic sequelae—children/teenagers	20.0%				
severe neurologic impairment for 20 year period		100%	$225	365.0	Institutional care (per year)
Chronic neurologic sequelae—adults	15.0%				
severe neurologic impairment for 10 year period		100%	$225	365.0	Institutional care (per year)
GENITAL					
Acute symptomatic infection	100.0%				
genital lesions, pain, fever		100%	$50	1.0	physician a
		100%	$50	1.0	medication b
		50%	$50	1.0	diagnostic a

Table A9-3 *Continued*

	% of Cases	% with Care	Cost per Unit	Units per Case	Form of Treatment
Minor recurrence	90.0%				
		100%	$50	1.0	physician a (per year)
		100%	$50	1.0	medication b (per year)
Serious recurrence	10.0%				
		100%	$50	4.0	physician a
		100%	$50	4.0	medication b
NEONATAL HSV					
Acute non-encephalitis	66.7%				
		100%	$7,000	1.0	hospitalization
		100%	$150	28	physician b
		100%	$500	4.0	diagnostic c
		100%	$1,000	1	additional delivery costs
Acute encephalitis	33.3%				
		100%	$12,000	1.0	hospitalization
		100%	150	28.0	physician c
		100%	$500	4.0	diagnostic c
		100%	$1,000	1.0	additional delivery costs
Chronic neurologic sequelae	13.3%				
		100%	$225	365.0	Institutional care (per year)

VACCINE PROGRAM CONSIDERATIONS

Target Population

For the purposes of the calculations in this report, it is assumed that the target population for this vaccine is all adolescents (age 12 years). It was assumed that 50% of the target population would utilize the vaccine.

Vaccine Schedule, Efficacy, and Costs

For the purposes of the calculations in this report, it was estimated that this vaccine would cost $50 per dose and that administration costs would be $10 per dose. Default assumptions of a 3-dose series and 75% efficacy were accepted. Table 4-1 summarizes vaccine program assumptions for all vaccines considered in this report.

RESULTS

If a vaccine program for HSV were implemented today and the vaccine was 100% efficacious and utilized by 100% of the target population, the annualized present value of the QALYs gained would be 28,000. Using committee assumptions of less-than-ideal efficacy and utilization and including time and monetary costs until a vaccine program is implemented, the annualized present value of the QALYs gained would be 7,500. Most of the disease burden is associated with genital and CNS infections due to the large number of genital infections and the serious, chronic sequelae associated with the relatively fewer cases of CNS HSV disease.

If a vaccine program for HSV were implemented today and the vaccine was 100% efficacious and utilized by 100% of the target population, the annualized present value of the health care costs saved would be $850 million. Using committee assumptions of less-than-ideal efficacy and utilization and including time and monetary costs until a vaccine program is implemented, the annualized present value of the health care costs saved would be $225 million.

If a vaccine program for HSV were implemented today and the vaccine was 100% efficacious and utilized by 100% of the target population, the annualized present value of the program cost would be $680 million. Using committee assumptions of less-than-ideal efficacy and utilization and including time and monetary costs until a vaccine program is implemented, the annualized present value of the program cost would be $240 million.

Using committee assumptions of time and costs until licensure, the fixed cost of vaccine development has been amortized and is $7.2 million for a HSV vaccine.

If a vaccine program were implemented today and the vaccine were 100% efficacious and utilized by 100% of the target population, the annualized present value of the cost per QALY gained is -$6,000. A negative value represents a saving in costs in addition to a saving in QALYs. Using committee assumptions of less-than-ideal utilization and including time and monetary costs until a vaccine program is implemented, the annualized present value of the cost per QALY gained is $3,000.

See Chapters 4 and 5 for details on the methods and assumptions used by the committee for the results reported.

READING LIST

Hirsch MS. Herpes Simplex Virus. In: Principles and Practice of Infectious Diseases. GL Mandell, JE Bennett, Dolin R eds. New York, NY: Churchill Livingstone, 1995, pp. 1336–1345.

Institute of Medicine. New Vaccines Development: Establishing Priorities, Volume 1. Diseases of Importance in the United States. Washington, DC: National Academy Press, 1985a.

Koelle DM, Benedetti J, Langenberg A, et al. Asymptomatic Reactivation of Herpes Simplex Virus in Women after the First Episode of Genital Herpes. Annals of Internal Medicine 1992; 116:433–437.

Kohl S. Postnatal Herpes Simplex Virus Infection. In: Textbook of Pediatric Infectious Diseases. RD Feigin and JD Cherry eds. Philadelphia, PA: WB Saunder Company, 1992, pp. 1558–1583.

U.S. Bureau of the Census. Statistical Abstract of the U.S.: 1995 (115th edition.) Washington, DC. 1995.

Ventura SJ, Martin JA, Mathews TJ, et al. Advance Report of Final Natality statistics, 1994. Monthly Vital Statistics Report 1996; 44.

APPENDIX 10

Histoplasma capsulatum

Histoplasmosis is a common pulmonary mycosis of humans and animals. It is caused by *Histoplasma capsulatum*, a dimorphic soil fungus that is isolated from soil with high nitrogen concentrations. It has a definite association with the droppings of bat and avian habitats.

Histoplasmosis occurs at highest incidence in central and eastern areas of the United States, in particular the Ohio River Valley and portions of the Mississippi Valley.

DISEASE BURDEN

Epidemiology

For the purposes of the calculations in this report, the committee estimated that there are 500,000 new infections with *Histoplasma capsulatum* each year in the United States. The incidence rate varies with age; the highest incidence is seen in people between 15 and 34 years of age. *H. capsulatum* infections are clustered geographically. The committee estimated that half of the infections occur in people born in the region and half occur in migrants into the area. The infections was associated with an average mortality rate of 0.05 per 100,000 (138 deaths per year). See Table A10-1.

See Appendix 28 for more information.

Table A10-1 Incidence and Mortality Rates for Histoplasma Infection

Age Groups	Population	Incidence Rates (per 100,000)	% Distribution of Cases
<1	3,963,000	79.28	0.0063
1-4	16,219,000	79.28	0.0257
5-14	38,056,000	105.11	0.0800
15-24	36,263,000	348.84	0.2530
25-34	41,670,000	325.17	0.2710
35-44	42,149,000	161.33	0.1360
45-54	30,224,000	163.78	0.0990
55-64	21,241,000	174.19	0.0740
65-74	18,964,000	102.83	0.0390
75-84	11,088,000	54.47	0.0121
85+	3,598,000	54.47	0.0039
Total	263,435,000	189.80	1.000

500,000 cases

Age Groups	Population	Mortality Rates (per 100,000)	% Distribution of Deaths
<1	3,963,000	0.04	0.0114
1-4	16,219,000	0.01	0.0093
5-14	38,056,000	0.01	0.0290
15-24	36,263,000	0.03	0.0918
25-34	41,670,000	0.03	0.0983
35-44	42,149,000	0.08	0.2467
45-54	30,224,000	0.08	0.1796
55-64	21,241,000	0.09	0.1342
65-74	18,964,000	0.10	0.1415
75-84	11,088,000	0.05	0.0438
85+	3,598,000	0.05	0.0142
Total	263,435,000	0.05	1.0000

138 deaths

Disease Scenarios

For the purposes of the calculation in this report, the committee assumed that most infections are asymptomatic. Half of symptomatic infections were presumed to be associated with a mild flu-like illness. Other manifestations include pneumonitis, disseminated disease, and chronic pulmonary disease. Outpatient treatment of pneumonitis was associated with both inpatient and outpatient treatment. Disseminated histoplasma was associated with an acute and severe phase of illness followed by a more moderate but lengthy recovery. Health utility indexes associated with histoplasma disease range from .9 for a mild flu-like illness to .39 for the acute illness associated with disseminated disease. Table A10-2 shows the HUI and duration associated with the disease scenarios used in the calculations for the report.

COST INCURRED BY DISEASE

Table A10-3 summarizes the health care costs incurred by histoplasma infections. For the purposes of the calculations in this report, it was assumed that all patients with flu-like illness associated with histoplasma infection require outpatient care of a physician and that half receive medications or diagnostics. All patients with pneumonitis were assumed to incur costs associated with specialist visits and diagnostics. Inpatient hospital costs are included for a small fraction of these patients. It was assumed that half of the patients with disseminated disease would require hospitalization. All patients with disseminated disease would require outpatient treatment lasting several months and including 8 visits to a specialist and expensive medication and diagnostic costs. Approximately 40% of patients with chronic pulmonary disease would require hospitalization and all of the patients would require outpatient treatment similar to that estimated for disseminated disease but for 3 times the duration and cost.

VACCINE DEVELOPMENT

The committee assumed that it will take 15 years until licensure of a histoplasma vaccine and that $360 million needs to be invested. Table 4-1 summarizes vaccine development assumptions for all vaccines considered in this report.

VACCINE PROGRAM CONSIDERATIONS

Target Population

For the purposes of the calculations in this report, it is assumed that the target population for this vaccine is all infants in endemic regions (approximately 900,000 annually) and migrants into the area (approximately 1,300,000 annually at an average age of 28.9 per migrant vaccinee). It was assumed that 90% of the infants born in the region and 10% of migrants would utilize the vaccine.

Vaccine Schedule, Efficacy, and Costs

For the purposes of the calculations in this report, it was estimated that this vaccine would cost $50 per dose and that administration costs would be $10 per dose. Default assumptions of a 3-dose series and 75% effectiveness were accepted. Table 4-1 summarizes vaccine program assumptions for all vaccines considered in this report.

Table A10-2 Disease Scenarios for Histoplasma Infection

	No. of Cases	% of Cases	Committee HUI Values	Duration (years)
Total Deaths	138			
Total Cases (new symptomatic and asymptomatic infections)	500,000			
Asymptomatic		90%	1.00	
Flu-like illness		5.0%	0.90	0.0384 (14 days)
Pneumonitis: outpatient only		3.5%	0.78	0.0384 (14 days)
Pneumonitis: w/ inpatient		0.9%		
inpatient care			0.67	0.0274 (10 days)
outpatient care			0.78	0.0384 (14 days)
Disseminated histoplasmosis		0.5%		
disseminated intravascular coagulation, splenomegaly, hepatomegaly, fever			0.39	0.0192 (7 days)
recovery			0.90	0.2500 (3 months)
Chronic pulmonary		0.1%		
symptomatic, untreated			0.90	0.1667 (2 months)
outpatient treatment			0.90	0.7500 (9 months)

RESULTS

If a vaccine program for *H. capsulatum* were implemented today and the vaccine was 100% efficacious and utilized by 100% of the target population, the annualized present value of the QALYs gained would be 1,200. Using committee assumptions of less-than-ideal efficacy and utilization and including time and monetary costs until a vaccine program is implemented, the annualized present value of the QALYs gained would be 35.

If a vaccine program for *H. capsulatum* were implemented today and the vaccine was 100% efficacious and utilized by 100% of the target population, the annualized present value of the health care costs saved would be $29.7 million. Using committee assumptions of less-than-ideal efficacy and utilization and including time and monetary costs until a vaccine program is implemented, the annualized present value of the health care costs saved would be $860,000.

If a vaccine program for *H. capsulatum* were implemented today and the vaccine was 100% efficacious and utilized by 100% of the target population, the annualized present value of the program cost would be $390 million. Using committee assumptions of less-than-ideal efficacy and utilization and including time and monetary costs until a vaccine program is implemented, the annualized present value of the program cost would be $12.7 million.

Table A10-3 Health Care Costs Associated with Histoplasma Disease

	% with Care	Cost per Unit	Units per Case	Form of treatment
Flu-like illness				
(single state)	100%	$50	2.0	physician a
	50%	$150	1.0	medication b, diagnostic b
Pneumonitis: outpatient only				
(single state)	100%	$350	1.0	outpatient treatment 2 physician b, medication b, diagnostic b
Pneumonitis: w/ inpatient				
inpatient care	100%	$5,000	1.0	hospitalization
outpatient care	100%	$350	1.0	outpatient treatment (same as above)
Disseminated histoplasmosis				
disseminated intravascular coagulation, splenomegaly, hepatomegaly, fever	50%	$5,000	1.0	hospitalization
outpatient only	50%	$1,250	1.0	outpatient—3 months (8 physician b, 3 medication c)
recovery	50%	$1,250	1.0	outpatient—3 months
Chronic pulmonary				
symptomatic (untreated, initial treatment)	40%	$5,000	1.0	hospitalization
outpatient treatment	100%	$1,250	3.0	outpatient (same as for disseminated disease)

Using committee assumptions of time and costs until licensure, the fixed cost of vaccine development has been amortized and is $10.8 million for a *H. capsulatum* vaccine.

If a vaccine program were implemented today and the vaccine were 100% efficacious and utilized by 100% of the target population, the annualized present value of the cost per QALY gained is $300,000. Using committee assumptions of less-than-ideal utilization and including time and monetary costs until a vaccine program is implemented, the annualized present value of the cost per QALY gained is $600,000.

See Chapters 4 and 5 for details on the methods and assumptions used by the committee for the results reported.

READING LIST

Bullock WE. Histoplasma Capsulatum. In: Principles and Practice of Infectious Diseases. GL Mandell, JE Bennett, Dolin R eds. New York, NY: Churchill Livingstone, 1995, pp. 2340–2353.

Byerly E, Deardorff K. National and State Population Estimates: 1990 to 1994, U.S. Bureau of the Census, Current Population Reports, pp. 25–1127, U.S. Government Printing Office, Washington, DC, 1995.

Hansen KA. Geographical Mobility: March 1993 to March 1994, U.S. Bureau of the Census, Current Population Reports, pp. 20–485, U.S. Government Printing Office, Washington, DC, 1995.

Leissa B, Widerman BL. Histoplasmosis. In: Textbook of Pediatric Infectious Diseases. RD Feigin and JD Cherry eds. Philadelphia, PA: WB Saunder Company, 1992, pp. 1952–1964.

Ventura SJ, Martin JA, Mathews TJ, et al. Advance Report of Final Natality Statistics, 1994. Monthly Vital Statistics Report 1996; 44.

APPENDIX 11

Human Papillomavirus

Human papillomavirus (HPV) infects stratified squamous, metaplastic squamous, and columnar epithelial cells. The majority of human papillomavirus cells are self-limited, but there is now a clear correlation between malignant tumors and the development of a subset of infections that involve oncogenic viruses. Specific types of HPV tend to infect different types of epithelia and produce different clinical and pathogenic manifestations. The two distinct types of cells are mucosal HPV infection and cutaneous HPV infection.

Genital tract HPV is thought to be currently the most common sexually transmitted viral infection in the United States. Genital warts occur on the vulva, vagina, cervix, penis, and anus. In addition to being a common STD, genital HPV infection is of considerable importance in the pathogenesis role of epithelial cancers of the female and male genital tracts.

DISEASE BURDEN

Epidemiology

For the purposes of the calculations in this report, the committee estimated that there are 1 million new infections of human papillomavirus (HPV) each year in the United States in males and females between the ages of 15 and 29 years of age. New infections are equally divided between males and females.

Disease Scenarios

For the purposes of the calculation in this report, the committee assumed that approximately half of women with HPV infection experience a 3-month episode of limited or severe genital warts and the other half experience recurrences of limited or severe genital warts. Health utility indices (HUI) associated with those episodes range from .85 to .95. It was assumed that 10% of women with HPV infections develop cervical dysplasia due to the infection. It was also assumed that cancers that develop secondary to HPV infection occur with an average lag of 25 years from time of infection. Cervical cancers were separately described as carcinoma in situ, locally invasive at diagnosis, and advanced at diagnosis. Treatment phases and follow-up phases are included, with HUI and duration of that state ranging from 4 months of treatment at an HUI of .8 to 16 years of life spent at an HUI of .9.

Sequelae of HPV infection of men was assumed to parallel to a great degree that in women: several scenarios of genital warts and penile cancers. HUI and duration of time in the specific disease states show the same ranges as for women. Table A11-1 shows the disease states for both men and women.

COST INCURRED BY DISEASE

Table A11-2 summarizes the health care costs incurred by HPV infections. For the purposes of the calculations in this report, it was assumed that women with genital warts incur costs associated with physician visits and diagnostics. More severe cases were assumed to involve more frequent physician visits. It was assumed that approximately half of women with mild recurrent warts and all of the women with extensive recurrent warts visit a physician four times per year. It was assumed that women with cervical dysplasia incur costs associated with specialist visits, diagnostics, and follow-up visits for 1.5 years.

It was assumed that cervical carcinoma in situ was associated with multiple visits, advanced diagnostics, and ambulatory surgery during the treatment phase. During the 2-year follow-up, it was assumed that all patients receive 3 follow-up visits; and diagnostics per year. Treatment for locally invasive cervical cancer was assumed to be associated with physician visits, diagnostics, hospitalization, including costs for surgeons/anesthesiologists; and radiation therapy. The 2-year follow-up phase was assumed to include quarterly physician and diagnostic evaluation. Advanced cervical cancer was associated with similar treatment costs as for locally invasive cancer, but with increased physician visits during both the treatment phase and the follow-up phase.

Treatment patterns for acute and chronic (recurring genital warts and penile cancers) sequelae of HPV infection in men were assumed to be similar to that of treatment patterns in women.

Table A11-1 Disease Scenarios for Women and Men for HPV Infection

	No. of Cases	% of Cases	Committee HUI Values	Duration (years)
WOMEN				
Genital warts, limited	237,500	47.5%		
minor physical discomfort			0.95	0.2500 (3 months)
Genital warts, limited but recurring	237,500	47.5%		
minor physical discomfort (2 recurrences per year for 10 years)			0.90	0.5000 (6 months/year)
Genital warts, extensive	12,500	2.5%		
same physical discomfort			0.85	0.2500 (3 months)
Genital warts, extensive and recurring	12,500	2.5%		
some physical discomfort (2 recurrences per year for 10 years)			0.85	0.5000 (6 months/year)
Cervical dysplasia	50,000	10.0%	0.97	1.5000 (18 months)
All Cancers: assume average 25-year lag from infection				
Cervical cancer—carcinoma in situ	25,000	5.0%		
treatment phase			0.80	0.3333 (4 months)
posttreatment phase (follow-up)			0.97	2.0000 (2 years)
Cervical cancer—locally invasive at diagnosis	5,000	1.0%		
treatment phase (surgery, radiation, chemotherapy)			0.79	0.3333 (4 months)
posttreatment phase (follow-up)			0.90	16.7349 (years remaining)
Cervical cancer—advanced at diagnosis	2,500	0.5%		
treatment phase (surgery, radiation, chemotherapy)			0.62	0.3333 (4 months)
posttreatment phase (follow-up and sequelae e.g., infertiity, sexual dysfunction, urinary dysfunction)			0.62	3.0000 (3 years)
premature death (by 3 years after diagnosis)			0.00	15.7265 (years lost)

Continued

Table A11-1 *Continued*

	No. of Cases	% of Cases	Committee HUI Values	Duration (years)
MEN				
Genital warts, limited	237,500	47.5%		
minor physical discomfort			0.90	0.2500 (3 months)
Genital warts, limited but recurring	237,500	47.5%		
minor physical discomfort (2 recurrences per year for 10 years)			0.90	0.5000 (6 months/ year)
Genital warts, extensive	12,500	2.5%		
some physical discomfort			0.85	0.2500 (3 months)
Genital warts, extensive and recurring	12,500	2.5%		
some physical discomfort (2 recurrences per year for 10 years)			0.85	0.5000 (6 months/ year)
All Cancers: assume average 25-year lag from infection				
Penile cancer—carcinoma in situ	25,000	5.0%		
treatment phase			0.80	0.3333 (4 months)
post-treatment phase (follow-up)			0.97	2.0000 (2 years)
Penile cancer—locally invasive at diagnosis	5,000	1.0%		
treatment phase (surgery, radiation, chemotherapy)			0.80	0.3333 (4 months)
post-treatment phase (follow-up)			0.90	16.7349 (years remaining)
Penile cancer—advanced at diagnosis	2,500	0.5%		
treatment phase (surgery, radiation, chemotherapy)			0.62	0.3333 (4 months)
post-treatment phase (follow-up and sequelae e.g., infertility, sexual dysfunction, urinary dysfunction)			0.62	3.0000 (3 years)
premature death (by 3 years after diagnosis)			0.00	15.7265 (years lost)

Table A11-2 Health Care Costs Associated with HPV Disease in Women and Men

	% with Care	Cost per Unit	Units per Case	Form of Treatment
WOMEN				
Genital warts, limited				
minor physical discomfort	100%	$50	3	physician a
	100%	$50	1	diagnostic a
Genital warts, limited but recurring				
minor physical discomfort	50%	$50	4	physician a/year
2 recurrences per year for 10 years	50%	$50	1	diagnostic a
Genital warts, extensive				
some physical discomfort	100%	$50	3	physician a
Genital warts, extensive and recurring				
some physical discomfort	100%	$50	4	physician a/year
2 recurrences per year for 10 years	100%	$50	1	diagnostic a
Cervical dysplasia				
treated precancerous condition	100%	$650	1	physician c plus diagnostic c
follow-up period	100%	$100	6	physician b
All Cancers: assume average 25-year lag from infection				
Cervical cancer—carcinoma in situ				
treatment phase	100%	$50	5	physician a
	100%	$500	1	diagnostic c
	100%	$1,000	1	ambulatory surgery
post-treatment phase (follow-up)	100%	$50	3	physician a/year
	100%	$50	3	diagnostic a/year
Cervical cancer-locally invasive at diagnosis				
treatment phase (surgery, radiation, chemotherapy)	100%	$100	2	physician b
	100%	$500	2	diagnostic c
	100%	$4,000	1	hospitalization
	100%	$500	2	surgeons/anesthesiologist
	100%	$5,000	1	radiation
follow-up	10%	$100	4	physician b/year
	10%	$50	4	diagnostic a/year

Table A11-2 *Continued*

	% with Care	Cost per Unit	Units per Case	Form of Treatment
Cervical cancer—advanced at diagnosis				
treatment phase (surgery, radiation, chemotherapy)	100%	$100	5	physician b
	100%	$500	2	diagnostic c
	100%	$4,000	1	hospitalization
	100%	$5,000	1	radiation
	100%	$500	2	surgeon/anesthesiologist
	100%	$50	12	physician a
	100%	$50	3	medication b
post-treatment phase (follow up and sequelae (e.g., infertility, sexual dysfunction, urinary dysfunction)	100%	$100	6	physician b/year
	100%	$50	6	diagnostic a/year
MEN				
Genital warts, limited				
minor physical discomfort	100%	$50	1	physician a
minor physical discomfort; recurrences for 10 years	100%	$50	2	physician a/year
Genital warts, extensive				
some physical discomfort	100%	$50	2	physician a
Genital warts, extensive and recurring				
some physical discomfort	100%	$50	2	physician a
2 recurrences per year for 10 years	100%	$50	2	physician a/year
All Cancers: assume average 25-year lag from infection				
Penile cancer—carcinoma in situ				
treatment phase	100%	$50	1	physician a
	50%	$1,000	1	ambulatory surgery
	100%	$100	1	diagnostic b
	50%	$4,000	1	hospitalization
	100%	$500	2	surgeon/anaesthiologist
post-treatment phase (follow-up)	100%	$100	2	physician b/year
Penile cancer—locally invasive at diagnosis				
treatment phase (surgery, radiation, chemotherapy)	100%	$100	1	physician b
	100%	$4,000	1	hospitalization
	100%	$500	2	surgeon/anesthesiologist
	50%	$5,000	1	radiation

Table A11-2 *Continued*

	% with Care	Cost per Unit	Units per Case	Form of Treatment
Penile cancer—locally invasive at diagnosis (*continued*)				
	50%	$5,000	1	chemotherapy
post-treatment phase (follow-up)	100%	$50	1	physician a/year
Penile cancer—advanced at diagnosis				
treatment phase (surgery, radiation, chemotherapy)	100%	$100	1	physician b
	100%	$4,000	1	hospitalization
	100%	$500	2	surgeon/anesthesiologist
	50%	$5,000	1	radiation
	50%	$5,000	1	chemotherapy
post-treatment phase (follow-up and sequelae (e.g., infertility, sexual dysfunction, urinary dysfunction)	100%	$100	6	physician b/year

VACCINE DEVELOPMENT

The committee assumed that it will take 7 years until licensure of a HPV vaccine and that $360 million needs to be invested. Table 4-1 summarizes vaccine development assumptions for all vaccines considered in this report.

VACCINE PROGRAM CONSIDERATIONS

Target Population

For the purposes of the calculations in this report, it is assumed that the target population for this vaccine male and female adolescents (age 12) . It was assumed that 50% of the target population would utilize the vaccine.

Vaccine Schedule, Efficacy, and Costs

For the purposes of the calculations in this report, it was estimated that this vaccine would cost $100 per dose and that administration costs would be $10 per dose. Default assumptions of a 3-dose series and 75% effectiveness were accepted. Table 4-1 summarizes vaccine program assumptions for all vaccines considered in this report.

RESULTS

If a vaccine program for HPV were implemented today and the vaccine was 100% efficacious and utilized by 100% of the target population, the annualized present value of the QALYs gained would be 180,000. Using committee assumptions of less than ideal efficacy and utilization and including time and monetary costs until a vaccine program is implemented, the annualized present value of the QALYs gained would be 48,000.

If a vaccine program for HPV were implemented today and the vaccine was 100% efficacious and utilized by 100% of the target population, the annualized present value of the health care costs saved would be $530 million. Using committee assumptions of less than ideal efficacy and utilization and including time and monetary costs until a vaccine program is implemented, the annualized present value of the health care costs saved would be $140 million.

If a vaccine program for HPV were implemented today and the vaccine was 100% efficacious and utilized by 100% of the target population, the annualized present value of the program cost would be $1.2 billion. Using committee assumptions of less than ideal efficacy and utilization and including time and monetary costs until a vaccine program is implemented, the annualized present value of the program cost would be $435 million.

Using committee assumptions of time and costs until licensure, the fixed cost of vaccine development has been amortized and is $10.8 million for a HPV vaccine.

If a vaccine program were implemented today and the vaccine were 100% efficacious and utilized by 100% of the target population, the annualized present value of the cost per QALY gained is $4,000. Using committee assumptions of less than ideal utilization and including time and monetary costs until a vaccine program is implemented, the annualized present value of the cost per QALY gained is $6,000.

See Chapters 4 and 5 for details on the methods and assumptions used by the committee for the results reported.

READING LIST

CDC, NCID. National Registry Established for Pediatric Recurrent Respiratory Papillomatosis. URL http://www.cdc.gov/ncidod/focus/vol6no2/dvrd.htm (accessed September 26, 1997).

Institute of Medicine. The Hidden Epidemic: Confronting Sexually Transmitted Diseases. Eng TR, Butler WT (eds.). Washington, DC: National Academy Press, 1997.

Miller BA, Kolonel LN, Bernstein L, et al. (eds). Racial/Ethnic Patterns of Cancer in the United States 1988–1992, National Cancer Institute. NIH Pub. No. 96-4104. Bethesda, MD, 1996.

Stoeckle MY. Human Herpesvirus 6 and Human Herpesvirus 7. In: Principles and Practice of Infectious Diseases. GL Mandell,, JE Bennett, Dolin R eds. New York, NY: Churchill Livingstone, 1995, pp. 1377–1400.

U.S. Bureau of the Census. Statistical Abstract of the U.S.: 1995 (115th edition). Washington, D.C. 1995.

Ventura SJ, Martin JA, Mathews TJ, et al. Advance Report of Final Natality statistics, 1994. Monthly Vital Statistics Report 1996; 44.

APPENDIX 12

Influenza A and B

The variability of the influenza virus can explain why reinfection is so common. The two major structural proteins, nucleoprotein (NP) and matrix protein (M), produce antigenic differences which classify the influenza virus as type A, B, or C. Influenza A and B are pleomorphic-enveloped viruses with a genome of 8 different (-)RNA nucleocapsid segments. The reassortment of these segments along with mutations enhance genetic diversity upon infection with two different strains (Murray, Kibosh, et. al., 620). Both types are covered with the glycoprotein spikes, hemagglutinin (HA) and neuraminidase (NA). Influenza A is further subtyped into groups based on the characteristics of the NA and HA (Murray et. al., 918).

The HA is responsible for viral attachment to sialic acid on epithelial cell surfaces, fusion of the envelope to the cell membrane, and agglutination of erythrocytes. Mutagenic changes in HA can induce an antigenic shift which is seen only with influenza A (Murray, Kibosh et. al., 620). This antigenic shift is a result of genome reassortment between different virus strains, including animal strains. The NA cleaves the sialic acid, removing it from the virus and infected cells to prevent clumping and to allow the release of the virus from infected cells (Murray, 919). Minor mutagenic alterations (usually brought about by accumulated point mutations) in HA and/or NA prompts an antigenic drift of both influenza A and B. These two types of antigenic variations (antigenic shift and drift) allow the influenza virus to evade preexisting immunity and evolve into pandemics and epidemics.

The highly contagious influenza virus accounts for many epidemics and pandemics of respiratory illnesses. Some of the milder symptoms of this illness include fever, pharyngitis, rhinitis, cough, myalgia, and malaise. In children, otitis media may develop with influenza. Influenza A has been associated primarily with increased mortality in the elderly population. Therefore, influenza encompasses a variety of clinical responses ranging from asymptomatic or mild respiratory infection to primary viral pneumonia or secondary bacterial pneumonia with fatal outcome.

Recently, epidemics have alternated between those caused primarily by type A and those caused by type B. Both are transmitted by sneezing, coughing, speaking, and also by direct contact through small-particle aerosols. Transmission usually occurs during the initial stages when infected individuals shed substantial amounts of the virus through respiratory secretions. The episodes of winter influenza are partly explained by the ability of small droplets to remain infectious in the cold and in low humidity.

DISEASE BURDEN

Epidemiology

For the purposes of the calculations in this report, the committee estimated that there are approximately 54,000,000 cases of influenza A and B each year in the United States. Incidence rates in children under 14 years of age are over twice that in adults 35 years of age and older. There were approximately 42,250 deaths each year due to influenza, with very high mortality in people 65 years of age and older. See Table A12-1.

Disease Scenarios

For the purposes of the calculation in this report, the committee assumed that 98% of influenza infections are associated with a moderate to severe respiratory illness not requiring hospitalization. It was assumed that most of these infections require only 3 days of bed rest and 2 weeks of mild recovery. Approximately 10% of infections are associated with a more serious sinusitis in conjunction with the 2-week recovery. It was assumed that approximately 5% of influenza infections are associated with a 3-month period of fatigue in addition to the scenario described above. It was assumed that 2% of influenza infections result in hospitalization for pneumonia. It was further assumed that a small number (.1%) of influenza infections exacerbate underlying cardiac or pulmonary conditions. This exacerbation of chronic disease was assumed to be associated with an extra disease burden of 8.5 days of an HUI of .53. See Table A12-2.

COST INCURRED BY DISEASE

Table A12-3 summarizes the health care costs incurred by influenza A and B infections. For the purposes of the calculations in this report, it was assumed

Table A12-1 Incidence and Mortality of Influenza A and B Disease

INCIDENCE RATES

5-Year Age Groups	Total Population	Incidence Rates (per 100,000) (5-yr age groups)	Cases	Age Groups	Population	Incidence Rates (per 100,000)	% Distribution of Cases
0-4	20,182,000	33,700	6,801,334	<1	3,963,000	33,700	0.0246
5-9	19,117,000	39,300	7,512,981	1-4	16,219,000	33,700	0.1006
10-14	18,939,000	30,200	5,719,578	5-14	38,056,000	34,771	0.2435
15-19	17,790,000	30,200	5,372,580	15-24	36,263,000	24,851	0.1658
20-24	18,473,000	19,700	3,639,181	25-34	41,670,000	15,500	0.1189
25-29	19,294,000	15,500	2,990,570	35-44	42,149,000	14,800	0.1148
30-34	22,376,000	15,500	3,468,280	45-54	30,224,000	14,800	0.0823
35-39	22,215,000	14,800	3,287,820	55-64	21,241,000	14,800	0.0579
40-44	19,934,000	14,800	2,950,232	65-74	18,964,000	14,800	0.0517
45-49	16,873,000	14,800	2,497,204	75-84	11,088,000	14,800	0.0302
50-54	13,351,000	14,800	1,975,948	• 85	3,598,000	14,800	0.0098
55-59	11,050,000	14,800	1,635,400				
60-64	10,191,000	14,800	1,508,268	**Total**	263,435,000	20,627	1.0000
65-69	10,099,000	14,800	1,494,652				
70-74	8,865,000	14,800	1,312,020				
75-79	6,669,000	14,800	987,012				
80-84	4,419,000	14,800	654,012				
• 85	3,598,000	14,800	532,504				
Total	263,435,000		54,339,576				

...

226

Table A12-1 *Continued*

MORTALITY RATES

5-Year Age Groups	Total Population	Incidence Rates (per 100,000) (5-yr age groups)	Cases
0-4	20,182,000	2.7	545
5-9	19,117,000	0.9	172
10-14	18,939,000	0.9	170
15-19	17,790,000	0.9	160
20-24	18,473,000	1.1	203
25-29	19,294,000	1.1	212
30-34	22,376,000	1.1	246
35-39	22,215,000	1.1	244
40-44	19,934,000	1.1	219
45-49	16,873,000	10.2	1,721
50-54	13,351,000	10.2	1,362
55-59	11,050,000	10.2	1,127
60-64	10,191,000	10.2	1,039
65-69	10,099,000	103.5	10,452
70-74	8,865,000	103.5	9,175
75-79	6,669,000	103.5	6,902
80-84	4,419,000	103.5	4,574
• 85	3,598,000	103.5	3,724
Total	263,435,000		42,250

Age Groups	Population	Incidence Rates (per 100,000)	% Distribution of Cases
<1	3,963,000	2.7	0.0025
1-4	16,219,000	2.7	0.0104
5-14	38,056,000	0.9	0.0081
15-24	36,263,000	1.0	0.0086
25-34	41,670,000	1.1	0.0108
35-44	42,149,000	1.1	0.0110
45-54	30,224,000	10.2	0.0730
55-64	21,241,000	10.2	0.0513
65-74	18,964,000	103.5	0.4646
75-84	11,088,000	103.5	0.2716
• 85	3,598,000	103.5	0.0881
Total	263,435,000	16.0	1.0000

Table A12-2 Disease Scenarios for Influenza A and B Infection

	No. of Cases	% of Cases	Committee HUI Values	Duration (years)
Moderate to severe respiratory illness	45,264,867	83.30%		
bed rest			0.75	0.0082 (3 days)
discomfort following bed rest			0.90	0.0384 (14 days)
Respiratory illness with sinusitis	5,325,278	9.80%		
bed rest			0.75	0.0082 (3 days)
sinusitis			0.75	0.0192 (7 days)
discomfort following bed rest			0.90	0.0192 (7 days)
Respiratory illness w/ post-influenza fatigue	2,662,639	4.90%		
bed rest			0.75	0.0082 (3 days)
discomfort following bed rest			0.90	0.0384 (14 days)
post-influenza fatigue			0.87	0.2466 (90 days)
Pneumonia	978,112	1.80%		
acute care hospitalization			0.65	0.0274 (10 days)
recuperation			0.90	0.0384 (14 days)
Pneumonia—ICU	108,679	0.20%		
ICU hospitalization			0.52	0.0274 (10 days)
recuperation			0.90	0.0384 (14 days)
Exacerbation of underlying asthma/heart disease	54,340	0.10%	0.53	0.0233 (8.5 days)

that everyone requiring bed rest for acute influenza infection incurs costs for an over-the-counter symptomatic treatment. The cost calculations include one visit to a physician and a prescription medication for 20% of the patients during the acute phase. Recovery phases were assumed to include costs for over-the-counter medications and physician visits for some of the patients with sinusitis and post-influenza fatigue. Hospitalization costs, diagnostics, inpatient and with outpatient physician visits, and medications were included costs for patients with pneumonia. There were no costs calculated for the exacerbation of underlying chronic disease states by influenza infection with pneumonia.

Table A12-3 Health Care Costs Associated with Influenza A and B Disease

	% with Care	Cost per Unit	Units per Case	Form of Treatment
Moderate to severe respiratory illness				
bed rest	50%	$50	1.0	physician a
	20%	$50	1.0	medication b
	100%	$10	1.0	medication a
discomfort following bed rest	50%	$10	1.0	medication a
Respiratory illness with sinusitis				
bed rest	50%	$50	1.0	physician a
	20%	$50	1.0	medication b
	100%	$10	1.0	medication a
sinusitis	50%	$50	1.0	medication b
	100%	$10	1.0	medication a
discomfort following bed rest	50%	$50	1.0	physician a
Respiratory illness with post-influenza fatigue				
bed rest	50%	$50	1.0	physician a
	50%	$50	1.0	medication b
	100%	$10	1.0	medication a
discomfort following bed rest	50%	$10	1.0	medication a
post-influenza fatigue	50%	$50	1.0	physician a
Pneumonia				
acute care and ICU together	100%	$50	1.0	physician a
percentage of cases adjusted	100%	$4,000	1.0	hospitalization
	100%	$100	1.0	physician b
	100%	$100	1.0	diagnostic b
recuperation	100%	$50	1.0	physician a
	100%	$50	1.0	medication b
	100%	$10	1.0	medication a

VACCINE DEVELOPMENT

The committee assumed that it will take 7 years until licensure of a influenza vaccine and that $360 million needs to be invested. The committee assumed that the licensed vaccine would most likely be a DNA vaccine requiring immunization every 5 years. Table 4-1 summarizes vaccine development assumptions for all vaccines considered in this report.

VACCINE PROGRAM CONSIDERATIONS

Target Population

For the purposes of the calculations in this report, it is assumed that the target population for this vaccine is one-fifth of the entire population every year. It was assumed that 30% of the target population would utilize the vaccine.

Vaccine Schedule, Efficacy, and Costs

For the purposes of the calculations in this report, it was estimated that this vaccine would cost $50 per dose and that administration costs would be $10 per dose. It was assumed that 1 dose would be required every 5 years. It is assumed that the current influenza immunization program would no longer be needed. Default assumption of 75% effectiveness were accepted. Table 4-1 summarizes vaccine program assumptions for all vaccines considered in this report.

RESULTS

If a vaccine program for influenza were implemented today and the vaccine was 100% efficacious and utilized by 100% of the target population, the annualized present value of the QALYs gained would be 800,000. Using committee assumptions of less-than-ideal efficacy and utilization and including time and monetary costs until a vaccine program is implemented, the annualized present value of the QALYs gained would be 125,000.

If a vaccine program for influenza were implemented today and the vaccine was 100% efficacious and utilized by 100% of the target population, the annualized present value of the health care costs saved would be $6.4 billion. Using committee assumptions of less-than-ideal efficacy and utilization and including time and monetary costs until a vaccine program is implemented, the annualized present value of the health care costs saved would be $1 billion.

If a vaccine program for influenza were implemented today and the vaccine was 100% efficacious and utilized by 100% of the target population, the annualized present value of the program cost would be $3.2 billion. Using committee assumptions of less-than-ideal efficacy and utilization and including time and monetary costs until a vaccine program is implemented, the annualized present value of the program cost would be $430 million.

Using committee assumptions of time and costs until licensure, the fixed cost of vaccine development has been amortized and is $10.8 million for an influenza vaccine.

If a vaccine program were implemented today and the vaccine were 100% efficacious and utilized by 100% of the target population, the annualized present value of the cost per QALY gained is -$4,000. A negative value represents a saving in costs in addition to a saving in QALYs. Using committee assumptions of less-than-ideal utilization and including time and monetary costs until a vaccine program is implemented, the annualized present value of the cost per QALY gained is -$4,500.

See Chapters 4 and 5 for details on the methods and assumptions used by the committee for the results reported.

READING LIST

Barker WH. Excess Pneumonia and Influenza Associated Hospitalization during Influenza Epidemics in the United States, 1970–78. American Journal of Public Health 1986; 76:761–765.

Betts RF. Influenza Virus. In: Principles and Practice of Infectious Diseases. GL Mandell, JE Bennett, Dolin R eds. New York, NY: Churchill Livingstone, 1995, pp. 1546–1567.

CDC. Influenza Surveillance—United States, 1992–3 and 1993–4. Morbidity and Mortality Weekly Report 1997; 46:1–12.

CDC. Prevention and Control of Influenza. Morbidity and Mortality Weekly Report 1996; 45:9–24.

CDC. Prevention and Control of Influenza. Morbidity and Mortality Weekly Report 1997; 46:1–25.

Glezen WP. Influenza in an urban area. Canadian Journal of Infectious Diseases 1993; 4:272–4.

Glezen WP, Cherry JD. Influenza Viruses. In: Textbook of Pediatric Infectious Diseases. RD Feigin and JD Cherry eds. Philadelphia, PA: WB Saunder Company, 1992, pp. 1688–1704.

Glezen WP, Couch RB. Influenza Viruses. In: Virus Infections of Humans. Evans AS, ed. 3rd ed. New York, NY: Plenum Medical Book Company, 1989.

Gruber WC, Belshe RB, King JC. Evaluation of Live Attenuated Influenza Vaccines in Children 6–18 Months of Age: Safety, Immunogenicity, and Efficacy. The Journal of Infectious Diseases 1996; 173:1313–1319.

Marwick C. Facing Inevitable Future Flu Seasons, Experts Set 1996 Vaccine and Plan for Unpredictable Pandemic. JAMA 1995; 273:1079–1080.

McBean AM, Babish JD, Warren JL. The Impact and Cost of Influenza in the Elderly. Archives of Internal Medicine 1993; 153:2105–2111.

Mullooly JP, Bennett MD, Hornbrook MC, et al. Influenza Vaccination Programs for Elderly Persons: Cost-effectiveness in a Health Maintenance Organization. Annals of Internal Medicine 1994; 121:947–952.

Nichol KL, Lind A, Margolis KL, et al. The Effectiveness of Vaccination Against Influenza in Healthy, Working Adults. The New England Journal of Medicine 1995; 333:889–893.

Nichol KL, Margolis KL, Wuorenma J, et al. The Efficacy and Cost Effectiveness of Vaccination Against Influenza Among Elderly Persons Living in the Community. The New England Journal of Medicine 1994; 331:778–784.

Patriarca PA, Strikas RA. Influenza Vaccine for Healthy Adults? The New England Journal of Medicine 1995; 333:933–934.

Sullivan KM, Monto AS, Longini IM. Estimates of the U.S. Health Impact of Influenza. American Journal of Public Health 1993; 83:1712–1716.

APPENDIX 13

Insulin-Dependent Diabetes Mellitus

Insulin-dependent diabetes mellitus (IDDM) is becoming one of the most studied autoimmune diseases. The pathogenesis of IDDM involves a sequence of events ultimately leading to the destruction of beta cells of the pancreas which normally function as the insulin-producing cells. First, there must be a genetic susceptibility to the disease. Next, an environmental event, possibly a virus, initiates the disease process. Once the disease has been triggered, an inflammatory response called "insulitis" begins in the pancreas. Insulitis is an inflammatory infiltrate composed mainly of T lymphocytes which invade the cells of the pancreas. The fourth step is a transformation in the surface of the beta cells causing the activation of the autoimmune response. This response occurs because the beta cell is no longer recognized as "self" but is targeted as a "nonself" foreign cell. As a result, the beta cells are destroyed, which leads to the appearance of diabetes mellitus.

DISEASE BURDEN

Epidemiology

For the purposes of the calculations in this report, the committee estimated that there are approximately 30,000 new cases of insulin-dependent diabetes mellitus (IDDM) each year in the United States. It was assumed that the incidence varies slightly with age, but that the highest incidence occurs in people between 5 and 34 years of age.

233

Disease Scenarios

For the purposes of the calculation in this report, the committee assumed that there are two phases of health states associated with IDDM. During the first 20 years, it is assumed that on average, patients experience minor discomforts and only occasional, serious health incidents. This phase was assumed to be associated with a health utility index (HUI) of .97. During the second phase, which lasts for the duration of the person's life, there are many possible complications with varying impacts on a HUI. On average, it was assumed that this phase was associated with an HUI of .79. It was assumed that patients with IDDM, on average, experience a decrease in life expectancy of approximately 12 years. This was calculated as one-third reduction of life expectancy at the time of onset of the disease.

COST INCURRED BY DISEASE

Table A13-1 summarizes the health care costs incurred by IDDM. For the purposes of the calculations in this report, it was assumed that 70% of patients receive conventional treatment for IDDM and 30% receive intensive treatment. It is assumed that there are costs associated with the diagnostic and very early phase of treatment, with the disease management during the 20-year period that was assumed to be free of chronic, serious sequelae, and with the disease management during the second phase, as well as costs associated with serious complications.

It will be assumed that a therapeutic vaccine strategy will only reduce costs associated with long-term management of disease and treatment of complications. The initial diagnostic phase will not be eliminated. Therefore, only the preventable costs will be described in detail. Costs incurred during the first 20 years of disease management include outpatient visits to specialists (endocrinologists and ophthalmologists, for example) and associated diagnostics, occasional visits to diabetes case managers/educators, and treatment for severe hypoglycemia in some patients. Self-care supplies are assumed to include insulin, syringes, and blood glucose monitoring supplies. It is assumed that patients in intensive treatment incur higher costs due to more frequent physician visits, diagnostics, and supplies.

Costs incurred due to serious complications associated with IDDM are also approximated for the calculations in the report. For example, it was assumed that 60% of people with IDDM will require treatment for retinopathy, renal evaluation and angiotensin-converting enzyme-inhibitor medication, and neurologic evaluation. It is assumed that 20% incur additional costs associated with blindness and end-stage renal disease. It was also assumed that a small percentage of patients will require amputation and associated costs.

The committee assumed that it will take 15 years until licensure of a therapeutic IDDM vaccine and that $360 million needs to be invested. Table 4-1 summarizes vaccine development assumptions for all vaccines considered in this report.

For the purposes of the calculations in this report, it is assumed that the costs associated with diagnostic phase would be incurred even with a treatment vaccine strategy. Therefore, only the costs of the treatment phase will be assumed to be averted with a vaccine strategy.

VACCINE DEVELOPMENT

The committee assumed that it will take 15 years until licensure of a therapeutic IDDM vaccine and that $360 million needs to be invested. Table 4-1 summarizes vaccine development assumptions for all vaccines considered in this report.

VACCINE PROGRAM CONSIDERATIONS

Target Population

For the purposes of the calculations in this report, it is assumed that the target population for this vaccine is all newly diagnosed cases of IDDM. It was assumed that 90% of the target population would utilize the vaccine.

Vaccine Schedule, Efficacy, and Costs

For the purposes of the calculations in this report, it was estimated that this vaccine would cost $500 per dose and that administration costs would be $10 per dose. Default assumptions for therapeutic vaccines of a 3-dose series and 40% effectiveness were accepted. Table 4-1 summarizes vaccine program assumptions for all vaccines considered in this report.

RESULTS

If a vaccine program for IDDM were implemented today and the vaccine was 100% efficacious and utilized by 100% of the target population, the annualized present value of the QALYs gained would be 170,000. Using committee assumptions of less-than-ideal efficacy and utilization and including time and monetary costs until a vaccine program is implemented, the annualized present value of the QALYs gained would be 38,000.

236

Table A13-1 Health Care Costs Associated with IDDM

	% of Cases	Duration (years)	% with Care	Cost per Unit	Units per Case	Form of Treatment
First 20 years	100%					
CONVENTIONAL THERAPY—70%						
Treatment phase						Yearly
Hypoglycemia		20.00	20%	$500	1.0	Treatment of severe hypoglycemia
		20.00	35%	$100	1.0	Treatment modification
Physician visits and diagnostics		20.00	35%	$150	4.0	Quarterly visit plus diagnostic
		20.00	35%	$150	2.0	Semiannual visit plus diagnostic
		20.00	35%	$150	1.0	Specialist visit plus diagnostic
		20.00	35%	$50	1.0	Case management, counseling
Self-management		20.00	70%	$15	18.0	Insulin
		20.00	70%	$100	12.0	Other supplies
INTENSIVE THERAPY—30%						
Treatment phase						Yearly
Hypoglycemia		20.00	15%	$500	1.0	Treatment of severe hypoglycemia
Physician visits and diagnostics		20.00	30%	$150	1.0	Quarterly visit (endocrinologist)
		20.00	30%	$500	1.0	Annual visit (e.g., ophthalmologist)
		20.00	30%	$50	2.0	Case management, counseling
Self-management		20.00	30%	$16	24.0	Insulin
		20.00	30%	$200	12.0	Other supplies
Remainder of life	100%					

CONVENTIONAL THERAPY					
Hypoglycemia	Treatment of severe hypoglycemia	15.00	15%	$500	1.0
	Treatment modification	15.00	5%	$220	1.0
Physician visits and diagnostics	Quarterly visit	15.00	70%	$80	2.0
	Semiannual visit	15.00	70%	$100	1.0
	Annual visit	15.00	70%	$250	1.0
	Case management, counseling	15.00	70%	$50	1.0
Self-management	Insulin	15.00	70%	$16	24.0
INTENSIVE THERAPY					
Hypoglycemia	Treatment of severe hypoglycemia	15.00	30%	$500	1.0
Physician visits and diagnostics	Monthly visit	15.00	30%	$70	8.0
	Quarterly visit	15.00	30%	$120	2.0
	Semiannual visit	15.00	30%	$120	1.0
	Annual visit	15.00	30%	$280	1.0
	Case management, counseling	15.00	30%	$50	1.0
Self-management	Insulin	15.00	30%	$16	24.0
	Other supplies	15.00	30%	$2,000	1.0
COMPLICATIONS (conventional and intensive treatment)					
Retinopathy					
Episodic	Photocoagulation		60%	$950	1.0
Chronic treatment	Blindness	7.00	20%	$1,900	1
Nephropathy					
Episodic	Renal evaluation		60%	$1,100	1.0
Chronic treatment	End-stage renal disease treatment (per year)	7.00	20%	$46,000	1
Neuropathy					
Episodic	Neurologic evaluation		60%	$125	1.0
	Lower extremity amputation		5%	$31,225	1.0

If a vaccine program for IDDM were implemented today and the vaccine was 100% efficacious and utilized by 100% of the target population, the annualized present value of the health care costs saved would be $2.5 billion. Using committee assumptions of less-than-ideal efficacy and utilization and including time and monetary costs until a vaccine program is implemented, the annualized present value of the health care costs saved would be $550 million.

If a vaccine program for IDDM were implemented today and the vaccine was 100% efficacious and utilized by 100% of the target population, the annualized present value of the program cost would be $45 million. Using committee assumptions of less-than-ideal efficacy and utilization and including time and monetary costs until a vaccine program is implemented, the annualized present value of the program cost would be $25 million.

Using committee assumptions of time and costs until licensure, the fixed cost of vaccine development has been amortized and is $10.8 million for an IDDM vaccine.

If a vaccine program were implemented today and the vaccine were 100% efficacious and utilized by 100% of the target population, the annualized present value of the cost per QALY gained is -$14,500. A negative value represents a saving in costs in addition to a saving in QALYs. Using committee assumptions of less-than-ideal utilization and including time and monetary costs until a vaccine program is implemented, the annualized present value of the cost per QALY gained is -$13,500.

See Chapters 4 and 5 for details on the methods and assumptions used by the committee for the results reported.

READING LIST

DERI Mortality Study Group. International Analysis of Insulin-Dependent Diabetes Mellitus Mortality: A Preventable Mortality Perspective. American Journal of Epidemiology 1995; 142:612–618.

Gorham ED, Garland FC, Barrett-Connor E, et al. Incidence of Insulin-Dependent Diabetes Mellitus in Young Adults: Experience of 1,587,630 US Navy Enlisted Personnel. American Journal of Epidemiology 1993; 138:984–987.

Metcalfe MA, Baum JD. Incidence of Insulin-Dependent Diabetes in Children Aged Under 15 years in the British Isles During 1988. BMJ 1991; 302:443–447.

Mølbak AG, Christau B, Marner B, et al. Incidence of Insulin-Dependent Diabetes Mellitus in Age Groups Over 30 years in Denmark. Diabetic Medicine 1994; 11:650–655.

National Institute of Diabetes and Digestive and Kidney Diseases. Diabetes Statistics [WWW document]. URL http://www.niddk.nih.gov/index.htm (accessed September 23, 1996).

Schoenle EJ, Molinari L, Bagot M, et al. Epidemiology of IDDM in Switzerland. Diabetes Care 1994; 17:955–960.

APPENDIX 14

Melanoma

Melanoma arises from melanocytes, which are pigment cells normally found in the epidermis and occasionally in the dermis. Melanocytes that invade the dermis and deeper tissues mark the development of invasive malignant melanoma.

Malignant melanoma can be clinically divided into four main types: superficial spreading melanoma, nodular melanoma, lentigo maligna melanoma, and acral lentiginous melanoma.

DISEASE BURDEN

Epidemiology

For the purposes of the calculations in this report, the committee estimated that there are approximately 35,000 new cases of melanoma every year in the United States. The incidence increases with age. See Table A14-1.

Disease Scenarios

For the purposes of the calculations in this report, the committee assumed that melanoma is represented by 4 disease scenarios by time of diagnosis: local disease (82% of new cases) and regional disease with no subsequent metastases (8% of new cases) from which there is recovery, regional disease with subsequent metastases (6% of new cases), and metastatic disease at diagnosis (4% of new cases). The latter two disease scenarios are associated with premature death. The health utility indexes associated with melanoma range from .93 for

Table A14-1 Incidence and Melanoma

Age Groups	Population	Incidence Rates (per 100,000)	% Distribution of Cases
<1	3,963,000	0.0	0.0000
1-4	16,219,000	0.0	0.0000
5-14	38,056,000	0.2	0.0022
15-24	36,263,000	2.7	0.0279
25-34	41,670,000	8.6	0.1030
35-44	42,149,000	14.9	0.1808
45-54	30,224,000	20.7	0.1798
55-64	21,241,000	27.4	0.1673
65-74	18,964,000	33.3	0.1815
75-84	11,088,000	36.1	0.1153
85+	3,598,000	40.8	0.0422
Total	263,435,000	13.2	1.0000
		Total Cases	34,753

23 months of recovery and follow-up from non-metastatic disease to 0.18 for 3 months of treatment for metastatic disease. See Table A14-2.

COST INCURRED BY DISEASE

Table A14-3 summarizes the health care costs incurred by melanoma. For the purposes of the calculations in this report, it was assumed that local disease is associated with costs for outpatient surgery, four specialist physician visits per year for 2 years and, for 75% of patients, 2 physician visits per year for 5 years. Regional disease with no subsequent metastases was associated with outpatient surgery and six specialist physician visits. The recovery phase for this scenario was assumed to involve slightly more physician visits and folllow-up surgery for 90% of patients.

Regional disease associated with development of metastatic disease was associated with costs including extensive surgery, follow-up treatment, multiple visits to a specialist physician and after-care treatment. Patients who present with metastatic melanoma at diagnosis are assumed to require in-home care and multiple visits with a physician for 3 months.

VACCINE DEVELOPMENT

The committee assumed that it will take 7 years until licensure of a therapeutic melanoma vaccine and that $360 million needs to be invested. Appendix 31 summarizes vaccine development assumptions for all vaccines considered in this report.

Table A14-2 Disease Scenarios for Melanoma

	No. of Cases	% of Cases	Committee HUI Values	Duration (years)
Local disease	28,498	82.00%		
surgery			0.84	0.0833 (1 month)
recovery			0.93	1.9167 (23 months)
Regional at diagnosis, no metastases	2,780	8.00%		
treatment phase			0.84	0.5000 (6 months)
recovery			0.93	1.5000 (18 months)
Regional at diagnosis, develop metastatic disease	2,088	6.00%		
treatment			0.63	1.0000 (1 year)
premature death			0.00	13.4023 (quality-adjusted life expectancy)
Metastatic at diagnosis	1,390	4.00%		
treatment			0.18	0.2500 (3 months)
premature death			0.00	13.5750 (quality-adjusted life expectancy) or 5.9855 (unadjusted life expectancy)

Table A14-3 Health Care Costs Associated with Melanoma

	% with Care	Cost per Unit	Units per Case	Form of Treatment
Local disease				
surgery	100%	$2,000	1.0	outpatient surgery
recovery	100%	$100	4.0	physician b/year
follow-up	75%	$50	2.0	physician a/year
Regional at diagnosis, no metastases				
treatment phase	100%	$2,000	1.0	outpatient surgery
	100%	$100	6.0	physician b
recovery	90%	$100	4.0	physician b/year
	90%	$2,000	1.0	follow-up treatment
follow-up	75%	$100	2.0	physician b/year
Regional at diagnosis, develop metastatic disease				
treatment	100%	$4,000	1.0	surgery
	100%	$2,000	1.0	follow-up treatment
	100%	$100	12.0	physician b
	100%	$3,000	1.0	aftercare
Metastatic at diagnosis				
	100%	100	6.0	physician b
treatment	100%	$3,000	1.0	aftercare

VACCINE PROGRAM CONSIDERATIONS

Target Population

For the purposes of the calculations in this report, it is assumed that the target population for this vaccine is all newly diagnosed cases of melanoma. It was assumed that 90% of the target population would utilize the vaccine.

Vaccine Schedule, Efficacy, and Costs

For the purposes of the calculations in this report, it was estimated that this vaccine would cost $500 per dose and that administration costs would be $10 per dose. Default assumptions for therapeutic vaccines of a 3-dose series and 40% effectiveness were accepted. Table 4-1 summarizes vaccine program assumptions for all vaccines considered in this report.

RESULTS

If a vaccine program for melanoma were implemented today and the vaccine was 100% efficacious and utilized by 100% of the target population, the annualized present value of the QALYs gained would be 51,000. Using committee assumptions of less-than-ideal efficacy and utilization and including time and monetary costs until a vaccine program is implemented, the annualized present value of the QALYs gained would be 14,000.

If a vaccine program for melanoma were implemented today and the vaccine was 100% efficacious and utilized by 100% of the target population, the annualized present value of the health care costs saved would be $130 million. Using committee assumptions of less-than-ideal efficacy and utilization and including time and monetary costs until a vaccine program is implemented, the annualized present value of the health care costs saved would be $36.1 million.

If a vaccine program for melanoma were implemented today and the vaccine was 100% efficacious and utilized by 100% of the target population, the annualized present value of the program cost would be $53.2 million. Using committee assumptions of less-than-ideal efficacy and utilization and including time and monetary costs until a vaccine program is implemented, the annualized present value of the program cost would be $36.7 million.

Using committee assumptions of time and costs until licensure, the fixed cost of vaccine development has been amortized and is $10.8 million for a melanoma vaccine.

If a vaccine program were implemented today and the vaccine were 100% efficacious and utilized by 100% of the target population, the annualized present value of the cost per QALY gained is -$1,500. A negative value represents a saving in costs in addition to a saving in QALYs. Using committee assumptions of less-than-ideal utilization and including time and monetary costs until a vaccine program is implemented, the annualized present value of the cost per QALY gained is $800.

See Chapters 4 and 5 for details on the methods and assumptions used by the committee for the results reported.

READING LIST

Miller BA, Kolonel LN, Bernstein L, et al. (eds). Racial/Ethnic Patterns of Cancer in the United States 1988-1992, National Cancer Institute. NIH Pub. No. 96-4104. Bethesda, MD, 1996.

Multiple Sclerosis

Multiple sclerosis (MS), the most common of the demyelinating diseases, is characterized by many scattered discrete areas of demyelination. These plaques are the pathologic hallmark of this disease appearing in the white matter areas of the central nervous system (CNS). MS has multiple presentations depending on the location foci of demyelination within the CNS. Some of the common signs of this disease include impaired vision, involuntary eye movements, speech impairments, weakened sense of vibration and position, ataxia and intention tremor, weakness or paralysis of one or more limbs, spasticity, and bladder complications.

At the site of active lesions are accumulations of T-lymphocyte and monocyte macrophages around venules and at plaque margins where myelin is being destroyed. The actual breakdown of myelin can be attributed to the soluble mediators (lymphokines and monokines) released by the inflammatory cells which invade the white matter.

DISEASE BURDEN

Epidemiology

For the purposes of the calculations in this report, the committee estimated that there are 8,000 new cases of multiple sclerosis per year in the United States. It was assumed that all new cases occur between the ages of 15 and 54 years of age.

Table A15-1 Health Care Costs Associated with Multiple Sclerosis

	% of Cases	Duration (years)	% with Care	Cost per Unit	Units per Case	Form of Treatment
Benign	15.00%					
Treatment per year		43.3484	100%	$100	2.0	Physician B
		43.3484	100%	$500	1.0	Diagnostic C
Relapsing/remitting (secondary progressive)	65%					
Treatment per year		43.3484	25%	$3,000	1.0	Hospitalization
		43.3484	25%	$150	4.0	Physician C
		43.3484	25%	$500	1.0	Diagnostic C
		43.3484	100%	$100	6.0	Physician B
		43.3484	100%	$500	1.0	Diagnostic C
Primary Progressive	15.00%					
Treatment per year		20.0000	25%	$225	365.0	Nursing home care
		20.0000	100%	$100	12.0	Physician B
		20.0000	100%	$500	1.0	Diagnostic C
		20.0000	50%	$3,000	1.0	Hospitalization or acute care/rehabilitation
		20.0000	50%	$150	4.0	Physician C
Fulminant	5.00%					
Treatment per year		5.0000	75%	$225	365.0	Nursing home care
		5.0000	100%	$100	12.0	Physician B
		5.0000	25%	$3,000	1.0	Hospitalization or acute care/rehabilitation
		5.0000	25%	$150	4.0	Physician C
		5.0000	100%	$500	1.0	Diagnostic C

Disease Scenarios

For the purposes of the calculation in this report, the committee assumed that there were four scenarios associated with MS. It was estimated that 15% of people with MS experience a lifelong, mild, intermittent disease, associated with an average health utility index (HUI) of .97. It was assumed that most (65%) cases of MS are associated with a relapsing, remitting MS that is associated with an average HUI of .61. 15% of patients were assumed to experience a chronic, progressive disease for 20 years until death from the disease. This is associated with an HUI of .47. The rapid, fulminant expression of MS was assumed to occur in 5% of patients and be associated with a 5-year period of an HUI of .31 until the time of death from the disease.

COST INCURRED BY DISEASE

Table A15-1 summarizes the health care costs incurred by MS. For the purposes of the calculations in this report, it was assumed that for all scenarios there is a diagnostic phase, followed by a treatment phase which lasts the duration of the patients lifetime. The diagnostic phase was estimated to be approximately the same for all patients with MS: hospitalization and associated inpatient physician costs, visits to a specialist, and extensive diagnostics. For the purposes of the calculations in this report, it was assumed that no costs associated with the diagnostic phase of MS would be averted with a therapeutic vaccine strategy and are not described here. Chronic, treatment costs would be averted by a vaccine strategy.

The costs and patterns of care incurred during treatment phase vary greatly depending on the type of MS experienced. For example, it was assumed that all patients with benign and with relapsing-remitting MS visit a specialist and receive a diagnostic work-up each year for the duration of their lifetime. It was assumed that on average, 25% of patients with relapsing-remitting MS but none of the patients with benign MS require hospitalization each year. Patients with primary progressive MS were assumed to incur annual costs over 20 years associated with diagnostics, multiple specialist visits, hospitalization (50% of patients per year), and nursing home care (25% of patients). Patients with fulminant MS were assumed to incur annual costs for 5 years associated with diagnostics, specialist visits, hospitalization (25% of patients per year) and nursing home care (for 75% of patients).

VACCINE DEVELOPMENT

The committee assumed that it will take 15 years until licensure of a therapeutic MS vaccine and that $360 million needs to be invested. Table 4-1 summarizes vaccine development assumptions for all vaccines considered in this report.

VACCINE PROGRAM CONSIDERATIONS

Target Population

For the purposes of the calculations in this report, it is assumed that the target population for this vaccine is all new cases of MS at time of diagnosis. It was assumed that 90% of the target population would utilize the vaccine.

Vaccine Schedule, Efficacy, and Costs

For the purposes of the calculations in this report, it was estimated that this vaccine would cost $500 per dose and that administration costs would be $10 per dose. Default assumptions of a 3-dose series was accepted. For therapeutic vaccines it was assumed that effectiveness is 40%. Table 4-1 summarizes vaccine program assumptions for all vaccines considered in this report.

RESULTS

If a vaccine program for MS were implemented today and the vaccine was 100% efficacious and utilized by 100% of the target population, the annualized present value of the QALYs gained would be 68,000. Using committee assumptions of less-than-ideal efficacy and utilization and including time and monetary costs until a vaccine program is implemented, the annualized present value of the QALYs gained would be 15,000.

If a vaccine program for MS were implemented today and the vaccine was 100% efficacious and utilized by 100% of the target population, the annualized present value of the health care costs saved would be $830 million. Using committee assumptions of less-than-ideal efficacy and utilization and including time and monetary costs until a vaccine program is implemented, the annualized present value of the health care costs saved would be $180 million.

If a vaccine program for MS were implemented today and the vaccine was 100% efficacious and utilized by 100% of the target population, the annualized present value of the program cost would be $12.2 million. Using committee assumptions of less-than-ideal efficacy and utilization and including time and monetary costs until a vaccine program is implemented, the annualized present value of the program cost would be $6.7 million.

Using committee assumptions of time and costs until licensure, the fixed cost of vaccine development has been amortized and is $10.8 million for a MS vaccine.

If a vaccine program were implemented today and the vaccine were 100% efficacious and utilized by 100% of the target population, the annualized present value of the cost per QALY gained is -$12,000. A negative value represents a saving in costs in addition to a saving in QALYs. Using committee assumptions of less-than-ideal utilization and including time and monetary costs until a vaccine program is implemented, the annualized present value of the cost per QALY gained is -$11,000.

See Chapters 4 and 5 for details on the methods and assumptions used by the committee for the results reported.

READING LIST

Anderson DW, Ellenberg JH, Leventhal CM, et al. Revised Estimate of the Prevalence of Multiple Sclerosis in the United States. Annals of Neurology 1992; 31:333–336.

Koch-Henriksen N. Incidence of Multiple Sclerosis in Denmark 1948–1982: A Descriptive Nationwide Study. Neuroepidemiology 1992; 11:1–10.

Miller CM, Hens M. Multiple Sclerosis: A Literature Review. Journal of Neuroscience Nursing 1993; 25:174–179.

Multiple Sclerosis Foundation. 1997. Multiple Sclerosis Statistics. URL http://www.msfacts.org/stats.htm (accessed September 26, 1997).

Warren S, Warren KG. Prevalence, Incidence, and Characteristics of Multiple Sclerosis in Westlock County, Alberta, Canada. Neurology 1993; 43:1760–1763.

APPENDIX 16

Mycobacterium tuberculosis

In the majority of infected individuals, the primary lesions of mycobacterium tuberculosis (TB) heal completely and leave no clinical evidence of prior infection except hypersensitivity to tuberculin. In some however, the primary infection progresses directly and evolves into a pneumonic process as the organisms spread through the bronchi or when a tuberculous node ruptures into a bronchus. Contiguous spread can cause infection in the pleural and pericardial spaces. At this stage, pleurisy, which is usually abrupt and resembles bacterial pneumonia with fever, chest pain, and shortness of breath are present.

Secondary tuberculosis is usually caused by organisms seeded in the apices of the lungs during the primary infection. These foci may evolve soon after seeding or after a long period of dormancy. Small patches of pneumonia develop around the foci. As the disease progresses, there is an insidious onset and development of nonspecific symptoms such as fatigue, fever, anorexia, night sweats, and general wasting. Cough and sputum denote more advanced disease.

Miliary tuberculosis occurs when the tubercle bacilli gain access to the lymphatics and bloodstream and seed distant organs. Miliary lesions may develop in almost any organ of the body, but of the most favored sites are bones and joints, the genitourinary tract, meninges, lymph nodes, and peritoneum. Miliary tuberculosis in its primary infection stage, when associated with meningitis, is responsible for deaths in young children.

See Appendix 28 for more information.

DISEASE BURDEN

Epidemiology

For the purposes of the calculations in this report, the committee estimated that there are approximately 23,000 new cases of mycobacterium tuberculosis (TB) in the United States each year. It was assumed that incidence of TB infection increases with age. It is assumed that half the cases occur in people belonging to a high-risk group and half occur in people in multi-drug resistant areas. It was estimated that there are approximately 1,500 deaths associated with TB annually. See Table A16-1.

Disease Scenarios

For the purposes of the calculation in this report, the committee assumed that most cases of TB infection result in pulmonary disease. Extrapulmonary disease is seen in the remaining 12% of infected people. The health utility index (HUI) was assumed to range from 1.0 for treatment of asymptomatic people (described below) to .89 for the 9-month treatment phase for pulmonary TB and .72 for 20 days of severe extrapulmonary TB (including hospitalization). See Table A16-2.

COST INCURRED BY DISEASE

Table 16-3 summarizes the health care costs incurred by TB infections. For the purposes of the calculations in this report, it was assumed that costs are incurred for both active and asymptomatic (suspected and latent) cases of TB. It is assumed that for every case of confirmed, active TB disease, treatment for 3 to 5 asymptomatic (suspected or latent) cases of TB is required until TB infection is confirmed. Asymptomatic, latent infections require additional treatment. These treatments are assumed to include two visits to a general physician, three visits to a nurse, diagnostic evaluation, and medications. Although the model assumes that all suspected cases of TB undergo the care described above, it is assumed that adherence to a 6-month treatment regime for latent infections is not complete (e.g., that 40% of patients take medications for only 3 months).

Health care costs incurred for pulmonary and extrapulmonary TB are assumed to involve hospitalization followed by 9 months of outpatient treatment. This follow-up involves monthly costs for a physician visit, diagnostic evaluation, and medication.

Table A16-1 Incidence and Mortality Rates of TB Infections

Age Groups	Population	Incidence Rates (per 100,000)	% Distribution of Cases	Cases
<1	3,963,000	2.66	0.0046	106
1-4	16,219,000	2.66	0.0189	432
5-14	38,056,000	2.66	0.0445	1,014
15-24	36,263,000	4.69	0.0746	1,700
25-34	41,670,000	9.82	0.1794	4,090
35-44	42,149,000	9.82	0.1815	4,137
45-54	30,224,000	11.63	0.1542	3,515
55-64	21,241,000	11.63	0.1084	2,470
65-74	18,964,000	15.85	0.1318	3,005
75-84	11,088,000	15.85	0.0771	1,757
85+	3,598,000	15.85	0.0250	570
Total	263,435,000	8.65	1.0000	22,795

Age Groups	Population	Mortality Rates (per 100,000)	% Distribution of Cases	Cases
<1	3,963,000	0.00	0.0000	0
1-4	16,219,000	0.02	0.0020	3
5-14	38,056,000	0.00	0.0007	1
15-24	36,263,000	0.04	0.0102	15
25-34	41,670,000	0.18	0.0495	73
35-44	42,149,000	0.33	0.0928	137
45-54	30,224,000	0.50	0.1030	152
55-64	21,241,000	0.96	0.1382	204
65-74	18,964,000	1.65	0.2121	313
75-84	11,088,000	3.22	0.2419	357
85+	3,598,000	6.14	0.1497	221
Total	263,435,000	0.56	1.0000	1,476

VACCINE DEVELOPMENT

The committee assumed that it will take 15 years until licensure of a TB vaccine and that $360 million needs to be invested. Table 4-1 summarizes vaccine development assumptions for all vaccines considered in this report.

VACCINE PROGRAM CONSIDERATIONS

Target Population

For the purposes of the calculations in this report, it is assumed that the target population for this vaccine is 500,000 high-risk people. 300,000 of those people are high-risk individuals in multi-drug-resistant areas. It was assumed that 90% of the selective high-risk population would utilize the vaccine and that

Table A16-2 Disease Scenarios for TB Infection

	No. of Cases	% of Cases	Committee HUI Values	Duration (years)
Total Deaths (from acute infection)	1,476			
Total Cases (reported)	22,795			
Asymptomatic—suspect suspect cases (treatment begun)	68,385	300.00%	1.0000	0.2500 (3 months)
Asymptomatic—latent infection preventive treatment for latent infection	113,975	500.00%	1.0000	0.5000 (6 months)
Pulmonary TB inpatient	20,060	88.00%	0.8700	0.0548 (20 days)
Pulmonary TB outpatient	19,057	83.60%	0.8900	0.7500 (9 months)
Extrapulmonary TB inpatient	2,735	12.00%	0.7200	0.0548 (20 days)
Extrapulmonary TB outpatient	2,462	10.80%	0.8600	0.7500 (9 months)

60% of the targeted population in multi-drug-resistant areas would receive the vaccine.

Vaccine Schedule, Efficacy, and Costs

For the purposes of the calculations in this report, it was estimated that this vaccine would cost $50 per dose and that administration costs would be $10 per dose. Default assumptions of a 3-dose series and 75% effectiveness were accepted. Table 4-1 summarizes vaccine program assumptions for all vaccines considered in this report.

RESULTS

If a vaccine program for TB were implemented today and the vaccine was 100% efficacious and utilized by 100% of the target population, the annualized present value of the QALYs gained would be $4,000. Using committee assumptions of less-than-ideal efficacy and utilization and including time and monetary costs until a vaccine program is implemented, the annualized present value of the QALYs gained would be 1,300.

Table A16-3 Health Care Costs Associated with TB Infection

	% with Care	Cost per Unit	Units per Case	Form of Treatment
Asymptomatic—suspect				
treated (detected in screening, etc.)				
suspect cases: 3 months treatment until culture results available	100%	$50	2.0	physician a
	100%	$25	3.0	nurse visit
	100%	$50	1.0	diagnostic a
	100%	$50	3.0	medication b
Asymptomatic—latent				
treated (detected in screening, etc.)	75%	$50	3.0	physician a
preventive treatment for latent infection: 6 months	75%	$25	6.0	nurse visit
estimated 60% complete treatment; rest complete half of treatment	100%	$50	1.0	diagnostic a
	60%	$50	6.0	medication b: completes course
	40%	$50	3.0	medication b: completes half course
Pulmonary TB				
inpatient	100%	$6,000	1.0	hospitalization
	100%	$100	3.0	physician b
	100%	$50	1.0	diagnostic a
	25%	$500	1.0	diagnostic c
Pulmonary TB				
outpatient	100%	$50	9.0	physician a
	100%	$50	9.0	diagnostic a
	100%	$50	9.0	medication b
Extrapulmonary TB				
inpatient	100%	$6,000	1.0	hospitalization
	100%	$100	3.0	physician b
	100%	$50	1.0	diagnostic b
	25%	$500	1.0	diagnostic c
Extrapulmonary TB				
outpatient	100%	$50	9.0	physician a
	100%	$50	9.0	diagnostic a
	100%	$50	9.0	medication b

If a vaccine program for TB were implemented today and the vaccine was 100% efficacious and utilized by 100% of the target population, the annualized present value of the health care costs saved would be $100 million. Using committee assumptions of less-than-ideal efficacy and utilization and including time and monetary costs until a vaccine program is implemented, the annualized present value of the health care costs saved would be $34.2 million.

If a vaccine program for TB were implemented today and the vaccine was 100% efficacious and utilized by 100% of the target population, the annualized present value of the program cost would be $90 million. Using committee assumptions of less-than-ideal efficacy and utilization and including time and monetary costs until a vaccine program is implemented, the annualized present value of the program cost would be $35.9 million.

Using committee assumptions of time and costs until licensure, the fixed cost of vaccine development has been amortized and is $10.8 million for a TB vaccine.

If a vaccine program were implemented today and the vaccine were 100% efficacious and utilized by 100% of the target population, the annualized present value of the cost per QALY gained is –$3,000. A negative value represents a saving in costs in addition to a saving in QALYs. Using committee assumptions of less-than-ideal utilization and including time and monetary costs until a vaccine program is implemented, the annualized present value of the cost per QALY gained is $9,500.

See Chapters 4 and 5 for details on the methods and assumptions used by the committee for the results reported.

READING LIST

Brewer TF, Heymann SJ, Colditz GA, et al. Evaluation of Tuberculosis Control Policies Using Computer Simulation. JAMA 1996; 276:1898–1903.

Brown RE, Miller B, Taylor WR, et al. Health-Care Expenditure for Tuberculosis in the United States. Archives of Internal Medicine 1995; 155:1595–1600.

CDC. The Role of BCG Vaccine in the Prevention and Control of Tuberculosis in the United States. Morbidity and Mortality Weekly Report 1996; 45:1–18.

CDC. Tuberculosis Morbidity—United States, 1995. Morbidity and Mortality Weekly Report 1996; 45: 365–370.

Haas DW, Des Prez RM. Mycobacterium Tuberculosis. In: Principles and Practice of Infectious Diseases. GL Mandell, JE Bennett, Dolin R eds. New York, NY: Churchill Livingstone, 1995, pp. 2213–2243.

Miller B, Castro KG. Sharpen Available Tools for Tuberculosis Control, but New Tools Needed for Elimination. JAMA 1996; 276:1916–1917.

Singh GK, Kochanek KD, MacDorman MF. Advance Report of Final Mortality Statistics, 1994. Monthly Vital Statistics Report 1996; 45.

Smith MHD, Starke JR, Marquis JR. Tuberculosis and Opportunistic Mycobacterial Infections. In: Textbook of Pediatric Infectious Diseases. RD Feigin and JD Cherry eds. Philadelphia, PA: WB Saunder Company, 1992, pp. 1321–1362.

APPENDIX 17

Neisseria gonorrhea

DISEASE BURDEN

Epidemiology

For the purposes of the calculations in this report, the committee estimated that there are 1 million new cases of gonorrhea infection each year in the United States. Slightly more than half of these occur in males. It was assumed that 90% of cases occur in people between 15 and 34 years of age. Mortality was presumed to be minimal; 5 deaths were included for women per year (consequences of serious sequelae, for example). See Table A17-1 for a summary of the age distribution of gonorrhea infections.

Disease Scenarios

For the purposes of the calculation in this report, the committee assumed that 50% of cases in women are asymptomatic, but that half of those cases are detected through screening programs and receive treatment. The other 50% of cases experience mild manifestations, such as cervicitis, urethritis, or endometritis. More serious acute health consequences associated with gonorrhea infections in women include pelvic inflammatory disease (PID), salpingitis, and perihepatitis. Consequences of PID are assumed to occur with a 5-year lag from infection and include ectopic pregnancy, chronic pelvic pain, and infertility. The health utility index and length of time spent in the health state range from .85 HUI for 7 days (cervicitis) to .46 HUI for 2 days (surgery for PID) to .6 HUI for more than 20 years (chronic pelvic pain).

257

Table A17-1 Incidence of *N. gonorrhea* Infection in Women and Men

Age Groups	Female Population	Incidence Rates (per 100,000)	% Distribution of Cases	Cases
<1	1,933,000	0.00	0.0000	0
1-4	7,905,000	29.10	0.0050	2,300
5-14	18,554,000	111.57	0.0450	20,700
15-24	17,747,000	1,555.19	0.6000	276,000
25-34	20,835,000	662.35	0.3000	138,000
35-44	21,238,000	75.81	0.0350	16,100
45-54	15,447,000	29.78	0.0100	4,600
55-64	11,140,000	20.65	0.0050	2,300
65-74	10,544,000	0.00	0.0000	0
75-84	6,814,000	0.00	0.0000	0
85+	2,593,000	0.00	0.0000	0
Total	134,750,000	341.37	1.0000	460,000
Age Groups	Male Population	Incidence Rates (per 100,000)	% Distribution of Cases	Cases
<1	2,030,000	0.00	0.0000	0
1-4	8,314,000	32.48	0.0050	2,700
5-14	19,502,000	124.60	0.0450	24,300
15-24	18,516,000	1,749.84	0.6000	324,000
25-34	20,835,000	777.54	0.3000	162,000
35-44	20,911,000	90.38	0.0350	18,900
45-54	14,777,000	36.54	0.0100	5,400
55-64	10,101,000	26.73	0.0050	2,700
65-74	8,420,000	0.00	0.0000	0
75-84	4,274,000	0.00	0.0000	0
85+	1,005,000	0.00	0.0000	0
Total	128,685,000	419.63	1.0000	540,000

For the purposes of the calculations in this report, the committee assumed that 15% of cases in men are asymptomatic and untreated. The overwhelming utility index and length of time spent in the health state range from .85 HUI for 7 days (cervicitis) to .46 HUI for 2 days (surgery for PID) to .6 HUI for more than 20 years (chronic pelvic pain).

For the purposes of the calculations in this report, the committee assumed that 15% of cases in men are asymptomatic and untreated. The overwhelming proportion of symptomatic cases involve urethritis, which was assumed to be associated with an HUI of .84 and 7 days duration. A small percentage of men infected with gonorrhea experience epididymitis. The HUI and length of time spent in the health state for these manifestations range from .84 HUI for 7 days (urethritis) to .3 HUI for 3 days (hospitalization for epididymitis).

A small fraction of both men and women infected with gonorrhea experience disseminated infections. Hospitalization for these patients is associated with an HUI of .52 for 4 days; outpatient treatment is associated with a week of a higher HUI state. See Table A17-2 for a summary of the disease states associated with gonorrhea infections.

Table A17-2 Disease Scenarios for *N. Gonorrhea* Infection in Women and Men

	% of Cases	Committee HUI Values	Duration (years)
WOMEN			
Total Cases	460,000		
Asymptomatic	50.0%	1.00	
untreated	25.0%		
treated (detected in screening, etc.)	25.0%		
Mild (cervicitis, urethritis, endometritis, bartholinitis)	50.0%		
outpatient		0.85	0.0192 (7 days)
Serious (PID, salpingitis, perihepatitis)—outpatient only	10.0%	0.63	0.0274 (10 days)
Serious (PID, salpingitis, perihepatitis)—inpatient			
inpatient—no surgery	7.5%	0.57	0.0110 (4 days)
inpatient with surgery	2.5%	0.46	0.0055 (2 days)
outpatient after inpatient	10.0%	0.83	0.0274 (10 days)
Serious (PID, etc.)	0.8%		
inpatient with bilateral salpingo-oophorectomy		0.40	0.0027 (1 day)
outpatient after inpatient		0.76	0.0274 (10 days)
infertility		0.82	23.6523 (remaining lifetime at onset)
ALL PID sequelae: 5-year lag from infection			
Ectopic Pregnancy— Outpatient only	3.3%	0.58	0.0767 (4 weeks)
Ectopic Pregnancy—Inpatient	3.3%		
inpatient		0.23	0.0082 (3 days)
outpatient after inpatient		0.66	0.0767 (4 weeks)
Chronic pelvic pain	6.6%	0.60	22.7313 (remaining lifetime at onset +5 years) discounted quality adjusted life expectancy at age 28.7
Infertility	4.0%	0.82	22.7313 (remaining lifetime at onset + 5 years); discounted quality adjusted life expectancy at age 28.7
Disseminated gonococcal infections (bacteremia, arthritis, etc.)—outpatient only	0.5%	0.60	0.0219 (8 days)

Continued

Table A17-2 *Continued*

	% of Cases	Committee HUI Values	Duration (years)
Disseminated gonococcal infections (bacteremia, arthritis, etc.)—inpatient	0.5%		
inpatient		0.52	0.0110 (4 days)
outpatient after inpatient		0.78	0.0192 (7 days)
MEN			
Total cases	540,000		
Asymptomatic	15.0%	1.00	
Urethritis	84.0%	0.84	0.0192 (7 days)
Epididymitis—outpatient	0.9%	0.46	0.0192 (7 days)
Epididymitis—inpatient	0.1%	0.30	0.0082 (3 days)
Disseminated gonococcal infections (bacteremia, arthritis, etc.)—outpatient	0.5%	0.60	0.0219 (8 days)
Disseminated gonococcal infections (bacteremia, arthritis, etc.)—inpatient	0.5%		
inpatient		0.52	0.0110 (4 days)
outpatient after inpatient		0.78	0.0192 (7 days)

COST INCURRED BY DISEASE

Table A17-3 summarizes the health care costs incurred by gonorrhea infections. For the purposes of the calculations in this report, it was assumed that for mild acute manifestations in both men and women (e.g., cervicitis and urethritis), health care costs include a limited visit with a physician and inexpensive diagnostics and medications.

Disseminated gonococcal infections in both women and men were assumed to be associated with inpatient costs (hospitalization, diagnostics, specialist physicians) and outpatient costs (similar to that required for inpatient treatment but slightly fewer physician visits).

Outpatient treatment in women of more serious manifestations include increased diagnostic costs above those for cervicitis. Inpatient treatment (e.g., for PID or salpingitis) includes hospitalization costs, physician services (including surgeons and anesthesiologists for those who require surgery) and diagnostics. Outpatient costs following hospitalization include follow-up care with a specialist. Half of the cases of ectopic pregnancy were assumed to be treated as inpatient and half as outpatient. Costs include hospital costs (more for inpatient), specialist physicians, surgeons and anesthesiologists, and diagnostics. A follow-up visit with a specialist was also included. Chronic pelvic pain was associated with numerous physician visits, diagnostics, and medication. 75% of women with chronic pelvic pain were presumed to undergo outpatient laparoscopy, and

Table A17-3 Health Care Costs Associated with *N. gonorrhea* Infection in Women and Men

	% with Care	Cost per Unit	Units per Case	Form of Treatment
WOMEN				
Asymptomatic				
untreated				
treated (detected in screening, etc.)	100%	$50	1	physician a
	100%	$50	1	diagnostic a
	100%	$50	1	medication b
Mild (cervicitis, urethritis, endometritis, bartholinitis)				
outpatient	100%	$50	1	physician a
	100%	$50	1	diagnostic a
	100%	$50	1	medication b
Serious (PID, salpingitis, perihepatitis)				
outpatient	100%	$50	1	physician a
	100%	$100	1	diagnostic b
	100%	$100	1	medication
Serious (PID, salpingitis, perihepatitis)				
inpatient—no surgery	100%	$4,000	1	hospitalization
	100%	$150	3	physician c
	100%	$100	1	diagnostic b
Serious (PID, salpingitis, perihepatitis)				
inpatient with surgery	100%	$4,000	1	hospitalization
	100%	$150	3	physician c
	100%	$500	4	surgical staff
	100%	$100	1	diagnostic b
Serious (PID, salpingitis, perihepatitis)				
outpatient after inpatient	100%	$100	1	physician b
Serious (PID, etc.)				
inpatient and outpatient	100%	$1,550	1	outpatient laparoscopy
ALL PID sequelae: 5-year lag from infection Ectopic Pregnancy— Outpatient PID sequela: 5-year lag				
outpatient only	100%	$1,000	1	laparoscopy
	100%	$500	1	surgical staff
	100%	$500	1	surgical staff
	100%	$50	1	diagnostic a
	100%	$100	1	physician b

Continued

Table A17-3 *Continued*

	% with Care	Cost per Unit	Units per Case	Form of Treatment
Ectopic Pregnancy— Inpatient PID sequela: 5-year lag				
inpatient	100%	$4,000	1	hospitalization
	100%	$150	3	physician c
	100%	$100	1	diagnostic b
	100%	$500	2	surgical staff
outpatient after inpatient	100%	$100	1	physician b
Chronic pelvic pain PID sequela: 5-year lag				
treatment assumed to occur 5 years after onset of infection	100%	$100	1	physician b
duration of condition: remaining lifetime	100%	$50	4	physician a
	100%	$50	1	medication b
	100%	$100	1	diagnostic b *outpatient laparoscopy*
	75%	$1,000	1	hospitalization
	75%	$500	1	surgical staff
	75%	$500	1	surgical staff *lower abdominal* *surgery*
	30%	$4,000	1	hospitalization
	30%	$500	1	surgical staff
	30%	$500	1	surgical staff
	30%	$150	3	physician c
Infertility PID sequela: 5-year lag	50%	$150	6	physician c
treatment assumed to occur 5 years after onset of infection				
duration of condition: remaining lifetime	50%	$500	1	diagnostic c
	50%	$250	1	procedure *outpatient laparoscopy* *(75% of those seeking* *treatment)*
	38%	$1,000	1	hospitalization
	38%	$500	1	surgical staff
	38%	$500	1	surgical staff *tubal surgery (30% of* *those seeking treatment)*
	15%	$1,000	1	outpatient surgery
	15%	$500	1	surgeon
	15%	$500	1	anesthesiology *in vitro fertilization* *(12% of those seeking* *treatment)*
	6%	$4,000	2	per trial

Table A17-3 *Continued*

	% with Care	Cost per Unit	Units per Case	Form of Treatment
Disseminated gonococcal infections (bacteremia, arthritis, etc.)—outpatient				
	100%	$100	2	physician b
	100%	$50	1	culture—gonorrhea
	100%	$50	1	medication
Disseminated gonococcal infections (bacteremia, arthritis, etc.)—inpatient				
	100%	$3,000	1	hospitalization
	100%	$150	3	physician c
	100%	$50	1	diagnostic a
	100%	$50	1	medication b
outpatient after inpatient		$100	1	physician b
MEN				
Asymptomatic (untreated) Urethritis				
	100%	$50	1	physician a
	100%	$50	1	diagnostic a
Epididymitis				
outpatient	100%	$100	1	physician b
	100%	$50	1	physician a
	100%	$50	1	diagnostic a
	100%	$50	1	medication b
Epididymitis				
inpatient	100%	$3,000	1	hospitalization
	100%	$150	3	physician c
	100%	$50	1	physician a
	100%	$50	1	medication b
	50%	$500	1	surgical staff
	50%	$500	1	surgical staff
Disseminated gonococcal infections (bacteremia, arthritis, etc.)—outpatient				
	100%	$100	2	physician b
	100%	$50	1	culture—gonorrhea
	100%	$50	1	medication
Disseminated gonococcal infections (bacteremia, arthritis, etc.)—inpatient				
	100%	$3,000	1	hospitalization
	100%	$150	3	physician c
	100%	$50	1	diagnostic a
	100%	$50	1	medication b
outpatient after inpatient		$100	1	physician b

30% were presumed to undergo abdominal surgery. For the purposes of the calculations in this report, it was assumed that half of women infertile due to gonorrhea infection seek some kind of medical care related to infertility. This includes hysterosalphoingography, outpatient laparoscopy, tubal surgery, and infertility treatment.

Epididymitis in men was estimated to be treated primarily on an outpatient basis and includes costs for both limited visits and specialist physician visits, diagnostics, and medications. For the few patients who undergo surgery, costs for surgeons and anesthesiologist are included.

VACCINE DEVELOPMENT

The committee assumed that it will take 15 years until licensure and that $360 million needs to be invested. Table 4-1 summarizes vaccine development assumptions for all vaccines considered in this report.

VACCINE PROGRAM CONSIDERATIONS

Target Population

For the purposes of the calculations in this report, it is assumed that the target population for this vaccine is adolescents (age 12 years). It was assumed that 50% of the target population would utilize the vaccine.

Vaccine Schedule, Efficacy, and Costs

For the purposes of the calculations in this report, it was estimated that this vaccine would cost $50 per dose and that administration costs would be $10 per dose. Default assumptions of a 3-dose series and 75% effectiveness were accepted. Table 4-1 summarizes vaccine program assumptions for all vaccines considered in this report.

RESULTS

If a vaccine program for *N. gonorrhea* were implemented today and the vaccine were 100% efficacious and utilized by 100% of the target population, the annualized present value of the QALYs gained would be 230,000. Using committee assumptions of less-than-ideal efficacy and utilization and including time and monetary costs until a vaccine program is implemented, the annualized present value of the QALYs gained would be 47,000. Although the proportion of cases are slightly higher in men than in women, the number of QALYs lost due to disease in women is over 200 fold that in men. The more severe nature of the sequelae of infection in women and the chronic nature of several of the sequelae account for this large difference.

If a vaccine program for *N. gonorrhea* were implemented today and the vaccine was 100% efficacious and utilized by 100% of the target population, the annualized present value of the health care costs saved would be $440 million. Using committee assumptions of less-than-ideal efficacy and utilization and including time and monetary costs until a vaccine program is implemented, the annualized present value of the health care costs saved would be $92.1 million.

If a vaccine program for *N. gonorrhea* were implemented today and the vaccine was 100% efficacious and utilized by 100% of the target population, the annualized present value of the program cost would be $680 million. Using committee assumptions of less-than-ideal efficacy and utilization and including time and monetary costs until a vaccine program is implemented, the annualized present value of the program cost would be $190 million.

Using committee assumptions of time and costs until licensure, the fixed cost of vaccine development has been amortized and is $10.8 million for a *N. gonorrhea* vaccine.

If a vaccine program were implemented today and the vaccine was 100% efficacious and utilized by 100% of the target population, the annualized present value of the cost per QALY gained is $1,000. Using committee assumptions of less-than-ideal utilization and including time and monetary costs until a vaccine program is implemented, the annualized present value of the cost per QALY gained is $2,300.

See Chapters 4 and 5 for details on the methods and assumptions used by the committee for the results reported.

READING LIST

Alexander LL, Treiman K, Clarke P. A National Survey of Nurse Practitioner Chlamydia Knowledge and Treatment Practices of Female Patients. Nurse Practitioner 1996; 21:48, 51–4.

Gutman, LT. Gonorrhea. In: Textbook of Pediatric Infectious Diseases. RD Feigin and JD Cherry eds. Philadelphia, PA: WB Saunder Company, 1992, pp. 540–552.

Handsfield HH, Sparling PF. Neisseria Gonorrhoeae. In: Principles and Practice of Infectious Diseases. GL Mandell, JE Bennett, Dolin R eds. New York, NY: Churchill Livingstone, 1995, pp. 1909–1926.

Magid D, Douglas JM, Schwartz JS. Doxycycline Compared with Azithromycin for Treating Women with Genital Chlamydia Trachomatis Infections: An Incremental Cost-Effectiveness Analysis. Annals of Internal Medicine 1996; 124:389–99.

U.S. Bureau of the Census. Statistical Abstract of the U.S.: 1995 (115th edition). Washington, D.C. 1995.

APPENDIX 18

Neisseria meningitidis B

DISEASE BURDEN

Epidemiology

For the purposes of the calculations in this report, the committee estimated that there are 1,200 new cases of *Neisseria meningitidis* B (NMB) infection each year in the United States. Approximately half of these occur in children and infants under 5 years of age. Overall mortality rate was estimated at 0.05 per 100,000, or just under 150 deaths per year in the United States. Table A18-1 illustrates the age distribution of new annual NMB infections.

Disease Scenarios

For the purposes of the calculations in this report, the committee estimated that 65% of new cases of NMB manifest as meningitis. The acute manifestations of meningitis require hospitalization (most often in the intensive care unit or ICU). The committee-estimated health utility index (HUI) associated with those states ranges from 0.24 to 0.39 for those requiring ICU and non-ICU hospitalization, respectively.

Just fewer than 10% of patients with NMB meningitis have acute complications, such as gangrene, arthritis, and cardiac involvement. These complications were associated with a HUI of 0.27. Approximately 3.25% of patients experi-

---

See Appendix 28 for more information.

Table A18-1 Incidence and Mortality Rates for *Neisseria meningitidis* B Epidemiology

Age Groups	Population	Incidence Rates (per 100,000)	% Distribution of Cases
<1	3,963,000	8.78	0.2900
1-4	16,219,000	1.48	0.2000
5-14	38,056,000	0.33	0.1057
15-24	36,263,000	0.33	0.1007
25-34	41,670,000	0.27	0.0927
35-44	42,149,000	0.20	0.0704
45-54	30,224,000	0.20	0.0505
55-64	21,241,000	0.20	0.0355
65-74	18,964,000	0.20	0.0317
75-84	11,088,000	0.20	0.0185
85+	3,598,000	0.20	0.0060
Total	263,435,000	0.46	1.0017
		Total cases	1,200

Age Groups	Population	Mortality Rates (per 100,000)	% Distribution of Cases
<1	3,963,000	1.05	0.2900
1-4	16,219,000	0.18	0.2000
5-14	38,056,000	0.04	0.1057
15-24	36,263,000	0.04	0.1007
25-34	41,670,000	0.03	0.0927
35-44	42,149,000	0.02	0.0704
45-54	30,224,000	0.02	0.0505
55-64	21,241,000	0.02	0.0355
65-74	18,964,000	0.02	0.0317
75-84	11,088,000	0.02	0.0185
85+	3,598,000	0.02	0.0060
Total	263,435,000	0.05	1.0017
		Total deaths	144

ence neurologic sequelae lasting a lifetime. These sequelae were estimated to be associated with an HUI of 0.6.

The committee estimated that 35% of new cases of NMB manifest as bacteremia and sepsis. Approximately half of these cases require ICU hospitalization, such as those with Waterhouse Friederichsen syndrome. The HUI associated with bacteremia range from 0.16 to 0.71. Approximately 5.25% of patients experience complications and just over 1% experiences sequelae, such as amputation, that last a lifetime.

Table A18-2 illustrates the estimated number of cases in each health state, the duration of time that state is experienced, and the HUI associated with each state.

Table A18-2 Disease Scenarios for *Neisseria meningitidis* B Infection

	No. of Cases	% of Cases	Committee HUI Values	Duration (years)
MENINGITIS	780	65.00%		
Meningitis (ICU)	624	52.00%		
ICU			0.24	0.0055 (2 days)
inpatient after ICU			0.28	0.0137 (5 days)
Meningitis (no ICU)	156	13.00%		
inpatient			0.39	0.0137 (5 days)
Meningitis—complications	117	9.75%		
acute complications (gangrene, arthritis, heart failure, etc.)			0.27	0.0274 (10 days)
Meningitis - sequelae	39	3.25%		
neurologic sequelae (cranial nerve damage, deafness, etc.)			0.60	23.2209 (discounted quality adjusted life expectancy at average age at onset) (average age at onset = 18.3)
BACTEREMIA/SEPSIS	420	35.00%		
Bacteremia/Sepsis	210	17.50%		
ICU (Waterhouse Friederichsen)			0.16	0.0110 (4 days)
inpatient after ICU			0.44	0.0274 (10 days)
Bacteremia/Sepsis (hospitalization; no ICU)	210	17.50%	0.71	0.0137 (5 days)
Bacteremia/Sepsis—complications acute complications (cardiac, DIC, pneumonia, etc.)	63	5.25%	0.59	0.0274 (10 days)
Bacteremia/Sepsis—sequelae	13	1.05%	0.63	23.2209 (discounted quality adjusted life expectancy at age 18) (average age at onset)

COST INCURRED BY DISEASE

Table A18-3 summarizes the health care costs incurred by NMB infections. For the purposes of the calculations in this report, it was assumed that patients with meningitis incur costs associated with hospitalization (hospital costs, specialist physicians, diagnostics). Patients who experience complications incur additional hospitalization costs. The small percentage of patients who

Table A18-3 Health Care Costs Associated with *Neisseria meningitidis* B Infection

	% with Care	Cost per Unit	Units per Case	Form of Treatment
Meningitis (ICU)				
uncomplicated	100%	$7,000	1.0	hospitalization
	100%	$150	3.0	physician b
	100%	$50	1.0	medication b
	100%	$100	1.0	diagnostic b
	10%	$500	1.0	diagnostic c
Meningitis—complications				
acute complications (gangrene, arthritis, heart failure, etc)	100%	$7,000	1.0	hospitalization
	100%	$150	6.0	physician b
	100%	$50	1.0	medication b
	100%	$100	1.0	diagnostic b
	100%	$500	1.0	diagnostic c
Meningitis—sequelae				
neurologic sequelae (cranial nerve damage, deafness, etc)	100%	$100	6.0	physician b (per year)
Bacteremia/Sepsis				
ICU (Waterhouse Friederichsen)	100%	$4,000	1.0	hospitalization
	100%	$100	3.0	physician b
Bacteremia/Sepsis (no ICU)				
inpatient	100%	$4,000	1.0	hospitalization
	100%	$100	3.0	physician b
	100%	$100	1.0	diagnostic b
Bacteremia/Sepsis—complications				
acute complications (cardiac, disseminated intravascular coagulation, pneumonia, etc.)	100%	$4,000	1.0	hospitalization
	100%	$100	3.0	physician b
	100%	$500	1.0	diagnostic c
	20%	$7,000	1.0	amputation
	20%	$500	2.0	surgical staff
	20%	$3,000	1.0	rehabilitation

experience neurologic sequelae incur costs associated with multiple visits per year to a specialist and therapists for the duration of their life.

Costs associated with NMB-related bacteremia and sepsis include hospitalization and related expenses (physicians, diagnostics). Those who experience complications incur additional costs associated with hospitalization and rehabilitation for the small number of patients who require amputation.

VACCINE DEVELOPMENT

The committee assumed that the development of an NMB vaccine is feasible and that licensure can occur within the middle of the time frame within the charge. The estimates for the model are that it will take 7 years until licensure and that $300 million needs to be invested. Table 4-1 summarizes vaccine development assumptions for all vaccines considered in this report.

VACCINE PROGRAM CONSIDERATIONS

Target Population

The committee's model assumes that immunization with this vaccine will occur only during infancy. It is estimated that 90% of infants will receive the immunization.

Vaccine Schedule, Efficacy, and Costs

The committee estimated that this would be a relatively low-cost vaccine, costing $50 per dose. Vaccine administration would cost an additional $10. The committee has accepted default assumptions that this vaccine will require a series of 3 doses and that effectiveness will be 75%. Table 4-1 summarizes vaccine program assumptions for all vaccines considered in this report.

RESULTS

If a vaccine program for *N. meningitidis* B were implemented today and the vaccine were 100% efficacious and utilized by 100% of the target population, the annualized present value of the QALYs gained would be 2,300. Using committee assumptions of less-than-ideal efficacy and utilization and including time and monetary costs until a vaccine program is implemented, the annualized present value of the QALYs gained would be 1,100. The mortality accounts for a large portion of the lost QALYs, due primarily to the deaths in children and infants. QALY loss associated with morbidity is largely due to the lifetime sequelae associated with both meningitis and bacteremia.

If a vaccine program for *N. meningitidis* B were implemented today and the vaccine was 100% efficacious and utilized by 100% of the target population, the annualized present value of the health care costs saved would be $6 million. Using committee assumptions of less-than-ideal efficacy and utilization and including time and monetary costs until a vaccine program is implemented, the annualized present value of the health care costs saved would be $2.9 million.

If a vaccine program for *N. meningitidis* B were implemented today and the vaccine was 100% efficacious and utilized by 100% of the target population, the annualized present value of the program cost would be $720 million. Using committee assumptions of less-than-ideal efficacy and utilization and including time and monetary costs until a vaccine program is implemented, the annualized present value of the program cost would be $450 million.

Using committee assumptions of time and costs until licensure, the fixed cost of vaccine development has been amortized and is $9 million for a *N. meningitidis* B vaccine.

If a vaccine program were implemented today and the vaccine was 100% efficacious and utilized by 100% of the target population, the annualized present value of the cost per QALY gained is $300,000. Using committee assumptions of less-than-ideal utilization and including time and monetary costs until a vaccine program is implemented, the annualized present value of the cost per QALY gained is $400,000.

See Chapters 4 and 5 for details on the methods and assumptions used by the committee for the results reported.

READING LIST

Adams AG, Deaver KA, Cochi SL, et al. Decline of Childhood *Haemophilus influenzae* Type b (Hib) Disease in the Hib Vaccine Era. JAMA 1993; 269:221–226.

Apicella MA. Neisseria Meningitidis. In: Principles and Practice of Infectious Diseases. GL Mandell, JE Bennett, Dolin R eds. New York, NY: Churchill Livingstone, 1995, pp. 1896–1908.

Bushore M, Marante AA. Emergency Department Stabilization of Pediatric Patients with Bacterial Meningitis—Current Advances. Emergency Medical Clinics of North America; 9:239–250.

Durand ML, Calderwood SB, Weber DJ, et al. Acute Bacterial Meningitis in Adults—A Review of 493 Episodes. The New England Journal of Medicine 1993; 328:21–28.

Frasch CE. Meningococcal Vaccines: Past, Present and Future. In: Meningococcal Disease. K Cartwright ed. New York, NY: John Wiley & Sons Ltd., 1995, pp. 245–283.

Glode MP, Smith AL. Meningococcal Disease. In: Textbook of Pediatric Infectious Diseases. RD Feigin and JD Cherry eds. Philadelphia, PA: WB Saunder Company, 1992, pp. 1185–1197.

Jackson LA, Wenger JD. Laboratory-Based Surveillance for Meningococcal Disease in Selected Areas, United States, 1989–1991. Morbidity and Mortality Weekly Report 1993; 42:21–30.

Milagres LG, Ramos SR, Sacchi CT, et al. Immune Response of Brazilian Children to a *Neisseria meningitidis* Serogroup B Outer Membrane Protein Vaccine: Comparison with Efficacy. Infection and Immunity 1994; 62:4419–4424.

APPENDIX 19

Parainfluenza Virus

DISEASE BURDEN

Epidemiology

For the purposes of the calculations in this report, the committee estimated that there are 2.5 million cases of parainfluenza virus (PIV) infection each year in the United States in children under 2 years of age. An additional 3.5 million infections occur in people greater than 2 years of age (25% of those in people 65 years of age or older). It is also assumed that there are 300 deaths per year in children 2 years of age and under and 140 deaths in people 65 years of age and older due to PIV disease.

Disease Scenarios

For the purposes of the calculation in this report, the committee assumed that PIV disease manifests as either a mild infection such as pharyngitis or otitis media, croup, or bronchiolitis/pneumonia. It was assumed that in children 2 years of age and under, the proportion of infections manifesting as those 3 disease scenarios is 70%, 20%, and 10% respectively. For people 2 years of age and older, it was assumed that the distribution is 90% as pharyngitis and 10% as bronchiolitis and pneumonia. The health utility index associated with PIV disease ranges from 0.9 (7 days of pharyngitis) to .5 (7 days of either croup or bronchiolitis). See Table A19-1.

Table A19-1 Disease Scenarios for Parainfluenza Virus Infection

	% of Cases	Committee HUI Values	Duration (years)
Upper Respiratory	70.00%		
pharyngitis, otitis media		0.90	0.0192 (7 days)
Croup	19.20%		
outpatient only		0.75	0.0274 (10 days)
Croup	0.80%		
inpatient		0.50	0.0192 (7 days)
outpatient		0.75	0.0082 (3 days)
Bronchiolitis/pneumonia	9.60%		
outpatient only		0.75	0.0274 (10 days)
Bronchiolitis/pneumonia	0.40%		
inpatient		0.50	0.0192 (7 days)
outpatient		0.75	0.0082 (3 days)
Upper Respiratory	90.00%	0.90	0.0192 (7 days)
Bronchiolitis/pneumonia	10.00%	0.75	0.0274 (10 days)
Upper Respiratory	90.00%	0.90	0.0192 (7 days)
Bronchiolitis/pneumonia	9.60%	0.75	0.0274 (10 days)
Bronchiolitis/pneumonia	0.40%		
inpatient		0.50	0.0192 (7 days)
outpatient		0.75	0.0082 (3 days)

COST INCURRED BY DISEASE

Table A19-2 summarizes the health care costs incurred by PIV infections. For the purposes of the calculations in this report, it was assumed that all children 2 years of age and under with PIV disease receive medical treatment. It was assumed that only 50% of people between the ages of 2 and 64 receive treatment for PIV disease. It was also assumed that only 50% of people 65 years of age and older receive treatment for mild (requiring only outpatient treatment if treated) pharyngitis and bronchiolitis. A small number of people age 65 years of age and older are hospitalized for bronchiolitis and pneumonia.

Pharyngitis, otitis media, croup, and outpatient treatment of bronchiolitis/pneumonia were assumed to be associated with physician visits, diagnostics and medications. The more serious disease incurred more visits to the physician. Hospitalization costs are included for the small number of people with PIV disease who require it.

Table A19-2 Costs of Care for Parainfluenza Virus Infection

	% with Care	Cost per Unit	Units per Case	Form of Treatment
AGE <2				
Upper Respiratory				
pharyngitis, otitis media	100%	$50	1.0	physician a
	100%	$50	1.0	diagnostic a
	100%	$50	1.0	medication b
Croup				
outpatient only	100%	$50	2.0	physician a
	100%	$50	1.0	diagnostic a
	100%	$50	1.0	medication b
inpatient	100%	$3000	1.0	hospitalization
	100%	$50	2.0	physician a
	100%	$50	1.0	diagnostic a
	100%	$50	1.0	medication b
Bronchiolitis/pneumonia				
outpatient only	100%	$50	2.0	physician a
	100%	$50	1.0	diagnostic a
	100%	$50	1.0	medication b
Bronchiolitis/pneumonia				
inpatient	100%	$4000	1.0	hospitalization
	100%	$50	2.0	physician a
	100%	$50	1.0	diagnostic a
	100%	$50	1.0	medication b
AGE 2-64				
Upper Respiratory				
pharyngitis, otitis media	50%	$50	1.0	physician a
	50%	$50	1.0	diagnostic a
	50%	$50	1.0	medication b
Bronchiolitis/pneumonia				
outpatient only	50%	$50	2.0	physician a
	50%	$50	1.0	diagnostic a
	50%	$50	1.0	medication b
AGE 65+				
Upper Respiratory				
pharyngitis, otitis media	50%	$50	1.0	physician a
	50%	$50	1.0	diagnostic a
	50%	$50	1.0	medication b
Bronchiolitis/pneumonia				
outpatient only	50%	$50	2.0	physician a
	50%	$50	1.0	diagnostic a
	50%	$50	1.0	medication b
Bronchiolitis/pneumonia				
inpatient	100%	$4000	1.0	hospitalization
	100%	$50	2.0	physician a
	100%	$50	1.0	diagnostic a
	100%	$50	1.0	medication b

VACCINE DEVELOPMENT

The committee assumed that it will take 7 years until licensure of a PIV vaccine and that $300 million needs to be invested for licensure for infants and another $360 million for a vaccine for pregnant women. Table 4-1 summarizes vaccine development assumptions for all vaccines considered in this report.

VACCINE PROGRAM CONSIDERATIONS

Target Population

For the purposes of the calculations in this report, it is assumed that the target population for this vaccine is all infants and all primiparas. It was assumed that 90% of infants and targeted pregnant women would receive the vaccine.

Vaccine Schedule, Efficacy, and Costs

For the purposes of the calculations in this report, it was estimated that this vaccine would cost $50 per dose and that administration costs would be $10 per dose. Default assumptions of a 3-dose series and 75% effectiveness were accepted. Table 4-1 summarizes vaccine program assumptions for all vaccines considered in this report.

RESULTS

If a vaccine program for PIV were implemented today and the vaccine were 100% efficacious and utilized by 100% of the target population, the annualized present value of the QALYs gained would be 21,000. Using committee assumptions of less-than-ideal efficacy and utilization and including time and monetary costs until a vaccine program is implemented, the annualized present value of the QALYs gained would be 10,000.

If a vaccine program for PIV were implemented today and the vaccine was 100% efficacious and utilized by 100% of the target population, the annualized present value of the health care costs saved would be $580 million. Using committee assumptions of less-than-ideal efficacy and utilization and including time and monetary costs until a vaccine program is implemented, the annualized present value of the health care costs saved would be $275 million.

If a vaccine program for PIV were implemented today and the vaccine was 100% efficacious and utilized by 100% of the target population, the annualized present value of the program cost would be $1 billion. Using committee assumptions of less-than-ideal efficacy and utilization and including time and monetary costs until a vaccine program is implemented, the annualized present value of the program cost would be $640 million.

Using committee assumptions of time and costs until licensure, the fixed cost of vaccine development has been amortized and is $19.8 million for a PIV vaccine.

If a vaccine program were implemented today and the vaccine was 100% efficacious and utilized by 100% of the target population, the annualized present value of the cost per QALY gained is $20,000. Using committee assumptions of less-than-ideal utilization and including time and monetary costs until a vaccine program is implemented, the annualized present value of the cost per QALY gained is $38,000. If only 10% of primiparas utilized the vaccine, the annualized present value of the cost per QALY gained is $50,000.

See Chapters 4 and 5 for details on the methods and assumptions used by the committee for the results reported.

READING LIST

Hall CB. Parainfluenza Viruses. In: Textbook of Pediatric Infectious Diseases. RD Feigin and JD Cherry eds. Philadelphia, PA: WB Saunder Company, 1992, pp. 1613–1624.

Henrickson K, Ray R, Belshe R. Parainfluenza Viruses. In: Principles and Practice of Infectious Diseases. GL Mandell, JE Bennett, Dolin R eds. New York, NY: Churchill Livingstone, 1995, pp. 1489–1496.

Karron RA, Wright PF, Newman FK, et al. A Live Human Parainfluenza Type 3 Virus Vaccine is Attenuated and Immunogenic in Healthy Infants and Children. The Journal of Infectious Diseases 1995; 172:1445–1450.

Ventura SJ, Martin JA, Mathews TJ, et al. Advance Report of Final Natality Statistics, 1994. Monthly Vital Statistics Report 1996; 44.

APPENDIX 20

Respiratory Syncytial Virus

DISEASE BURDEN

Epidemiology

For the purposes of the calculations in this report, the committee estimated that there are approximately 5 million infections with respiratory syncytial virus (RSV) each year in the United States. It was assumed that 1 million RSV infections occur in children under 1 year of age, 2 million RSV infections in children between the ages of 1 and 4 years of age, and 2 million RSV infections in people 5 years of age and greater. The number of deaths due to RSV infection in those three age groups is 300, 200, and 20, respectively. The mortality in the third age group is seen in those 65 years of age and older. See Table A20-1.

Disease Scenarios

For the purposes of the calculation in this report, the committee described disease states associated with RSV infection as either a mild upper respiratory or related condition (pharyngitis/otitis media) or as bronchiolitis/pneumonia. It was assumed that in children 4 years of age and under the relative distribution of cases between those two scenarios is 60% and 40% respectively. In people 5 years of age and older, it was assumed that 80% of infections manifest as pharyngitis/otitis media and 20% as the more severe lower respiratory disease. The health utility index (HUI) and time in that state range from 7 days at an HUI of .9 (pharyngitis) to 7 days at an HUI of .5 (inpatient treatment of bronchiolitis/pneumonia). See Table A20-2.

Table A20-1 Incidence Rate for Respiratory Syncytial Virus Infection

Age Groups	Population	Incidence Rates (per 100,000)	Cases
<1	3,963,000	25,233.41	1,000,000
1-4	16,219,000	12331.22	2,000,000
5-14	38,056,000	822.19	312,892
15-24	36,263,000	822.19	298,150
25-34	41,670,000	822.19	342,606
35-44	42,149,000	822.19	346,545
45-54	30,224,000	822.19	248,498
55-64	21,241,000	822.19	174,641
65-74	18,964,000	822.19	155,920
75-84	11,088,000	822.19	91,164
85+	3,598,000	822.19	29,582
Total	263,435,000		

COST INCURRED BY DISEASE

Table A20-3 summarizes the health care costs incurred by RSV infections. For the purposes of the calculations in this report, it was assumed that treatment of pharyngitis and otitis media are associated with physician visit, diagnostic, and medication (over-the-counter, symptomatic treatment). It was estimated that 100% of children 4 years of age and under incur such treatment but that approximately 50% of people 5 years of age and older seek such medical treatment.

It was assumed that the majority of cases of lower respiratory infections are treated as an outpatient and involve costs similar to that for pharyngitis, but with the addition of an extra physician visit. For the small number of cases of lower respiratory disease which is treated as an inpatient, hospitalization costs are added to the costs similar to that incurred as outpatient treatment. It was assumed that while 100% of children 4 years of age and under receive treatment for lower respiratory infections, only 50% of people 5 years of age or older who are not hospitalized for lower respiratory RSV infections seek medical treatment.

VACCINE DEVELOPMENT

The committee assumed that it will take 7 years until licensure of a RSV vaccine and that $360 million needs to be invested. It was assumed that the same vaccine would be used in infants and in adolescent girls. Table 4-1 summarizes vaccine development assumptions for all vaccines considered in this report.

Table A20-2 Disease Scenarios for RSV

	No. of Cases	% of Cases	Committee HUI Values	Duration (years)
AGE <1				
Total Deaths	300			
Total Cases	1,000,000			
Upper Respiratory pharyngitis, otitis media	600,000	60.00%	0.90	0.0192 (7 days)
Bronchiolitis/pneumonia outpatient only	340,000	34.00%	0.75	0.0274 (10 days)
Bronchiolitis/pneumonia	60,000	6.00%		
inpatient			0.50	0.0192 (7 days)
outpatient			0.75	0.0082 (3 days)
AGE 1-4				
Total Deaths (from acute infection)	200			
Total Cases	2,000,000			
Upper Respiratory pharyngitis, otitis media	1,200,000	60.00%	0.90	0.0192 (7 days)
Bronchiolitis/pneumonia outpatient only	760,000	38.00%	0.75	0.0274 (10 days)
Bronchiolitis/pneumonia	40,000	2.00%		
inpatient			0.50	0.0192 (7 days)
outpatient			0.75	0.0082 (3 days)
AGE 5+				
Total Deaths (from acute infection)	20			
Total Cases	2,000,000			
Upper Respiratory pharyngitis, otitis media	1,600,000	80.00%	0.90	0.0192 (7 days)
Bronchiolitis/pneumonia outpatient only	396,000	19.80%	0.75	0.0274 (10 days)
Bronchiolitis/pneumonia	4,000	0.20%		
inpatient			0.50	0.0192 (7 days)
outpatient			0.75	0.0082 (7 days)

VACCINE PROGRAM CONSIDERATIONS

Target Population

For the purposes of the calculations in this report, it is assumed that the target population for this vaccine is all adolescent girls (age 12 years) and all infants. For this example, the committee included adolescent girls in order to induce immunity that would protect the neonate. Infants are immunized to protect against disease after 1 year of age. It was assumed that 50% of adolescent females and 90% of infants would utilize the vaccine.

Table 20-3 Health Care Costs Associated with RSV Infections

	% with Care	Cost per Unit	Units per Case	Form of Treatment
AGE <5				
Upper Respiratory				
pharyngitis, otitis media	100%	$50	1.0	physician a
	100%	$50	1.0	diagnostic a
	100%	$50	1.0	medication b
Bronchiolitis/pneumonia				
outpatient only	100%	$50	1.0	physician a
	100%	$50	1.0	diagnostic a
	100%	$50	1.0	medication b
Bronchiolitis/pneumonia				
inpatient	100%	$4,000	1.0	hospitalization
	100%	$50	2.0	physician a
	100%	$50	1.0	diagnostic a
	100%	$50	1.0	medication b
AGE 5+				
Upper Respiratory				
pharyngitis, otitis media	100%	$50	1.0	physician a
	100%	$50	1.0	diagnostic a
	100%	$50	1.0	medication b
Bronchiolitis/pneumonia				
outpatient only	100%	$50	1.0	physician a
	100%	$50	1.0	diagnostic a
	100%	$50	1.0	medication b
Bronchiolitis/pneumonia				
inpatient	100%	$4,000	1.0	hospitalization
	100%	$50	2.0	physician a
	100%	$50	1.0	diagnostic a
	100%	$50	1.0	medication b

Vaccine Schedule, Efficacy, and Costs

For the purposes of the calculations in this report, it was estimated that this vaccine would cost $50 per dose and that administration costs would be $10 per dose. Default assumptions of a 3-dose series and 75% effectiveness were accepted. Table 4-1 summarizes vaccine program assumptions for all vaccines considered in this report.

RESULTS

If a vaccine program for RSV were implemented today and the vaccine were 100% efficacious and utilized by 100% of the target population, the annualized present value of the QALYs gained would be 33,000. Using committee assumptions of less-than-ideal efficacy and utilization and including time and monetary costs until a vaccine program is implemented, the annualized present value of the QALYs gained would be 14,000. Slightly over half of the loss is accounted for by disease in children under 1 year of age. Deaths of very young infants contribute substantially to loss of QALYs.

If a vaccine program for RSV were implemented today and the vaccine was 100% efficacious and utilized by 100% of the target population, the annualized present value of the health care costs saved would be $1.15 billion. Using committee assumptions of less-than-ideal efficacy and utilization and including time and monetary costs until a vaccine program is implemented, the annualized present value of the health care costs saved would be $490 million.

If a vaccine program for RSV were implemented today and the vaccine was 100% efficacious and utilized by 100% of the target population, the annualized present value of the program cost would be $1.05 billion. Using committee assumptions of less-than-ideal efficacy and utilization and including time and monetary costs until a vaccine program is implemented, the annualized present value of the program cost would be $570 million.

Using committee assumptions of time and costs until licensure, the fixed cost of vaccine development has been amortized and is $10.8 million for a RSV vaccine.

If a vaccine program were implemented today and the vaccine was 100% efficacious and utilized by 100% of the target population, the annualized present value of the cost per QALY gained is -$3,000. A negative value represents a saving in costs in addition to a saving in QALYs. Using committee assumptions of less-than-ideal utilization and including time and monetary costs until a vaccine program is implemented, the annualized present value of the cost per QALY gained is $6,500.

See Chapters 4 and 5 for details on the methods and assumptions used by the committee for the results reported.

READING LIST

CDC. Update: Respiratory Syncytial Virus Activity—United States, 1996–7 Season. Morbidity and Mortality Weekly Report 1996; 45:1053–1055.

Committee on Infectious Diseases and Committee on Fetus and Newborn of the American Academy of Pediatrics. Respiratory Syncytial Virus Immune Globulin Intravenous: Indications for Use. Pediatrics 1997; 99:645–650.

Dowell SF, Anderson LJ, Gary HE, et al. Respiratory Syncytial Virus Is an Important Cause of Community-Acquired Lower Respiratory Infection among Hospitalized Adults. The Journal of Infectious Diseases 1996; 174:456–462.

Fisher RG, Gruber WC, Edwards KM, et al. Twenty Years of Outpatient Respiratory Syncytial Virus. Pediatrics 1997; 99:E7.

Hall CB. Respiratory Syncytial Virus. In: Textbook of Pediatric Infectious Diseases. RD Feigin and JD Cherry eds. Philadelphia, PA: WB Saunder Company, 1992, pp. 1633–1656.

Hall CB, McCarthy CA. Respiratory Syncytial Virus. In: Principles and Practice of Infectious Diseases. GL Mandell, JE Bennett, Dolin R eds. New York, NY: Churchill Livingstone, 1995, pp. 1501–1519.

Meissner HC, Groothuis JR. Immunoprophylaxis and the Control of RSV Disease. Pediatrics 1997; 100:260–263.

Paradise JL, Rockette HE, Colborn DK, et al. Otitis Media in 2253 Pittsburgh-Area Infants: Prevalence and Risk Factors During the First Two Years of Life. Pediatrics 1997; 99:318–333.

Prober CG, Wang EEL. Reducing the Morbidity of Lower Respiratory Tract Infections Caused by Respiratory Syncytial Virus: Still No Answer. Pediatrics 1997; 99:472–475.

Rodriguez WJ, Gruber WC, Welliver RC, et al. Respiratory Syncytial Virus (RSV) Immune Globulin Intravenous Therapy for RSV Lower Respiratory Tract Infection in Infants and Young Children at High Risk for Severe RSV Infections. Pediatrics 1997; 99:454–461.

Ventura SJ, Martin JA, Mathews TJ, et al. Advance Report of Final Natality Statistics, 1994. Monthly Vital Statistics Report 1996; 44.

APPENDIX 21

Rheumatoid Arthritis

Rheumatoid arthritis (RA) is a chronic multisystem disease which can have a variety of systemic manifestations. Persistent inflammatory synovitis, however, is the characteristic feature of RA, which usually involves the peripheral joints. Most often, the joints of the hands, wrists, knees, and feet are involved and are usually affected in a symmetrical fashion. The synovial inflammation can potentially destroy the cartilage and cause bone erosion, which subsequently leads to joint deformities. The destructive nature of this disease ranges from a brief oligoarticular illness with minimal joint damage to a more chronic, progressive polyarthritis with major joint deformity.

DISEASE BURDEN

Epidemiology

For the purposes of the calculations in this report, the committee estimated that there are approximately 65,000 new cases of rheumatoid arthritis each year in the United States. The incidence is highest in people 55 years of age and older, but new cases were included for people between the ages of 15 and 54 years of age as well. See Table A21-1.

Disease Scenarios

For the purposes of the calculation in this report, the committee assumed that there are four disease scenarios associated with RA. A relatively benign

Table A21-1 Incidence Rate for Rheumatoid Arthritis

Age Groups	Population	Incidence Rates (per 100,000)	Cases
<1	3,963,000	0.0	-
1-4	16,219,000	0.0	-
5-14	38,056,000	0.0	-
15-24	36,263,000	2.0	725
25-34	41,670,000	9.0	3,750
35-44	42,149,000	17.0	7,165
45-54	30,224,000	38.5	11,636
55-64	21,241,000	74.0	15,718
65-74	18,964,000	80.0	15,171
75-84	11,088,000	71.0	7,872
85+	3,598,000	71.0	2,555
Total	263,435,000	24.5	64,594

form experienced by 15% of people with RA is associated with a health utility index (HUI) of .91 for 1 year. A moderate form of RA experienced by 65% of the patients was associated with lifelong disease at an HUI of .72. It was assumed that there was premature death by 3 years in these patients.

For 15% of RA patients who experience a progressive disease, it was assumed that the remainder of life was spent in an average HUI of .49. Life expectancy was shortened by 5 years in these patients. For 5% of patients, RA manifests with severe systemic manifestations and is associated with an HUI of .33. Life expectancy was assumed to be decreased by 7 years in these patients. See Table A21-2.

COST INCURRED BY DISEASE

Table A21-3 summarizes the health care costs incurred by RA. For the purposes of the calculations in this report, it was assumed that initial treatment for all RA patients includes 4 visits to a physician (half will seek the attention of a specialist), medication, and diagnostic evaluation. Patients with a limited, benign course seek no further treatment. Yearly health care costs for patients experiencing chronic, moderate disease were assumed to include semi-annual visits to a physician (50% to a specialist) and medication. It was assumed that on average, each year 10% of patients would require hospitalization and rehabilitation services. Annual care for patients with progressive, serious disease was assumed to include quarterly visits to a specialist, medication, and hospitalization and rehabilitation services for 25% of patients. Annual care for patients with severe systemic disease was assumed to be associated with bimonthly visits to a

Table A21-2 Disease Scenarios for Rheumatoid Arthritis

	No. of Cases	% of Cases	Committee HUI Values	Duration (years)
Benign	9,689	15.00%		
short-term pain, resolved within 1 year			0.91	1.0000
Moderate disability	41,986	65.00%		
joint involvement			0.72	19.4924 (life expectancy at onset)
premature death: reduction in life expectancy by 3 years			0.00	3.0000
Progressive	9,689	15.00%		
seriously affected within 5-10 years of diagnosis			0.49	17.4924 (life expectancy at onset)
premature death: reduction in life expectancy by 5 years			0.00	5.0000
Severe systemic manifestations	3,230	5.00%		
joint involvement; complications may include pulmonary and cardiac involvement			0.33	15.4924 (life expectancy at onset)
premature death: reduction in life expectancy by 7 years			0.00	7.0000

specialist, medication, and hospitalization and rehabilitation services for 50% of patients.

VACCINE DEVELOPMENT

The committee assumed that it will take 15 years until licensure of a therapeutic RA vaccine and that $360 million needs to be invested. Table 4-1 summarizes vaccine development assumptions for all vaccines considered in this report.

Table A21-3 Health Care Costs Associated with Rheumatoid Arthritis

	% with Care	Cost per Unit	Units per Case	Form of Treatment (per year)
Benign				
short-term pain, resolved within 1 year	50%	$50	4.0	physician a
	50%	$100	4.0	physician b
	100%	$50	12.0	medication b
	100%	$500	1.0	diagnostic c
Moderate disability				
initial treatment	50%	$50	4.0	physician a
	50%	$100	4.0	physician b
	100%	$50	1.0	medication b
	100%	$500	1.0	diagnostic c
annual care	50%	$50	2.0	physician a
	50%	$100	2.0	physician b
	100%	$50	12.0	medication b
	10%	$3,000	1.0	hospitalization
	10%	$3,000	1.0	rehabilitation or other care
Progressive				
initial treatment	50%	$50	4.0	physician a
	50%	$100	4.0	physician b
	100%	$50	1.0	medication b
	100%	$500	1.0	diagnostic c
annual care	100%	$100	4.0	physician b
	100%	$50	12.0	medication b
	25%	$3,000	1.0	hospitalization
	25%	$3,000	1.0	rehabilitation or other care
Severe systemic manifestations				
initial treatment	50%	$50	4.0	physician a
	50%	$100	4.0	physician b
	100%	$50	1.0	medication b
	100%	$500	1.0	diagnostic c
annual care	100%	$100	6.0	physician b
	100%	$50	12.0	medication b
	50%	$3,000	1.0	hospitalization
	50%	$3,000	1.0	rehabilitation or other

VACCINE PROGRAM CONSIDERATIONS

Target Population

For the purposes of the calculations in this report, it is assumed that the target population for this vaccine is all new cases of RA. It was assumed that 90% of the target population would utilize the vaccine.

Vaccine Schedule, Efficacy, and Costs

For the purposes of the calculations in this report, it was estimated that this vaccine would cost $500 per dose and that administration costs would be $10 per dose. Default assumptions for a therapeutic vaccine of a 3-dose series and 40% effectiveness were accepted. Table 4-1 summarizes vaccine program assumptions for all vaccines considered in this report.

RESULTS

If a vaccine program for rheumatoid arthritis were implemented today and the vaccine were 100% efficacious and utilized by 100% of the target population, the annualized present value of the QALYs gained would be 275,000. Using committee assumptions of less-than-ideal efficacy and utilization and including time and monetary costs until a vaccine program is implemented, the annualized present value of the QALYs gained would be 60,000. Most of the QALY loss was attributed to the moderate form of the disease, due to the proportion of cases experiencing that scenario and the long time spent at a moderately decreased HUI.

If a vaccine program for rheumatoid arthritis were implemented today and the vaccine was 100% efficacious and utilized by 100% of the target population, the annualized present value of the health care costs saved would be $1.4 billion. Using committee assumptions of less-than-ideal efficacy and utilization and including time and monetary costs until a vaccine program is implemented, the annualized present value of the health care costs saved would be $300 million.

If a vaccine program for rheumatoid arthritis were implemented today and the vaccine was 100% efficacious and utilized by 100% of the target population, the annualized present value of the program cost would be $100 million. Using committee assumptions of less-than-ideal efficacy and utilization and including time and monetary costs until a vaccine program is implemented, the annualized present value of the program cost would be $53.8 million.

Using committee assumptions of time and costs until licensure, the fixed cost of vaccine development has been amortized and is $10.8 million for a rheumatoid arthritis vaccine.

If a vaccine program were implemented today and the vaccine was 100% efficacious and utilized by 100% of the target population, the annualized present value of the cost per QALY gained is -$5,000. A negative value represents a saving in costs in addition to a saving in QALYs. Using committee assumptions of less-than-ideal utilization and including time and monetary costs until a vaccine program is implemented, the annualized present value of the cost per QALY gained is -$4,000.

See Chapters 4 and 5 for details on the methods and assumptions used by the committee for the results reported.

READING LIST

Chan KW, Felson DT, Yood RA, et al. Incidence of Rheumatoid Arthritis in Central Massachusetts. Arthritis and Rheumatism 1993; 36:1691–6.

Prashker MJ, Meenan RF. The Total Costs of Drug Therapy for Rheumatoid Arthritis: A Model Based on Costs of Drug, Monitoring, and Toxicity. Arthritis and Rheumatism 1995; 38:318–25.

APPENDIX 22

Rotavirus

DISEASE BURDEN

Epidemiology

For the purposes of the calculations in this report, the committee estimated that there are approximately 3,500,000 new infections of rotavirus in the United States each year. It was assumed that all infections occur in infants and children between birth and 4 years of age and that the incidence in infants under 1 year of age (30,000 per 100,000) is twice that in children between 1 and 4 years of age. It was assumed that rotavirus infection leads to 100 deaths per year in the United States.

Disease Scenarios

For the purposes of the calculation in this report, the committee assumed that rotavirus infection is associated with 8 days of acute diarrhea and a health utility index of .75.

COST INCURRED BY DISEASE

Table A22-1 summarizes the health care costs incurred by rotavirus infections. For the purposes of the calculations in this report, it was assumed that all infants and children with rotavirus infection incur modest costs for over-the-counter treatment (e.g., oral rehydration) or extra diapers. It was also assumed

Table A22-1 Health Care Costs Associated with Rotavirus Infection

	% with Care	Cost per Unit	Units per Case (or per year)	Form of Treatment
Acute diarrhea	100%	$10	2.0	oral rehydration therapy
	15%	$50	1.0	physician a
	2%	$2,000	1.0	hospitalization
	2%	$150	1.0	physician c

that 15% of infants and children receive medical attention. It is further assumed that a small percentage of children with rotavirus infection are hospitalized.

VACCINE DEVELOPMENT

The committee assumed that it would take 3 years until licensure of a rotavirus vaccine and that $120 million needed to be invested. During the time the committee report was in final stages of analysis and preparation, the rotavirus vaccine was approved for licensure. Table 4-1 summarizes vaccine development assumptions for all vaccines considered in this report.

VACCINE PROGRAM CONSIDERATIONS

Target Population

For the purposes of the calculations in this report, it is assumed that the target population for this vaccine is the annual birth cohort of infants. It was assumed that 90% of the target population would utilize the vaccine.

Vaccine Schedule, Efficacy, and Costs

For the purposes of the calculations in this report, it was estimated that this vaccine would cost $50 per dose and that administration costs would be $10 per dose. Default assumptions of a 3-dose series and 75% effectiveness were accepted. Table 4-1 summarizes vaccine program assumptions for all vaccines considered in this report.

RESULTS

If a vaccine program for rotavirus were implemented today and the vaccine were 100% efficacious and utilized by 100% of the target population, the annualized present value of the QALYs gained would be 27,000. Using committee assumptions of less-than-ideal efficacy and utilization and including time and monetary costs until a vaccine program is implemented, the annualized present value of the QALYs gained would be 14,000.

If a vaccine program for rotavirus were implemented today and the vaccine was 100% efficacious and utilized by 100% of the target population, the annualized present value of the health care costs saved would be $225 million. Using committee assumptions of less-than-ideal efficacy and utilization and including time and monetary costs until a vaccine program is implemented, the annualized present value of the health care costs saved would be $120 million.

If a vaccine program for rotavirus were implemented today and the vaccine was 100% efficacious and utilized by 100% of the target population, the annualized present value of the program cost would be $720 million. Using committee assumptions of less-than-ideal efficacy and utilization and including time and monetary costs until a vaccine program is implemented, the annualized present value of the program cost would be $510 million.

Using committee assumptions of time and costs until licensure, the fixed cost of vaccine development has been amortized and is $3.6 million for a rotavirus vaccine.

If a vaccine program were implemented today and the vaccine was 100% efficacious and utilized by 100% of the target population, the annualized present value of the cost per QALY gained is $20,000. Using committee assumptions of less-than-ideal utilization and including time and monetary costs until a vaccine program is implemented, the annualized present value of the cost per QALY gained is $30,000.

See Chapters 4 and 5 for details on the methods and assumptions used by the committee for the results reported.

During the time the data for this report was being analyzed and written, a rotavirus vaccine was licensed. The calculated cost per QALY saved for a vaccine strategy for a currently licensed rotavirus vaccine (assuming 75% effectiveness and 90% utilization and all other disease burden and costs as described above) decreases slightly to approximately $26,500.

READING LIST

Glass RI, Kilgore PE, Holman RC, et al. The Epidemiology of Rotavirus Diarrhea in the United States: Surveillance and Estimates of Disease Burden. The Journal of Infectious Diseases 1996; 174:S5–11.

Matson DO. Potential Impact of Rotavirus Vaccines. URL http://rotavirus.com/ potential_impact_of_rota.html (accessed August 8, 1996).

Offit PA, Clark HF. Rotavirus. In: Principles and Practice of Infectious Diseases. GL Mandell, JE Bennett, Dolin R eds. New York, NY: Churchill Livingstone, 1995, pp. 1448–1455.

Orenstein WA, Hadler S, Kuritsky JN, et al. Rotavirus Vaccines—from Licensure to Disease Reduction. The Journal of Infectious Diseases 1996; 174:S118–24.

Smith JC, Haddix AC, Teutsch SM, et al. Cost-effectiveness Analysis of a Rotavirus Immunization Program for the United States. Pediatrics 1995; 96:609–615.

Ventura SJ, Martin JA, Mathews TJ, et al. Advance Report of Final Natality Statistics, 1994. Monthly Vital Statistics Report 1996; 44.

APPENDIX 23

Shigella

DISEASE BURDEN

Epidemiology

For the purposes of the calculations in this report, the committee estimated that there are approximately 30,000 new cases of *shigella* disease each year in the United States. It is assumed that the highest incidence is in children between the ages of 1 and 4 years of age. Children under one year of age and between 5 and 14 years of age also contribute heavily to the number of cases. It is assumed that there are no deaths associated with *shigella* infection in the United States. It was assumed that 25% of cases are in travelers from the United States to other countries.

Disease Scenarios

For the purposes of the calculation in this report, the committee assumed that *shigella* manifests as acute diarrhea lasting 6 days and associated with a health utility index of .51.

COST INCURRED BY DISEASE

For the purposes of the calculations in this report, it was assumed that 25% of people with *shigella* incur costs associated only with over-the-counter treatment, such as oral rehydration or anti-diarrheals. It was assumed that 75% of people with *shigella* infection seek the care of a physician and receive medication. See Table A23-1.

VACCINE DEVELOPMENT

The committee assumed that it will take 7 years until licensure of a *shigella* vaccine and that $240 million needs to be invested. It was assumed that research into the development of a *shigella* vaccine would lead to increased knowledge of mucosal immunity, which would benefit research and development of many vaccines in the future. Table 4-1 summarizes vaccine development assumptions for all vaccines considered in this report.

VACCINE PROGRAM CONSIDERATIONS

Target Population

For the purposes of the calculations in this report, two scenarios are discussed: a target population of travelers only and a target population of travelers and infants. It is assumed that 90% of infants and 30% of travelers will accept the vaccine.

Vaccine Schedule, Efficacy, and Costs

For the purposes of the calculations in this report, it was estimated that this vaccine would cost $50 per dose and that administration costs would be $10 per dose. Default assumptions of a 3-dose series and 75% effectiveness were accepted. Table 4-1 summarizes vaccine program assumptions for all vaccines considered in this report.

RESULTS

If a vaccine program for *Shigella* were implemented today and the vaccine were 100% efficacious and utilized by 100% of the target population, the annualized present value of the QALYs gained would be 160. Using committee assumptions of less-than-ideal efficacy and utilization and including time and monetary costs until a vaccine program is implemented, the annualized present value of the QALYs gained would be 57.

If a vaccine program for *Shigella* were implemented today and the vaccine was 100% efficacious and utilized by 100% of the target population, the annualized present value of the health care costs saved would be $1.7 million.

Table A23-1 Health Care Costs Associated with *Shigella* Infection

	% of Cases	Cost per Unit	Units per Case	Form of Treatment
Acute diarrhea	25%	$10	2.0	oral rehydration therapy
	75%	$50	1.0	physician a
	75%	$50	1.0	medication b

Using committee assumptions of less-than-ideal efficacy and utilization and including time and monetary costs until a vaccine program is implemented, the annualized present value of the health care costs saved would be $620,000.

If a vaccine program for *Shigella* were implemented today and the vaccine was 100% efficacious and utilized by 100% of the target population, the annualized present value of the program cost would be $1.2 billion. Using committee assumptions of less-than-ideal efficacy and utilization and including time and monetary costs until a vaccine program is implemented, the annualized present value of the program cost would be $550 million.

Using committee assumptions of time and costs until licensure, the fixed cost of vaccine development has been amortized and is $7.2 million for a *Shigella* vaccine.

If a vaccine program were implemented today and the vaccine was 100% efficacious and utilized by 100% of the target population, the annualized present value of the cost per QALY gained is $7 million. Using committee assumptions of less-than-ideal utilization and including time and monetary costs until a vaccine program is implemented, the annualized present value of the cost per QALY gained is $9 million. If the vaccine were utilized by 90% of travelers (and no infants) the annualized present value of the cost per QALY gained is $11 million.

See Chapters 4 and 5 for details on the methods and assumptions used by the committee for the results reported.

READING LIST

Ashkenazi S, Cleary TG. *Shigella* Infections. In: Textbook of Pediatric Infectious Diseases. RD Feigin and JD Cherry eds. Philadelphia, PA: WB Saunder Company, 1992, pp. 637–646.

CDC. Summary of Notifiable Diseases, United States 1994. Morbidity and Mortality Weekly Report 1994; 43:1–80.

DuPont HL. *Shigella* Species (Bacillary Dysentery). In: Principles and Practice of Infectious Diseases. GL Mandell, JE Bennett, Dolin R eds. New York, NY: Churchill Livingstone, 1995, pp. 2033–2039.

APPENDIX 24

Streptococcus, Group A

DISEASE BURDEN

Epidemiology

For the purposes of the calculations in this report, the committee estimated that there are 4,000,000 new cases of noninvasive Group A Streptococcus (GAS) per year in the United States. These cases were assumed to occur in people 24 years of age and under, with the highest incidence rate in children between the ages of 5 and 14 years. It was assumed that there was no mortality associated with noninvasive GAS disease. It was estimated that there, an additional 15,000 cases of invasive GAS disease and that the incidence rate of approximately 5.7 per 100,000 is the same in all age groups. It was assumed that 10% of invasive GAS disease is fatal. See Table A24-1.

Disease Scenarios

For the purposes of the calculation in this report, the committee assumed that 100% of noninvasive GAS infections result in a limited morbidity lasting 4 days and associated with a health utility index (HUI) of 0.9. The committee estimated that a small percentage of these patients (2,000) develop acute rheumatic fever and experience a more prolonged (28 days) illness associated with an HUI of .54. A very small number of those patients then go on to experience a chronic morbidity associated with an HUI of .82 for the duration of their lifetime.

See Appendix 28 for more information.

Table A24-1 Incidence Rate for Noninvasive and Invasive Group A
Streptococcus Infections

Age Groups	Population	Incidence Rates (per 100,000)	Cases
NONINVASIVE INFECTIONS			
<1	3,963,000	1,009.34	40,000
1-4	16,219,000	2,466.24	400,000
5-14	38,056,000	8,408.66	3,200,000
15-24	36,263,000	992.75	360,000
25-34	41,670,000	0.00	0
35-44	42,149,000	0.00	0
45-54	30,224,000	0.00	0
55-64	21,241,000	0.00	0
65-74	18,964,000	0.00	0
75-84	11,088,000	0.00	0
85+	3,598,000	0.00	0
Total	263,435,000	1,518.4	4,000,000
INVASIVE INFECTIONS			
<1	3,963,000	5.69	226
1-4	16,219,000	5.69	924
5-14	38,056,000	5.69	2,167
15-24	36,263,000	5.69	2,065
25-34	41,670,000	5.69	2,373
35-44	42,149,000	5.69	2,400
45-54	30,224,000	5.69	1,721
55-64	21,241,000	5.69	1,209
65-74	18,964,000	5.69	1,080
75-84	11,088,000	5.69	631
85+	3,598,000	5.69	205
Total	263,435,000	5.69	15,000

For the purposes of this report, the committee assumed that invasive GAS
disease manifests as necrotizing fasciitis (with and without lifetime sequelae) in
10% of cases and toxic shock (lasting 15 days and associated with HUIs of .16
during hospitalization and .58 following hospitalization) for 10% of cases. 80%
of the invasive forms of the disease are associated with 2 weeks of illness and
HUIs of .62 and .73 for the time spent inpatient and outpatient, respectively. See
Table A24-2.

COST INCURRED BY DISEASE

Table A24-3 summarizes the health care costs incurred by GAS infections.
For the purposes of the calculations in this report, it was assumed that all pa-

Table A24-2 Disease Scenarios for Group A Streptococcus Infection

	No. of Cases	% of Cases	Committee HUI Values	Duration (years)
NONINVASIVE				
Acute Infection pharyngitis, skin infections, etc.	4,000,000	100.00%	0.90	0.0110 (4 days)
Acute Rheumatic Fever	2,000	0.05%	0.54	0.0767 (28 days)
Chronic Rheumatic Fever	100	0.0025%	0.82	25.6422 (discounted quality adjusted life expectancy at onset)
INVASIVE				
Necrotizing Fasciitis: Severe	1,200	8.00%		
ICU			0.16	0.0274 (10 days)
Post-ICU			0.45	0.0274 (10 days)
Necrotizing Fasciitis: Moderate	300	2.00%	0.51	0.0274 (10 days)
Necrotizing Fasciitis: Sequelae	1,050	7.00%	0.61	19.2128 (discounted quality adjusted life expectancy at onset)
Toxic Shock	1,500	10.00%		
inpatient			0.16	0.0137 (5 days)
outpatient following hospitalization			0.58	0.0274 (10 days)
Other Invasive Forms	12,000	80.00%		
inpatient			0.62	0.0192 (7 days)
outpatient after inpatient			0.73	0.0192 (7 days)

tients with acute, noninvasive GAS disease seek outpatient medical attention (physician, diagnostics, medication). It was also assumed that all patients experiencing acute rheumatic fever require hospitalization and associated costs. The small number of patients with chronic rheumatic disease require 2 physician visits per year for the duration of their lifetime.

For the purposes of this report, it was also assumed that all patients with fasciitis require hospitalization. The costs for severe fasciitis are approximately twice that for moderate fasciitis. Lifelong sequelae associated with necrotizing fasciitis were presumed to occur in most patients and were associated with yearly aftercare costs in approximately half of the patients.

Table 24-3 Health Care Costs Associated with Group A Streptococcus Infection

	% with Care	Cost per Unit	Units per Case	Form of Treatment
Acute Infection				
pharyngitis, skin infections, etc	100%	$150	1.0	outpatient treatment
Acute Rheumatic Fever	100%	$3,400	1.0	hospitalization
Chronic Rheumatic Fever				
duration = life expectancy at onset	100%	$50	2.0	physician visit (2/year)
Necrotizing fasciitis: severe	100%	$7,000	1.0	hospitalization
	100%	$150	1.0	physician c
Necrotizing fasciitis: moderate				
hospitalization	100%	$3,000	1.0	hospitalization
	100%	$150	1.0	physician c
Necrotizing fasciitis: sequelae	50%	$3,000	1.0	aftercare per year
Toxic shock				
hospitalization	90%	$3,000	1.0	hospitalization
	10%	$15,000	1.0	ventilator support
outpatient after hospitalization	100%	$250	1.0	physician b plus medication c
Other invasive forms				
inpatient	100%	$4,000	1.0	hospitalization
outpatient after inpatient	100%	$250	1.0	physician b plus medication c

Patients with toxic shock from GAS were presumed to require hospitalization, with 10% requiring ventilator support and more expensive care. All patients with toxic shock were presumed to also require outpatient visits to a specialist and additional medication. Other forms of invasive disease were presumed to be associated with a hospitalization and subsequent outpatient visits to a specialist and additional medication.

VACCINE DEVELOPMENT

The committee assumed that it will take 15 years until licensure of a GAS vaccine and that $400 million needs to be invested. Table 4-1 summarizes vaccine development assumptions for all vaccines considered in this report.

VACCINE PROGRAM CONSIDERATIONS

Target Population

For the purposes of the calculations in this report, it is assumed that the target population for a GAS vaccine is all infants. It was assumed that 90% of the target population would utilize the vaccine.

Vaccine Schedule, Efficacy, and Costs

For the purposes of the calculations in this report, it was estimated that this vaccine would cost $50 per dose and that administration costs would be $10 per dose. Default assumptions of a 3-dose series and 75% effectiveness were accepted. Table 4-1 summarizes vaccine program assumptions for all vaccines considered in this report.

RESULTS

If a vaccine program for group A streptococci were implemented today and the vaccine were 100% efficacious and utilized by 100% of the target population, the annualized present value of the QALYs gained would be 16,500. Using committee assumptions of less-than-ideal efficacy and utilization and including time and monetary costs until a vaccine program is implemented, the annualized present value of the QALYs gained would be 6,200.

If a vaccine program for group A streptococci were implemented today and the vaccine was 100% efficacious and utilized by 100% of the target population, the annualized present value of the health care costs saved would be $495 million. Using committee assumptions of less-than-ideal efficacy and utilization and including time and monetary costs until a vaccine program is implemented, the annualized present value of the health care costs saved would be $185 million.

If a vaccine program for group A streptococci were implemented today and the vaccine was 100% efficacious and utilized by 100% of the target population, the annualized present value of the program cost would be $720 million. Using committee assumptions of less-than-ideal efficacy and utilization and including time and monetary costs until a vaccine program is implemented, the annualized present value of the program cost would be $360 million.

Using committee assumptions of time and costs until licensure, the fixed cost of vaccine development has been amortized and is $12 million for a group A streptococci vaccine.

If a vaccine program were implemented today and the vaccine was 100% efficacious and utilized by 100% of the target population, the annualized present value of the cost per QALY gained is $14,000. Using committee assumptions of less-than-ideal utilization and including time and monetary costs until a vaccine program is implemented, the annualized present value of the cost per QALY gained is $30,000.

See Chapters 4 and 5 for details on the methods and assumptions used by the committee for the results reported.

READING LIST

Bisno AL. Streptococcus Pyogenes. In: Principles and Practice of Infectious Diseases. GL Mandell, JE Bennett, Dolin R eds. New York, NY: Churchill Livingstone, 1995, pp. 1786–1799.

Kaplan EL. Group A Streptococcal Infections. In: Textbook of Pediatric Infectious Diseases. RD Feigin and JD Cherry eds. Philadelphia, PA: WB Saunder Company, 1992, pp. 1296–1305.

APPENDIX 25

Streptococcus, Group B

DISEASE BURDEN

Epidemiology

For the purposes of the calculations in this report, the committee estimated that there are approximately 7,000 new infections with streptococcus, group B (GBS) and 430 deaths in infants and 4,000 new GBS infections (and no deaths) in pregnant women each year. It is also assumed that there are approximately 11,000 new GBS infections and 2,300 deaths in nonpregnant adults. The highest incidence of disease in nonpregnant adults is in people 65 years of age and older. See Table A25-1.

Disease Scenarios

For the purposes of the calculations in this report, the committee assumed that 90% of GBS disease in neonates is early-onset disease and 20% is late-onset disease. Disease associated with neonatal GBS infections includes bacteremia (86%) and meningitis (14%). Approximately 72% of neonatal GBS infections are early-onset bacteremia, 14% are late-onset bacteremia, 8% are early-onset meningitis, and 6% are late-onset meningitis.

For the purposes of the calculations in the report, the committee assumed that all pregnant women infected with GBS experience chorioamnionitis, endometritis, or bacteremia. These infections are assumed to be associated with 7 days at an HUI of .68. It was assumed that all nonpregnant adults infected

Table A25-1 Incidence of Group B Streptococcus Infection in Noninfants and Nonpregnant Women

Age Groups	Population	Incidence Rates (per 100,000)	Cases
<1	3,963,000	0.00	0
1-4	16,219,000	0.92	149
5-14	38,056,000	0.91	347
15-24	36,263,000	1.70	616
25-34	41,670,000	1.76	731
35-44	42,149,000	1.68	708
45-54	30,224,000	4.84	1,464
55-64	21,241,000	8.31	1,766
65-74	18,964,000	11.57	2,194
75-84	11,088,000	22.69	2,516
85+	3,598,000	22.70	817
Total	263,435,000	4.29	11,308

with GBS experience invasive disease (e.g., bacteremia, sepsis, soft tissue infections) associated with 19 days at an HUI of .66. See Table A25-2.

COST INCURRED BY DISEASE

Table A25-3 summarizes the health care costs incurred by GBS infections. For the purposes of the calculations in this report, it was assumed that GBS infections in pregnant women are associated with additional hospitalization at the time of delivery and associated inpatient and outpatient physician visits and medication. Costs are also included for screening for GBS and chemoprophylaxis of pregnant women. It was estimated that all nonpregnant adults with invasive GBS disease require hospitalization (including inpatient physician visits) and outpatient services as well.

For the calculation in this report, it was assumed that all infants with GBS require hospitalization, including multiple inpatient physician visits and diagnostics. It was assumed that a small percentage of infants with GBS meningitis will require long-term care for 10 years until death.

VACCINE DEVELOPMENT

The committee assumed that it will take 7 years until licensure of a GBS vaccine and that $300 million needs to be invested for approval for use in nonpregnant people, and an additional $100 million needs to be invested for that same vaccine to be used in pregnant women. Special considerations regarding

Table 25-2 Disease Scenarios for Group B Streptococcus Infection in Infants and Adults

	% of Cases	Committee HUI Values	Duration (years)
INFANTS			
Bacteremia—NICU	36.0%	0.24	0.027 (10 days)
Bacteremia—Non-NICU	36.0%	0.24	0.027 (10 days)
Meningitis	6.4%	0.27	0.047 (17 days)
Meningitis with impairment	1.1%		
acute care (50% NICU; 50% Level 2)		0.27	0.047 (17 days)
permanent impairment— normal lifespan		0.53	26.804 (discounted quality adjusted life expectancy at birth)
Meningitis with early death	0.5%		
acute care		0.27	0.047 (17 days)
permanent impairment		0.53	10.000 (10 years)
death by age 10		0.00	25.690 (discounted quality adjusted life expectancy at age 10)
LATE ONSET DISEASE—20% of infant cases			
Bacteremia	14.0%	0.69	0.027 (10 days)
Meningitis	4.8%	0.27	0.047 (17 days)
Meningitis with impairment	0.8%		
acute care		0.27	0.047 (17 days)
permanent impairment— normal lifespan		0.53	26.804 (discounted quality adjusted life expectancy at birth)
Meningitis with early death	0.4%		
acute care		0.27	0.047 (17 days)
permanent impairment		0.53	10.000 (10 years)
death by age 10		0.00	25.690 (discounted quality adjusted life expectancy at age 10)
ADULTS			
Maternal Infection	100%		
inpatient		0.68	0.0192 (7 days)
outpatient treatment			0.0137 (5 days)
NONPREGNANT ADULTS			
Invasive disease	100.0%		
soft tissue, bone infection; bacteremia; urosepsis; pneumonia		0.66	0.052 (19 days)

Table 25-3 Health Care Costs Associated with GBS Disease in Infants and Adults

	% with Care	Cost per Unit	Units per Case	Form of Treatment
INFANTS				
EARLY ONSET DISEASE— 80% of infant cases				
Bacteremia—NICU				
bacteremia, sepsis, pneumonia	100%	$12,000	1.0	hospitalization NICU
	100%	$150	10.0	physician c
	100%	$500	1.0	diagnostic c
Bacteremia—Level 2 care				
bacteremia, sepsis, pneumonia	100%	$7,000	1.0	hospitalization non-NICU
	100%	$150	10.0	physician c
	100%	$500	1.0	diagnostic c
Meningitis				
acute care	50%	$12,000	1.0	hospitalization NICU
	50%	$7,000	1.0	hospitalization
	100%	$150	17.0	physician c
	100%	$500	1.0	diagnostic c
Meningitis with impairment				
acute care	50%	$12,000	1.0	hospitalization NICU
	50%	$7,000	1.0	hospitalization
	100%	$150	17.0	physician c
	100%	$500	1.0	diagnostic c
permanent impair-ment normal lifespan*	100%	$225	365.0	long-term care*/per year
Meningitis with early death				
acute care	50%	$12,000	1.0	hospitalization NICU
	50%	$7,000	1.0	hospitalization
	100%	$150	17.0	physician c
	100%	$500	1.0	diagnostic c
permanent impair-ment for 10-year period**	100%	$225	365.0	long-term care*/per year
LATE ONSET DISEASE—20% of infant cases				
Bacteremia				
bacteremia, sepsis, pneumonia	100%	$7,000	1.0	hospitalization
	100%	$150	10.0	physician c
	100%	$500	1.0	diagnostic c
Meningitis				
acute care	50%	$12,000	1.0	hospitalization NICU
	50%	$7,000	1.0	hospitalization
	100%	$150	17.0	physician c
	100%	$500	1.0	diagnostic c
Meningitis with impairment				
acute care	50%	$1,200	1.0	hospitalization NICU
	50%	$7,000	1.0	hospitalization
	100%	$150	10.0	physician c

Continued

Table 25-3 *Continued*

	% with Care	Cost per Unit	Units per Case	Form of Treatment
	100%	$500	1.0	diagnostic c
permanent impairment normal lifespan*	100%	$225	365.0	long-term care*/per year
Meningitis with early death				
acute care	50%	$12,000	1.0	hospitalization NICU
	50%	$7,000	1.0	hospitalization NICU
	50%	$150	10.0	physician c
	50%	$500	1.0	diagnostic c
permanent impairment for 10-year period**	100%	$225	365.0	long-term care*/per year
PREGNANT WOMEN				
Maternal Infection (chorioamnionitis, endometritis, bacteremia)				
additional inpatient treatment at time of delivery	100%	$1,000	1.0	hospitalization (in addition to normal delivery)
	100%	$150	1.0	physician c
	100%	$50	1.0	medication b
outpatient treatment	100%	$100	1.0	physician b
screening	90%	$50	1.0	diagnostic a
intrapartum chemoprophylaxis	25%	$50	1.0	medication b
NONPREGNANT ADULTS				
Invasive disease				
soft tissue, bone infection bacteremia; urosepsis; pneumonia	100%	$4,000	1.0	hospitalization
	100%	$150	19.0	physician c
	100%	$500	1.0	diagnostic c
outpatient	100%	$100	2.0	physician b

NOTE: *long-term care—$225/ day is maintenance expenditure per resident for residential facilities for persons with mental retardation.

 **cost per case is calculated as "present value" of annual cost for remaining life time (life expectancy at birth or 10 years, depending on scenario); additional discounting for immunization interval

development of a vaccine for use in pregnant women is discussed within the body of the report. Table 4-1 summarizes vaccine development assumptions for all vaccines considered in this report.

VACCINE PROGRAM CONSIDERATIONS

Target Population

The results of two vaccine strategies will be described. Both strategies involve annual immunization of 2,600,000 high-risk, nonpregnant adults (65 years of age or with specific chronic diseases). Both strategies involve immunization of younger females. One strategy involves annual immunization of pregnant women (approximately 1,630 primiparas). The other strategy involves annual immunization of 1,840,000 12-year-old girls. For the purposes of the calculations in this report, it is assumed that 30% of high-risk adults, 50% of 12-year-old girls, will utilize the vaccine. Additionally, it was assumed that utilization of the vaccine by pregnant women will either be 10% or 90%.

Vaccine Schedule, Efficacy, and Costs

For the purposes of the calculations in this report, it was estimated that this vaccine would cost $50 per dose and that administration costs would be $10 per dose. Default assumptions of a 3-dose series and 75% effectiveness were accepted. Table 4-1 summarizes vaccine program assumptions for all vaccines considered in this report.

RESULTS

Immunization of Pregnant Women and At-Risk Adults

If a vaccine program for group B streptococci were implemented today and the vaccine were 100% efficacious and utilized by 100% of the target population, the annualized present value of the QALYs gained would be 37,400. Using committee assumptions of less-than-ideal efficacy and utilization and including time and monetary costs until a vaccine program is implemented, the annualized present value of the QALYs gained would be 10,200 for 90% utilization by pregnant women and 4,500 for 10% utilization by pregnant women.

If a vaccine program for group B streptococci were implemented today and the vaccine was 100% efficacious and utilized by 100% of the target population, the annualized present value of the health care costs saved would be $630 million. Using committee assumptions of less-than-ideal efficacy and utilization and including time and monetary costs until a vaccine program is implemented, the annualized present value of the health care costs saved would be $310 million for 90% utilization by pregnant women and $45 million for 10% utilization by pregnant women.

If a vaccine program for group B streptococci were implemented today and the vaccine was 100% efficacious and utilized by 100% of the target population, the annualized present value of the program cost would be $760 million. Using committee assumptions of less-than-ideal efficacy and utilization and including time and monetary costs until a vaccine program is implemented, the annualized present value of the program cost would be $285 million for 90% utilization by pregnant women and $120 million for 10% utilization by pregnant women.

Using committee assumptions of time and costs until licensure, the fixed cost of vaccine development has been amortized and is $12 million for a group B streptococci vaccine.

If a vaccine program were implemented today and the vaccine was 100% efficacious and utilized by 100% of the target population, the annualized present value of the cost per QALY gained is $3,400. Using committee assumptions of less-than-ideal utilization and including time and monetary costs until a vaccine program is implemented, the annualized present value of the cost per QALY gained is -$1,500 for 90% utilization by pregnant women and $20,000 for 10% utilization by pregnant women. A negative value represents a saving in costs in addition to a saving in QALYs.

See Chapters 4 and 5 for details on the methods and assumptions used by the committee for the results reported.

Immunization of Girls at Puberty and At-Risk Adults

If a vaccine program for group B streptococci were implemented today and the vaccine was 100% efficacious and utilized by 100% of the target population, the annualized present value of the QALYs gained would be 33,000. Using committee assumptions of less-than-ideal efficacy and utilization and including time and monetary costs until a vaccine program is implemented, the annualized present value of the QALYs gained would be 6,200.

If a vaccine program for group B streptococci were implemented today and the vaccine was 100% efficacious and utilized by 100% of the target population, the annualized present value of the health care costs saved would be $435 million. Using committee assumptions of less-than-ideal efficacy and utilization and including time and monetary costs until a vaccine program is implemented, the annualized present value of the health care costs saved would be $125 million.

If a vaccine program for group B streptococci were implemented today and the vaccine was 100% efficacious and utilized by 100% of the target population, the annualized present value of the program cost would be $800 million. Using committee assumptions of less-than-ideal efficacy and utilization and including time and monetary costs until a vaccine program is implemented, the annualized present value of the program cost would be $215 million.

Using committee assumptions of time and costs until licensure, the fixed cost of vaccine development has been amortized and is $9 million for a group B streptococci vaccine.

If a vaccine program were implemented today and the vaccine was 100% efficacious and utilized by 100% of the target population, the annualized present value of the cost per QALY gained is $11,000. Using committee assumptions of less-than-ideal utilization and including time and monetary costs until a vaccine program is implemented, the annualized present value of the cost per QALY gained is $16,000.

See Chapters 4 and 5 for details on the methods and assumptions used by the committee for the results reported.

READING LIST

Anthony BF. Group B Streptococcal Infections. In: Textbook of Pediatric Infectious Diseases. RD Feigin and JD Cherry eds. Philadelphia, PA: WB Saunder Company, 1992, pp. 1305–1316.

Blumberg HM, Stephens DS, Modansky M, et al. Invasive Group B Streptococcal Disease: The Emergence of Serotype V. Journal of Infectious Diseases 1996; 173:365–73.

CDC. Prevention and control of influenza: recommendations of the Advisory Committee on Immunization Practices (ACIP). Morbidity and Mortality Weekly Report 1996; 45:1–24.

CDC. Prevention of perinatal group B streptococcal disease: a public health perspective. Morbidity and Mortality Weekly Report 1996; 45:1–24.

Edwards MS, Baker CJ. Streptococcus Agalactiae (Group B Streptococcus). In: Principles and Practice of Infectious Diseases. GL Mandell, JE Bennett, Dolin R eds. New York, NY: Churchill Livingstone, 1995, pp. 1835–1845.

Farley MM. A Population–Based Assessment of Invasive Disease Due to Group B Streptococcus in Nonpregnant Adults. The New England Journal of Medicine 1993; 328:1807–1811.

Farley MM. Group B Streptococcal Infection in Older Patients. Drugs & Aging 1995; 6:293–300.

Jackson LA, Hilsdon R, Farley MM, et al. Risk Factors for Group B Streptococcal Disease in Adults. Annals of Internal Medicine 1995; 123:415–420.

U.S. Bureau of the Census. Statistical Abstract of the U.S.: 1995 (115th edition). Washington, DC, 1995.

Ventura SJ, Martin JA, Mathews TJ, et al. Advance Report of Final Natality Statistics, 1994. Monthly Vital Statistics Report 1996; 44.

APPENDIX 26

Streptococcus pneumoniae

DISEASE BURDEN

Epidemiology

For the purposes of the calculations in this report, the committee estimated that there are approximately 6.4 million cases of *Streptococcus pneumoniae* in children 4 years of age and under each year in the United States. An additional 1 million cases were assumed to occur in people between the ages of 5 and 64 years of age and 400,000 cases in people 65 years of age and older. The number of deaths in those 3 age groups were estimated to be 1,450, 16,000, and 30,000, respectively. See Table A26-1.

Disease Scenarios

For the purposes of the calculation in this report, the committee assumed that *S. pneumoniae* disease manifests as bacteremia and sepsis, pneumonia, otitis media/sinusitis/bronchitis, and meningitis. The percentage of cases in the 3 age groups who experience these disease states can be found in Table A26-2. The health utility index (HUI) associated with these various scenarios ranges from .9 for sinusitis (10 days duration) to .16 for hospitalization for severe bacteremia and sepsis and .6 for neurologic sequelae of meningitis (lasting for the lifetime).

Table A26-1 Incidence of *Streptococcus pneumoniae* for Age Groups <5, 5–64, and >65

Age Groups	Population	Incidence rates (per 100,000)	% Distribution of Cases	Cases
LESS THAN 5 YEARS				
<1	3,963,000	18,167.74	0.1128	719,987
1-4	16,219,000	34,905.47	0.8872	5,661,319
Total		2,422.35	1.0000	6,381,306
5-64 YEARS				
5-14	38,056,000	467.19	0.1676	177,796
15-24	36,263,000	467.19	0.1597	169,419
25-34	41,670,000	467.19	0.1835	194,680
35-44	42,149,000	467.19	0.1856	196,918
45-54	30,224,000	467.19	0.1331	141,205
55-64	21,241,000	852.19	0.1706	181,015
Total		402.77	1.0000	1,061,032
GREATER THAN 65 YEARS				
65-74	18,964,000	1,182.19		224,191
75-84	11,088,000	1,182.19		131,082
85+	3,598,000	1,182.19		42,535
Total		151.01		397,808

COST INCURRED BY DISEASE

Table A26-3 summarizes the health care costs incurred by *S. pneumoniae* infections. For the purposes of the calculations in this report, it was assumed that general patterns of health care are the same for each age group in a scenario. Outpatient care for bacteremia/sepsis and for pneumonia was assumed to involve two physician visits, prescription medication, and an inexpensive diagnostic test. Hospitalization costs are also assumed in be incurred for some patients. For more severe cases (e.g., those requiring hospitalization), specialist physicians are included instead of generalists, who would be utilized for less severe infections.

Milder manifestations of *S. pneumoniae* (e.g., otitis media in children under 5 years of age and sinusitis/bronchitis in people over 5 years of age) were assumed to be associated with costs for general physician visits, prescription mediation, and (in half the cases) a diagnostic procedure (culture).

Acute treatment of meningitis was assumed to require hospitalization, specialist physicians, and expensive diagnostic procedures. It was assumed that a small percentage of patients with meningitis experience lifelong neurologic sequelae requiring multiple visits to a specialist and some sort of physical or other rehabilitative therapies for the disability.

Table A26-2 Disease Scenarios for *Streptococcus pneumoniae* Infection

	No. of Cases	% of Cases	Committee HUI Values	Duration (years)
<5 YEARS OF AGE				
Total Deaths (from acute infection)	1,450			
Total Cases	6,381,306			
BACTEREMIA/SEPSIS	6,216	0.10%		
Bacteremia/Sepsis	1,243	0.02%		
outpatient care only			0.93	0.0274 (10 days)
ICU			0.16	0.0055 (2 days)
inpatient after ICU			0.46	0.0137 (5 days)
Bacteremia/Sepsis— inpatient (no ICU)	3,730	0.06%	0.71	0.0110 (4 days)
Bacteremia/Sepsis— inpatient; complications	1,243	0.02%	0.59	0.0137 (5 days)
PNEUMONIA	62,161	0.97%		
Pneumonia—outpatient care only	6,216	0.10%	0.82	0.0274 (10 days)
Pneumonia	55,944	0.88%		
inpatient			0.71	0.0137 (5 days)
outpatient after inpatient			0.81	0.0137 (5 days)
Pneumonia with emphysema	932	0.01%		
inpatient			0.64	0.0384 (14 days)
outpatient after inpatient			0.82	0.0384 (14 days)
OTHER RESPIRATORY	6,312,729	98.93%		
Otitis Media			0.74	0.0110 (4 days)
Sinusitis, bronchitis			0.90	0.0274 (10 days)
MENINGITIS	200	0.0031%		
Meningitis	160	0.003%		
ICU			0.24	0.0055 (2 days)
inpatient after ICU			0.28	0.0274 (10 days)
Meningitis—inpatient (no ICU)	40	0.001%	0.39	0.0137 (5 days)
Meningitis—inpatient acute complications	30	0.0005%	0.27	0.0384 (14 days)
Meningitis—neurologic sequelae	60	0.001%	0.60	26.6824 (quality-adjusted life expectancy); 73.4869 (unadjusted life expectancy)
5-64 YEARS OF AGE				
Total Deaths (from acute infection)	15,584			
Total Cases	1,061,032			
BACTEREMIA/SEPSIS	17,915	1.6884%		
Bacteremia/Sepsis— outpatient care only	3,583	0.34%	0.93	0.0274 (10 days)
Bacteremia/Sepsis	3,583	0.34%		
ICU			0.16	0.0055 (2 days)
inpatient after ICU			0.46	0.0137 (5 days)

Table A26-2 *Continued*

	No. of Cases	% of Cases	Committee HUI Values	Duration (years)
Bacteremia/Sepsis—inpatient (no ICU)	10,749	1.01%	0.71	0.0110 (4 days)
Bacteremia/Sepsis—inpatient, complications	3,583	0.34%	0.59	0.0137 (5 days)
PNEUMONIA	179,145	16.8840%		
Pneumonia—outpatient care only	71,658	6.75%	0.82	0.0274 (10 days)
Pneumonia	107,487	10.13%		
inpatient			0.71	0.0137 (5 days)
outpatient after inpatient			0.81	0.0137 (5 days)
Pneumonia with emphysema	2,687	0.25%		
inpatient			0.64	0.0384 (14 days)
outpatient after inpatient			0.82	0.0384 (14 days)
OTHER RESPIRATORY	861,667	81.2103%		
Sinusitis, bronchitis			0.90	0.0274 (10 days)
MENINGITIS	2,306	0.2173%		
Meningitis	1,845	0.17%		
ICU			0.24	0.0055 (2 days)
inpatient after ICU			0.28	0.0274 (10 days)
Meningitis—inpatient (no ICU)	461	0.04%	0.39	0.0137 (5 days)
Meningitis—inpatient, acute complications	346	0.03%	0.27	0.0384 (14 days)
Meningitis—neurologic sequelae	692	0.07%	0.60	19.8289 (quality adjusted life expectancy at onset); 43.3814 (unadjusted life expectancy at onset)
65 YEARS AND OLDER				
Total Deaths (from acute infection)	29,592			
Total Cases	397,808			
BACTEREMIA/SEPSIS	23,555	5.92%		
Bacteremia/Sepsis	4,711	1.18%		
outpatient care only			0.93	0.0274 (10 days)
ICU			0.16	0.0055 (2 days)
inpatient after ICU			0.46	0.0137 (5 days)
Bacteremia/Sepsis	14,133	3.55%		
inpatient (no ICU)			0.71	0.0110 (4 days)
Bacteremia/Sepsis—inpatient; complications	4,711	1.18%	0.59	0.0137 (5 days)
PNEUMONIA	235,550	59.21%		
Pneumonia— outpatient care only	141,330	35.53%	0.82	0.0274 (10 days)

Table A26-2 *Continued*

	No. of Cases	% of Cases	Committee HUI Values	Duration (years)
Pneumonia	94,220	23.68%		
inpatient			0.71	0.0137 (5 days)
outpatient after inpatient			0.81	0.0137 (5 days)
Pneumonia with emphysema	3,533	0.89%		
inpatient			0.64	0.0384 (14 days)
outpatient after inpatient			0.82	0.0384 (14 days)
OTHER RESPIRATORY	138,333	34.77%		
Sinusitis, bronchitis			0.90	0.0274 (10 days)
MENINGITIS	370	0.09%		
Meningitis	296	0.07%		
ICU			0.24	0.0055 (2 days)
inpatient after ICU			0.28	0.0274 (10 days)
Meningitis—inpatient (no ICU)	74	0.02%	0.39	0.0137 (5 days)
Meningitis—inpatient, acute complications	56	0.01%	0.27	0.0384 (14 days)
Meningitis—neurologic sequelae	111	0.03%	0.60	6.9071 (remaining quality adjusted life expectancy); 11.2664 (unadjusted life expectancy at onset)

VACCINE DEVELOPMENT

The committee assumed that it will take 3 years until licensure of an *S. pneumoniae* vaccine and that $240 million needs to be invested. Table 4-1 summarizes vaccine development assumptions for all vaccines considered in this report.

VACCINE PROGRAM CONSIDERATIONS

Target Population

For the purposes of the calculations in this report, it is assumed that the target population for this vaccine is the annual birth cohort and people 65 years of age. It was assumed that utilization would be 90% and 60% respectively.

Table A26-3 Health Care Costs Associated with *Streptococcus pneumoniae* Infection

	Cost per Case	Cost per Unit	Units per Case	Form of Treatment
<5 YEARS OF AGE				
Bacteremia/Sepsis				
outpatient care only	$100	$50	2.0	physician a
	$50	$50	1.0	medication b
	$50	$50	1.0	diagnostic a
ICU and post-phase	$4,000	$4,000	1.0	hospitalization
	$300	$100	3.0	physician b
	$100	$100	1.0	diagnostic b
inpatient (no ICU)	$4,000	$4,000	1.0	hospitalization
	$300	$100	3.0	physician b
	$100	$100	1.0	diagnostic b
inpatient; complications	$4,000	$4,000	1.0	hospitalization
	$300	$100	3.0	physician b
	$500	$500	1.0	diagnostic c
Pneumonia				
outpatient care only	$100	$50	2.0	physician a
	$50	$50	1.0	diagnostic a
	$50	$50	1.0	medication b
inpatient	$4,000	$4,000	1.0	hospitalization
	$300	$100	3.0	physician b
	$100	$100	1.0	diagnostic b
outpatient after inpatient	$100	$50	2.0	physician a
	$50	$50	1.0	medication b
	$50	$50	1.0	diagnostics
Other Respiratory				
otitis media	$50	$50	1.0	physician visits
	$50	$50	1.0	medication b
	$50	$50	1.0	diagnostic a
Meningitis				
ICU and non-ICU	$7,000	$7,000	1.0	hospitalization
combine meningitis for costs	$450	$150	3.0	physician b
	$50	$50	1.0	medication b
	$100	$100	1.0	diagnostic b
	$500	$500	1.0	diagnostic c
inpatient, acute complications	$7,000	$7,000	1.0	hospitalization
	$900	$150	6.0	physician b
	$50	$50	1.0	medication b
	$100	$100	1.0	diagnostic b
	$500	$500	1.0	diagnostic c
Meningitis: sequelae				
lifelong annual costs	$600	$100	6.0	physician b
	$300	$50	6.0	physical therapy, other services

Table A26-3 *Continued*

	Cost per Case	Cost per Unit	Units per Case	Form of Treatment
5-64 YEARS OF AGE				
Bacteremia/Sepsis				
outpatient care only	$100	$50	2.0	physician visits
	$50	$50	1.0	medication b
	$50	$50	1.0	diagnostic a
ICU and post- phase	$4,000	$4,000	1.0	hospitalization
	$300	$100	3.0	physician b
	$100	$100	1.0	diagnostic b
inpatient (no ICU)	$4,000	$4,000	1.0	hospitalization
	$300	$100	3.0	physician b
	$100	$100	1.0	diagnostic b
inpatient; complications	$4,000	$4,000	1.0	hospitalization
	$300	$100	3.0	physician b
	$500	$500	1.0	diagnostic c
Pneumonia				
outpatient care only	$200	$100	2.0	physician b
	$100	$50	2.0	diagnostic a
	$50	$50	1.0	medication b
Pneumonia with and without emphysema				
inpatient	$4,000	$4,000	1.0	hospitalization
	$450	$150	3.0	physician c
	$100	$100	1.0	diagnostic b
	$50	$50	1.0	medication b
outpatient after inpatient	$100	$50	2.0	physician visits
	$50	$50	1.0	medication b
sinusitis, bronchitis				
	$100	$50	2.0	physician a
	$50	$50	1.0	medication b
	$50	$50	1.0	diagnostic b
Meningitis				
ICU, post-ICU, and non-ICU	$7,000	$7,000	1.0	hospitalization
	$450	$150	3.0	physician c
	$50	$50	1.0	medication b
	$100	$100	1.0	diagnostic b
	$500	$500	1.0	diagnostic c
Meningitis: sequelae				
cost per year for life	$300	$50	6.0	physical therapy
	$600	$100	6.0	physician b
>65 YEARS OF AGE+				
Bacteremia/Sepsis				
outpatient care only	$100	$50	2.0	physician a
	$50	$50	1.0	medication b
	$50	$50	1.0	diagnostic a
ICU and post ICU phase: inpatient	$4,000	$4,000	1.0	hospitalization
	$300	$100	3.0	physician b
	$100	$100	1.0	diagnostic b

Continued

Table A26-3 *Continued*

	Cost per Case	Cost per Unit	Units per Case	Form of Treatment
inpatient (no ICU)	$4,000	$4,000	1.0	hospitalization
	$300	$100	3.0	physician b
	$100	$100	1.0	diagnostic b
inpatient; complications	$4,000	$4,000	1.0	hospitalization
	$300	$100	3.0	physician b
	$500	$500	1.0	diagnostic c
Pneumonia				
outpatient care only	$100	$50	2.0	physician a
	$50	$50	1.0	medication b
	$50	$50	1.0	diagnostic a
inpatient	$4,000	$4,000	1.0	hospitalization
	$300	$100	3.0	physician b
	$100	$100	1.0	diagnostic b
outpatient after inpatient	$100	$50	2.0	physician a
	$50	$50	1.0	medication b
	$50	$50	1.0	diagnostic a
Sinusitis, bronchitis				
	$100	$50	2.0	physician a
	$50	$50	1.0	medication b
	$50	$50	1.0	diagnostic b
Meningitis				
all meningitis combined	$7,000	$7,000	1.0	hospitalization
% cases now corrected	$450	$150	3.0	physician c
	$50	$50	1.0	medication b
	$100	$100	1.0	diagnostic b
	$500	$500	1.0	diagnostic c
annual costs for life	$300	$50	6.0	physical therapy

Vaccine Schedule, Efficacy, and Costs

For the purposes of the calculations in this report, it was estimated that this vaccine would cost $50 per dose and that administration costs would be $10 per dose. Default assumptions of a 3-dose series and 75% effectiveness were accepted. Table 4-1 summarizes vaccine program assumptions for all vaccines considered in this report.

RESULTS

If a vaccine program for *S. pneumoniae* were implemented today and the vaccine were 100% efficacious and utilized by 100% of the target population, the annualized present value of the QALYs gained would be 265,000. Using committee assumptions of less-than-ideal efficacy and utilization and including time and monetary costs until a vaccine program is implemented, the annualized present value of the QALYs gained would be 120,000.

Although the number of cases of disease are much higher in children under 5 years of age, the largest number of lost QALYs are associated with disease in people 65 years of age and older. This discrepancy is caused by the much higher mortality rate and more severe morbidity in the older individuals compared to younger people.

If a vaccine program for *S. pneumoniae* were implemented today and the vaccine was 100% efficacious and utilized by 100% of the target population, the annualized present value of the health care costs saved would be $1.6 billion. Using committee assumptions of less-than-ideal efficacy and utilization and including time and monetary costs until a vaccine program is implemented, the annualized present value of the health care costs saved would be $815 million.

If a vaccine program for *S. pneumoniae* were implemented today and the vaccine was 100% efficacious and utilized by 100% of the target population, the annualized present value of the program cost would be $1.1 billion. Using committee assumptions of less-than-ideal efficacy and utilization and including time and monetary costs until a vaccine program is implemented, the annualized present value of the program cost would be $675 million.

Using committee assumptions of time and costs until licensure, the fixed cost of vaccine development has been amortized and is $7.2 million for a *S. pneumoniae* vaccine.

If a vaccine program were implemented today and the vaccine was 100% efficacious and utilized by 100% of the target population, the annualized present value of the cost per QALY gained is -$2,000. A negative value represents a saving in costs in addition to a saving in QALYs. Using committee assumptions of less-than-ideal utilization and including time and monetary costs until a vaccine program is implemented, the annualized present value of the cost per QALY gained is $1,000.

See Chapters 4 and 5 for details on the methods and assumptions used by the committee for the results reported.

READING LIST

Baron RC, Dicker RC, Bussell, KE, et al. Assessing Trends in Mortality in 121 U.S. Cities, 1970–79, from All Causes and from Pneumonia and Influenza. Public Health Reports 1988; 103:120–128.

Breiman RF, Spika JS, Navarro VJ, et al. Pneumococcal Bacteremia in Charleston County, South Carolina: A Decade Later. Archives of Internal Medicine 1990; 150: 1401–1405.

CDC. Defining the Public Health Impact of Drug-Resistant *Streptococcus pneumoniae*: Report of a Working Group. Morbidity and Mortality Weekly Report 1996; 45:1–2.

CDC. Increasing Pneumococcal Vaccination Rates Among Patients of a National Health-Care Alliance—United States, 1993. Morbidity and Mortality Weekly Report 1995; 44:741–742.

322 *VACCINES FOR THE 21ST CENTURY*

CDC. Pneumococcal and Influenza Vaccination Levels Among Adults Aged Over 65 Years—United States, 1995. Morbidity and Mortality Weekly Report 1997; 46:913–926.

CDC. Prevention of Pneumococcal Disease. Morbidity and Mortality Weekly Report 1997; 46:1–24.

Fedson DS. Pneumococcal Vaccination in the Prevention of Community-Acquired Pneumonia: An Optimistic View of Cost-Effectiveness. Seminars in Respiratory Infections 1993; 8:285–293.

Fedson DS, Shapiro ED, LaForce FM, et al. Pneumococcal Vaccine After 15 Years of Use—Another View. Archives of Internal Medicine; 154:2531–2535.

Institute for Advanced Studies in Immunology and Aging. Improving the Performance of Influenza and Pneumococcal Vaccines in Adults. Working Group Meeting—November 1995; Washington, DC.

King JC, Vink PE, Farley JJ, et al. Safety and Immunogenicity of Three Doses of a Five-Valent Pneumococcal Conjugate Vaccine in Children Younger Than Two Years With and Without Human Immunodeficiency Virus Infection. Pediatrics 1997; 99:575–580.

Kronenberger CB, Hoffman RE, Lezotte DC, et al. Invasive Penicillin-Resistant Pneumococcal Infections: A Prevalence and Historical Cohort Study. Emerging Infectious Diseases 1996; 2:121–124.

Lave JR, Fine MJ, Sankey SS, et al. Hospitalized Pneumonia—Outcomes, Treatment Patterns, and Costs in Urban and Rural Areas. Journal of General Internal Medicine 1996; 11:415–421.

Loughlin AM, Marchant CD, Lett SM. The Changing Epidemiology of Invasive Bacterial Infections in Massachusetts Children, 1984 through 1991. American Journal of Public Health 1995; 85:392–394.

Markowitz JS, Pashko S, Gutterman EM, et al. Death Rates among Patients Hospitalized with Community-Acquired Pneumonia: A Reexamination with Data from Three States. American Journal of Public Health 1996; 86:1152–1154.

Sisk JE, Moskowitz AJ, Whang W, et al. Cost-effectiveness of Vaccination Against Pneumococcal Bacteremia Among Elderly People. JAMA 1997; 278:1333–1339.

Tuomanen EI, Austrian R, Masure HR. Pathogenesis of Pneumococcal Infection. The New England Journal of Medicine 1995; 332:1280.

U.S. Bureau of the Census. Statistical Abstract of the U.S.: 1995 (115th edition). Washington, DC, 1995.

Wenger JD, Hightower AW, Facklam RR, et al. Bacterial Meningitis in the United States, 1986: Report of a Multistate Surveillance Study. The Journal of Infectious Diseases 1990; 162:1316–1323.

APPENDIX 27

Information on Accessing Electronic Spreadsheets

To access the electronic files for the vaccine appendixes and the modeling spreadsheets go to the following web site:

http://www4.nationalacademies.org/IOM/IOMHome.nsf/Pages/HPDP+Reports

Under the listing for the report *Vaccines for the 21st Century: A Tool for Decisionmaking*, is a link to the "Hypothetical Vaccine X" spreadsheets and the Excel spreadsheets that contain the data for the vaccine candidates discussed in the report. Click on the icon to download the Microsoft Excel spreadsheet.

APPENDIX 28

Summary of Workshops

Herpes Simplex 326
Epstein-Barr Virus 329
Hepatitis C Virus 334
Human Papillomavirus 338
Dengue Hemorrhagic Fever 342
Chlamydia trachomatis 347
Tuberculosis 351
Histoplasmosis and Coccidioidomycosis 355
Group A Streptococci 359
Helicobacter pylori 363
Neisseria gonorrhoea 367
Adjuvants 372
Antigen Delivery Systems 377
DNA Vaccines 381
Preventive Vaccine for Diabetes 386
Cytokine Modification of Autoreactivity 389
T-Cell Subset Choice on the Outcome of Autoimmune Disease 392
Antigen-Induced Programmed T-Cell Death as a New Approach to
  Immune Therapy 395
Induction, Propagation, and Immunoregulation of Autoimmune Diseases
  of the Central Nervous System 399
Peptide-Mediated Regulation of Autoimmunity 403
Stimulation and Costimulation 407
Viral Therapeutic Vaccines—Hepatitis B 412
CD8 CTL to Mutated Oncoproteins and Fusion Proteins 415
CTL Screening for Tumor Antigens 420
Immunity to Oncogenic Self-Proteins 425
Cytokines and Their Local Environments 429

HERPES SIMPLEX[1]

Pathobiology. Primary herpes simplex virus (HSV) infection occurs through mucosal surfaces, followed by Kaposi's varicelliform eruption. Immune host responses control this primary infection within 14 to 21 days. What is unique is the retrograde neuronal transport of the virus to the dorsal root ganglia, where a cycle of replication occurs and the virus becomes latent until a provocative stimulus leads to reactivation. At that time, anterior grade transport returns the virus to the mucosal surfaces, where replication ensues.

Incidence and Burden. By adulthood, about 80 percent of the U.S. population has been exposed to nongenital HSV type 1 and is at risk for reactivation, leading to herpes simplex labialis. There are about 750,000 new cases of genital infection per year in the United States, and overall seroprevalence of HSV-2 is about 60 million individuals. Genital herpes generates about 600,000 physician visits and 20,000 unnecessary caesarian sections annually. Two more serious infections are herpes simplex encephalitis and neonatal herpes, each with about 1,500 cases per year. The cost of neonatal herpes is at least $750 million per year, primarily in indirect costs for the long-term management of neurological sequelae from which these babies suffer.

Seroprevalence of HSV type 2 is increasing rapidly. In 1992, seroprevalence for the U.S. population at large was about 31 percent; for persons of color, between 50 and 55 percent. Acquisition is a function of the number of sexual partners to whom an individual is exposed: for heterosexual men with greater than 50 partners, the probability of acquiring HSV-2 is 80 percent or higher; for heterosexual women with more than 50 partners, over 90 percent. Women are more likely to acquire HSV-2 than men. As with other genital ulcerative disease, there is also a four- or fivefold increase in the risk of acquiring HIV infection.

Rationale and Goals of Vaccine. Studies of couples with discordant serostatus suggest that prior HSV-1 infection confers some degree of protection from acquiring HSV-2 infection. When the male is positive for HSV-2 and the female is seronegative, her probability of acquiring HSV-2 is 20 percent during the calendar year. This becomes particularly significant if she becomes pregnant during that year. If the female is seropositive for HSV-1, however, the probability drops to 10 percent. (The reverse also holds: if the male is positive for HSV-1 rather than seronegative, his probability of acquiring HSV-2 drops from 10 percent to 5 percent.) These findings suggest that a vaccine that could seroconvert the mother from at-risk to lower-risk could lower the probability of transmission to the newborn.

The goal of this vaccine would be to prevent or at least reduce the severity of primary infection, and possibly to reduce the frequency and clinical symptoms of reoccurrences. We know that exogenous reinfection is extremely

---

[1] Based on a presentation by Richard J. Whitley, M.D.

uncommon in the immune-competent host, and that HSV-1 antibodies reduce both the probability and the clinical symptoms of primary HSV-2 infection. Similarly, fetal transmission is 10 times less likely when there are preexisting HSV-2 antibodies, compared with primary infection. And the duration of primary HSV-2 infections are reduced in seropositive individuals from 21-28 days to 10-14 days.

Approaches to Vaccine Development. Four approaches have been attempted in developing such a vaccine. *Live virus by autoinoculation* has been defined as a failure in studies over the past 100 years. HSV has 13 glycoproteins in its envelope, two of which (B and D) are required for infectivity and potent inducers of neutralizing antibodies. *Subunit vaccines* for glycoprotein B, glycoprotein D, and a combination of B and D are under investigation. *Vector glycoprotein genes* using either canary pox or a vaccinia vector have been. *Engineered herpes simplex virus* is a potential future candidate for clinical trials.

Subunit Vaccines. Clinical trials are currently evaluating monoclonal antibody therapy using glycoprotein B and D combinations to treat neonatal HSV infection and HSV encephalitis. Other subunit trials underway include one therapeutic trial of approximately 800 volunteers and 2 primary prevention trials of approximately 500 couples each. In the latter prophylactic trial, one partner in each monogamous relationship has recurrent HSV-2 and the other is HSV-2-seronegative. The former, therapeutic trial is based on the results of a preliminary trial of 100 volunteers between the ages 18 and 55, who averaged 4 to 14 outbreaks per year and had not received acyclovir for 3 months prior to therapy. Half received 100 micrograms of glycoprotein D-2 with alum adjuvant; half received placebo; and there was a booster at 2 months. In those who received the vaccine, the average number of recurrences dropped from 0.5 to 0.42 per month, and the median from 6 to 4 per year.

Genetically Engineered HSV Virus. Genetic stability is a concern in all genetically engineered vaccines; reversions to or recombinations with wild-type viruses, when they do occur, should be less virulent than the current strain. In addition, live attenuated viruses abdicated the ability to become latent and therefore, under some circumstances, might be reactivated. This is why deletions in the gamma 134.5 gene are particularly promising: they debilitate the virus' ability to become latent and subsequently reactivate (see below).

The herpes simplex virus has a genome that is only 150,000 base pairs (150 kB) long, in an architecture consisting of a unique long segment and a unique short segment. There are internal repeats bonding the unique long and short segments so that the virus could invert upon itself, leaving four equimotor isomers in any population. There is a 70-percent homology between HSV-1 and HSV-2.

The starting point for an engineered vaccine is an intratypic hybrid identified as R-70-20 and was developed about 10 years ago. It consists of the unique long segment of HSV-1, a segment of the unique long segment of HSV-

2, and the unique short segment of HSV-2. A 12-kB deletion of internal repeats from the HSV-2 short domain, mapping for a series of glycoproteins (including G, J, GD, GI, and GE), was inserted. This vaccine considerably reduces virulence in rodent models, is stable upon serial passage in mouse brains, and is safe and efficacious in aotis monkeys at concentrations up to 10^7 PFU administered by any route, including intracerebrally. It was safe in humans at up to $10^{4.5}$ PFU (higher doses were not studied). This vaccine required two doses, implying that it was overly attenuated for administration to humans.

HSV can also be attenuated through deletions and stop codes. The gamma 134.5 gene resides in the inverted repeats in two copies on the unique long segment of the HSV-2 genome; when 134.5 is deleted, it leaves a virus with an LD-50 upon inoculation directly into the central nervous system of a mouse of 10^6 PFU, compared with 10^2 PFU for the restored wild-type virus. A stop-code on the carboxy terminus of the genome can similarly attenuate the virus.

Using the latter technique with HSV-2, a recombinant vaccine was generated that also deleted the structural components of UL-55 and UL-56. This vaccine has significantly reduced neurovirulence in mice—LD-50 is 5.6 X 10^5 PFU, compared with less than 50 PFU for the wild type in that circumstance—and is safe in the aotis monkey at up to 10^6 PFU. In terms of efficacy, the vaccine appears to protect guinea pigs from disease at dosages in the range of 10^4 to 10^5 PFU. Immunized aotis monkeys survive challenges with wild-type virus at up to 10^5 PFU when given intravaginally. These results suggests that this is, at least potentially, a genetically engineered vaccine that will provide a broader immune response than is encountered with subunit vaccines.

Both the method of attenuation and the route of administration seem to influence the efficacy of these candidate vaccines. When mice were inoculated intranasally and then challenged intranasally with either wild virus or HSV-2, there was a reduction of mortality of 20 percent for those inoculated with 134.5-deletion mutants, and 13 percent when a stop code is place at the carboxy terminus. When mice are immunized intranasally and challenged intravaginally, however, the effect is not as great. Researchers are currently looking for IgA and IgG2a in the vaginal secretions of these mice to learn more about these immune responses.

Animal Models. Two new animal models have emerged from this work. The first is a test of the virulence of the virus; the aotis monkey is exquisitely sensitive for the evaluation of genetically engineered viruses, which are inoculated directly into the eye. The second is a rodent model to establish the genetic stability of attenuated vaccines. It involves inoculating virus into the mouse brain, harvesting tissue, raising the virus again, and reinoculating virus into mouse brains on subsequent occasions; nine passages will usually select unstable variants or a reversion to wild type. Inoculation into mouse brain can also be used to evaluate the virulence of attenuated virus.

In response to questions from the audience, Dr. Whitley added the following:

• Researchers do not at present have a marker of host immune response that is predictive of vaccine efficacy. Both neutralizing antibodies and cell-mediated immune responses have been investigated and eliminated.

• Gamma-134.5-deletion vaccines will eventually be tested in immuno-compromised models.

• Subunit vaccines currently require three doses to provide persistent antibody levels, although the duration and intensity of immune response may increase with a new adjuvant. R-70-20 acted more like a dead vaccine, requiring two doses. There are hopes that replication-competent viruses like the 134.5-deletion mutants will provide enhanced immunogenic effects with one shot rather than two.

• There has been little work on cellular responses to these vaccines or indeed to primary and recurrent herpes at all. Some researchers are doing CTLs on mice, and others are looking at T-cell responses in humans who are seropositive but have no clinical recurrences. T-cell responses following primary infection are robust, but no one has done comprehensive CTLs or tried to dissect out specific T-cell response in all of these human populations.

• The target population for HSV-2 immunization is adolescents as they are about to begin sexual activity, perhaps 10 or 12 years old, and the vaccine should provide at least 10 years of resistance to the wild-type virus. It will probably be impractical to test for serologic status for HSV-1 or HSV-2 prior to immunization.

EPSTEIN-BARR VIRUS[2]

Epstein-Barr virus (EBV) is another extremely common virus, but it is linked to a growing list of pathologies. Unlike HSV, there have been few vaccine trials, but a great deal is known about the disease processes. This knowledge could be used to generate partial or complete immunity to block these diseases.

Incidence and Burden. Worldwide, about 95 percent of the adult population is infected with EBV. If the primary infection comes in late adolescence, about 50 percent of seronegatives will develop the clinical manifestation called infectious mononucleosis (IM). IM is a significant disease, with at least 125,000 new cases recorded each year in the United States. About 70 percent of patient will resolve their symptoms in 2 to 4 weeks and is the major cause of lost time for new Army recruits. However, 30 percent develop more extensive impairment that may not resolve for 3 to 4 months. About 1 percent of cases develop complications, including neurological, bone marrow, liver involvement, and

---

[2] Based on a presentation by Nancy Raab-Traub, M.D.

even fatal IM. This extensive morbidity might be decreased by appropriate immunotherapy, but there is at present no effective antiviral therapy.

In most cases EBV establishes latency in the B-lymphocytes. However, EBV is associated with a variety of aplastic diseases, including 80 percent of AIDS-related lymphomas. Among post-transplant proliferative disorders, anywhere from 25 percent to 100 percent (depending on organ) occur in patients who are having a primary EBV infection. Similarly, there are many similarities between IM and Hodgkin's disease—patients with a history of IM are 2 to 3 times more likely to develop Hodgkin's lymphoma, and 70 percent of Hodgkin's-like lymphocytes are EBV-positive. EBV is also associated with Burkitt's lymphoma, which is relatively rare in the United States but is endemic in Africa. EBV is associated with the vast majority of nasopharyngeal carcinoma, which occurs when the virus is reactivated in mucosal lymphocytes and infects epithelial cells, which develop abnormalities and rapidly becomes dysplasia or carcinoma in situ. EBV is now being described in an increasing number of T-cell lymphomas, a significant proportion of Hodgkin's disease, and in discrete substantive gastric carcinomas. Other related diseases include hairy leukoplakia, which was originally described in AIDS patients.

Pathobiology. EBV can establish both permissive infection in epithelial cells and lymphocytes and latent, nonpermissive transforming infections in lymphocytes. Pathogenesis involves introduction of the virus into the oral epithelial cells, which are usually permissive to viral infection, and virus is then secreted into the saliva. Secondarily to this epithelial infection, virus enters the B-lymphocyte, where it circularizes, forming an extra chromosomal episome in the nucleus. One week after the initial infection, as many as 5 percent to 20 percent of peripheral blood lymphocytes are infected with EBV, including a wide variety of cell types: B-lymphocytes, Reed-Sternberg-like cells, plasmacytoid cells, and even a small percentage of T-lymphocytes. This is basically a latent infection: most of these cells do not make viruses but instead begin to express viral gene products that are associated with the process of cellular transformation. Many of these gene products are very potent targets of cytotoxic T-lymphocytes (CTLs), which must be generated to control the infection and the transformed lymphocytes. In the absence of T-cell response, these lymphocytes grow uncontrolled and eventually develop into a lymphoma.

Viral Genome. Analysis of the viral genome can distinguish latent from replicative infection and is informative in other ways. Like HSV, the EBV genome is a double-stranded DNA molecule with variants, but with a simpler structure. It is about 190 kB long, but instead of inverted repeats, it has multiple copies of a 500-base-pair direct repeat at each end of the genome. Variants are highly heterogenous, with anywhere from 1 to 20 copies of the terminal fragments at either end of the genome. This assay was able to distinguish between the variant form from the larger episomal form, but it also revealed that (within each cell) each of the up to 100 copies of the EBV episome was identical with regard to the number of terminal repeats. This also suggested that every cell within a tumor would be identical, from which researchers deduced that the epithelial tumors associated with EBV (e.g., nasopharyngeal and salivary gland carcinomas) were also clonal. This was confirmed by comparing the clonality predicted by EBV terminal studies and the clonality found in immunoglobulin rearrangements.

This indicated that most of the tumors associated with EBV were clonal proliferations and, more importantly, that these proliferations had developed from a single EBV-infected progenitor cell. This has been confirmed in post-transplant proliferative disorders, Hodgkin's lymphoma, Burkitt's lymphoma, gastrocarcinomas, cancers of the salivary gland, and the new T-cell lymphomas that are being reported in Taiwan and Japan. In nasopharyngeal carcinoma, patients have extremely high titers to replicative antigens and, while the Southern blot test does show a single clonal EBV fragment, there is also a faint ladder array indicating that at least a few cells go into permissive infection and make additional virus. The principal exception is hairy leukoplakia, for which the tests show no evidence of a fused band representing an episomal compartment, but rather an abundant ladder array indicating that this is a permissive infection. In the majority of cases, however, the diseases associated with EBV are associated with latent infection.

EBV Gene Functions. As noted, EBV gene products are expressed by infected cells, and researchers have identified the function of many of these products. One of the most important is Epstein-Barr nuclear antigen type one (EBNA-1), which binds to a specific DNA sequence in the EBV genome (the origin of plasma replication) and allows replication by DNA prolimerase. As a result, these infections are not susceptible to any kind of antiviral therapy directed toward the prolimerase. EBNA-1 also has the ability to induce the expression of the rad genes, which may be critical in some of the genomic rearrangements that have been described in Burkitt's lymphoma. No CTLs have been identified that are specific for EBNA-1, apparently due to a unique sequence in the EBNA-1 gene that mimics a cellular gene and prevents it from being recognized by class one antigens.

Five additional nuclear antigens (EBNA-2 through 6) have viral regulatory functions. Three of them are essential for transformation of B-lymphocytes. EBNA-2 transactivates these other genes, and three of them regulate the expression of latent membrane protein one (LMP-1) in the transformed lymphocytes. Almost all of the CTL targets are in these genes, which are expressed uniquely in B-lymphocytes.

LMP-1 is considered to be the viral oncogene: it promotes transformation and cellular division; it is the only gene that transforms rodent cells and cultures; and it is essential to the activation of a B-lymphocyte. As a result, it is able to inhibit apoptosis both in B-lymphocytes (by inducing expression of BCL-2) and in epithelial cells (through a p53-dependent mechanism that occurs through the induction of the A-20 gene). The LMP-1 gene is expressed in post-transplant lymphomas and other malignancies associated with EBV; it appears to be a critical gene for neoplastic growth. LMP-2 associates with LMP-1 in transformed cells and appears to block activation of the B-lymphocyte by interfering with the signals that would induce antibody synthesis. In doing so, LMP-2 helps to maintain the latent infection.

A last set of EBV genes expressed in infected cells are called Epstein-Barr encoded RNAs (EBERs). They are RNA polymerase-3 transfers, but their function is not yet known. They are not essential for transformation, but they are extremely abundant (50,000 to 1 million copies per infected cell) and very stable. EBERs can be very useful for identifying infected tissues, and because they are not expressed in hairy leukoplakia (a permissive infection) they may be useful in identifying repositories of latent infection.

Levels of Latency. Research on the actual behavior of EBV in each of the associated pathologies has shown that there are actually three levels of latency. Type one latency is a minimal level of expression, characteristic of Burkitt's lymphoma. Only EBNA-1 and the EBERs are expressed, so the infected cells do not become targets for cytotoxic T-cells. The peripheral blood lymphocytes of normal individuals who have been exposed to EBV also express EBNA-1 and EBERs, and they are also believed to express LMP-2, helping to maintain them in a state of latent infection.

In type two latency, additional genes are expressed. Specifically, LMP-1 and LMP-2, two genes that are regulated by the EBNAs, are expressed in the absence of the EBNAs. In other words, the critical transforming genes are being expressed but not the key CTL targets, which may be important in the development of disease for which this is the characteristic state of latency, including nasopharyngeal carcinoma, Hodgkin's disease, and T-cell lymphoma.

In type three latency, the entire array of EBV latent genes are expressed, including not only the oncogenes but also EBNAs 2 through 6, which are the key CTL targets, as well as high levels of EBERs whose function is as yet unknown. This type of infection, which is typical of peripheral blood lymphocytes in infectious mononucleosis and most of the cells in post-transplant proliferative disease, should be very amenable to control by the immune system.

In replicative infection, one vital gene called ZEBRA is the replication activator that turns on the expression of the viral replicative antigens (including polymerase and thymidine kinase) and the structural proteins (including the viral caps antigen, or VCA, and glycoproteins 350/220, 110, 85, 42, and 27). The glycoproteins of EBV are much less complex than those of HSV, and one in particular—gp350/220—is the main target of neutralizing antibodies and hence the principal focus of research attention.

Approaches for Vaccine Development. One approach that is being pursued is recombinant gp350, which does induce antibody-dependent cytotoxicity. In cotton-top tamarinds, this vaccine protects against lymphoma after a parenteral challenge. This approach would probably protect humans in pathologies that are dependent on replication, such as IM and nasopharyngeal carcinoma. In a very limited trial in China, 10 children were infected with gp350 in vaccinia and 10 got placebo; after a year, all 10 on placebo became infected with EBV, but only 2 of the 10 who got gp350 were infected. Much has been done in terms of designing gp350 to be produced in the cells and working on a strategy for clarification in high quantities. Abnormal viral response in the absence of antibodies to fusion protein is a concern.

T-cell epitope vaccines are also being investigated, because researchers have identified so many of the CTL epitopes that are critical for EBV infections. Experiments with SCID mice indicate that it is possible to transfer CTLs and thereby control viral proliferations. Such a vaccine might provide prophylactic protection for transplant recipients and (in combination with gp350) in nasopharyngeal carcinoma. Tumors may not express key antigens, or viral functions may impair peptide presentation.

Ultimately, however, the goal would be to make a genetically altered EBV vaccine. This would be essential to protect against EBV-related malignancies such as Burkitt's lymphoma and nasopharyngeal carcinoma, where the infection would have to be eliminated to prevent the disease. As detailed above, many of the necessary steps have been taken in this direction. Many people are infected with both type 1 and type 2 EBV, suggesting that wild-type infection is not protective.

Animal Models. Animal models are somewhat limited. Cotton-top tamarinds develop lymphomas when EBV is injected parenterally, and they can be protected with gp350 vaccine. SCID-human chimeric mice also develop EBV lymphoproliferative diseases, and can be protected with transferred CTLs; but they may not be very useful for evaluating vaccines because of transient T-cell function and the absence of appropriate lymphokine synthesis.

A new and promising prototype is a mouse EBV homologue, although it might be more similar to *herpes saimiri*. You can induce infection by internasal inoculation, and the mice develop lymphoid proliferations that have some similarities to EBV infection. However, the most encouraging animal model is a rhesus EBV that is highly homologous to EBV, and has identical patterns of mucosal infection and disease. Also, SIV-infected animals develop lymphomas. This may be the ideal system to test a genetically altered EBV virus.

In response to questions from the audience, Dr. Raab-Traub added the following:

• No research is being done to analyze the mucosal infection or to induce mucosal immune response. There have been anecdotal reports of defective viral genomes in some seronegative subjects. These genomes, which lack the transforming EBV genes that generated immunoglobulin-A response in saliva, might offer some protection.

• 100 percent of infected B-lymphocytes become immortalized.

• Recombinant gp350 vaccine should be ready for testing in a small seronegative population soon. It would be effective against both type 1 and type 2 EBV.

HEPATITIS C VIRUS[3]

Hepatitis C virus (HCV) is a recent field of research but a major cause of disease. What used to be known as "non-A and non-B hepatitis" was recognized in the mid-1970s with the development of serological tests for the hepatitis A and B viruses, and the cause was identified and named in 1988. Researchers are only beginning to understand the interaction of HCV with the host and the ensuing immune responses. With the technology now available in the areas of recombinant antigen production, adjuvants, and genetic immunization, researchers hope to have at least some impact on transmission and disease development at some point in the future.

Burden and Epidemiology. HCV is a truly global problem and is the major infectious disease problem in Japan. In the United States, there have been 150,000 new cases of HCV infection per year for the past decade. From 50 percent to 60 percent of these infections progress to persistent viremia and chronic persistent hepatitis. Of patients with chronic hepatitis, about 20 percent will progress to cirrhosis, and about 20 percent of cirrhotics with HCV will undergo liver failure. As a result, HCV is most common cause for liver transplantation in the United States. In addition, it is now clear that hepatocellular carcinoma is associated with HCV, with cirrhosis as a precondition, and that about 10 percent of cirrhotics with HCV will develop cancer over a period of time.

Research in Japan indicates that mean time from infection to cirrhosis is 20 years, and to cancer 30 years, so this is a very indolent type of disease. At the same time, research at NIH indicates that in a minority of patients cirrhosis can develop in a few years. Conversely, around 15 percent of post-transfusion HCV infections become negative over the long term, so there are some spontaneous resolvers.

The biggest risk factor for contracting hepatitis C is intravenous drug use, constituting about half of U.S. infections. About 30 percent to 40 percent of cases have no known risk factor. Transfusion is now a negligible risk, with the introduction of a blood screening test. There is a measurable incidence in health care workers who are exposed to infected blood, and data from Japan indicated that mothers can transmit the virus to their babies. The issue of sexual transmission is controversial, but studies show that multiple heterosexual partners are a risk factor, while the incidence in homosexual men is extremely low; apparently HCV can be transmitted sexually, but it is inefficiently transmitted that way.

Viral Genome. HCV belongs to the Flaviviridae family, along with flavivirus and pestiviruses. It is an RNA virus that does not integrate into cellular DNA, and instead replicates only through RNA replication intermediates. The virus is highly heterogenous: it can change rapidly in the infected host, and at

---

[3] Based on a presentation by Michael Houghton, M.D.

least 6 major types and 40 subtypes have been identified around the world. The 1A and 1B subtypes account for most infections in the United States.

The genome consists of about 10,000 nucleotides, with a 5' terminal iris and an internal ribosome entry site. It makes a large polyprotein that is cleaved post-translationally and co-translationally by a combination of host enzymes and viral proteases. It seems that the host signal peptidase is primarily involved in processing the nuclear capsid and the two envelope glycoproteins (gpE1 and gpE2). The presumed nonstructural proteins (NS) appear to be processed by the action of two viral proteases, one in the NS3 domain that is a trypsin-like protease, and another that spans the NS2 and NS3 genes that appears to be a metallic protease.

Immunology. Preliminary work on the correlates of immunity have shown that peripheral CD4-positive T-cells respond to HCV nonstructural protein 3 (NS3) very early in the infection, and that this response persists following recovery. In chronic patients, however, there is very little T-cell response. There is evidence that the protective immune response is short-lived and weak, at best. For example, a study of polytransfused thalassemic children found that patients who normalized after an initial episode of acute hepatitis nevertheless developed a second infection that progressed to chronic persistent hepatitis. Both infections involved the HCV-1-B subtype.

Viral Persistence. HCV is remarkably adept at persisting in the host in the face of an apparently substantial immune response. In the livers of about 50 percent of patients with chronic hepatitis, researchers are able to identify CTLs of varying specificity to either structural protein or to nonstructural proteins in the polyprotein precursor. CTLs also infiltrate the livers of chimpanzees with chronic infections. It is not known how the virus persists in the face of such a response. One theory is that HCV has evolved a mechanism for abrogating a lymphokine action; another is that the virus inhibits CTL induction in vivo. It is possible that there may be immune-privilege sites in the host that have not been identified.

Another theory is based on recent work suggesting that there are CTL escape mutants in chronically infected chimpanzees. An otherwise conserved epitope in nonstructural protein 3 (NS3), which is the target for a strong CTL response, mutated over time, leading researchers to speculate that escape variants might emerge.

Immune Escape. Virtually every patient with chronic non-A and non-B hepatitis, whether from transfusion or IV drug use, has circulating levels of antibodies to the envelope glycoproteins gpE1 and gpE2. HCV can be difficult to grow in vitro, but work done in Japan suggests that the virus mutates over time to evade this humeral immune response. Using an RNA binding assay, researchers were able to show that serum taken from 1978 to 1982 contained antibodies that would neutralize HCV taken in 1977. In the same patient, however, the antibodies that neutralized the 1977 virus did not neutralize virus taken in 1990. By 1991, the patient did have antibodies to neutralize the 1990 virus.

This finding was consistent with the process of immune escape. Further research revealed that there were multiple mutations between the 1977 and 1990 virus, as would be expected from an RNA virus. The rate of mutation is at the level of about .01 percent per nucleotide per year, but there was a cluster of mutations in a very small region at the terminus of gpE2. These mutations, between residues 395 and 487, resulted in a variety of nonconservative amino acid changes.

This region appears to be under severe immune pressure, and isolates of HCV from patients around the world show that the end terminal region of gpE2 is different in virtually every isolate, often involving nonconservative neoacid changes. This region is a target for B-lymphocytes, and a recent study in Germany indicates that antibodies to this end-terminal hypervariable region prevented binding of HCV inoculum to human fibroblasts. This leads researchers to speculate that the end terminus of gpE2 may be the principal neutralizing domain of the virus. Given the difficulty of growing HCV in vitro, it will take some time to confirm this.

Vaccine Development. Many of the approaches that might be pursued aren't yet possible because of the early stage of the research on HCV.

The virus is very difficult to grow in tissue culture, and the only animal model is the chimpanzee, so it will also be difficult to attenuate the virus. There are few subunits circulating in these patients. As a result, there are only three approaches available at present: *recombinant subunit vaccines, naked DNA vaccines,* and *vector DNA vaccines.* Researchers are pursuing all three approaches in order to produce a very complete immune response. The following discussion focuses on subunit vaccines.

The subunit vaccine that has been tested in chimpanzees was derived by expressing the viral gpE1, gpE2, and NS-2 genes in mammalian cells, initially through the use of recombinant vaccinia donated by NIH. The pure subunits are combined with an adjuvant called MF-59 that has been used extensively in the herpes clinical trials. Usually the chimpanzee was immunized first with wild-type vaccinia, to rule out any residual live recombinant vaccinia in any subsequent protection, and then given up to 40 micrograms of subunits at months 0, 1, and 7. A total of 3 weeks after the final boost the animal was challenged with 10 infectious doses of homologous virus.

Out of 12 experimental chimpanzees, 5 were completely protected—there was no trace of viral RNA in the plasma, in the liver, or in the PBLs. Of the other 7 animals, 5 went through acute infection and resolved, after which there was no trace of virus. Only 2 experimental chimpanzees went on to develop chronic infection, and one of these had ameliorated acute hepatitis. By contrast, out of 7 unimmunized controls that were challenged with virus, 6 developed chronic infection following acute hepatitis and only one experienced resolution of the infection.

These results suggest that the vaccine not only gives some protection against infection but also causes resolution of infection when it does occur. Vaccination achieved a high level of immune response: antibody titers prior to challenge were higher than those usually seen in infected blood donors and patients with chronic hepatitis. Further analysis showed that complete protection against infection was correlated with antibody levels, but not with antibodies to the hypervariable region at the end terminus of gpE2.

However, researchers don't know how efficient this subunit vaccine, based on HCV subtype 1A, would be against heterologous viral isolates. Initial experiments with a related viral isolate produced rather low levels of antibodies following reboost, and a slight inhibition of the onset of viremia. But it was impossible to conclude from this study that a vaccine based on HCV-1 antigens can prevent chronic infection by heterologous virus. Additional studies are ongoing.

Goals and Problems. The objective for a prophylactic vaccine would be to prime the humeral immune response, using recombinant gpE1 and gpE2 subunits to produce neutralizing antibodies that will restrict viral spread and load and thereby allow cell-mediated immune (CMI) response to clear the infection. In addition, it should also prime the CMI response using antigens to conserved viral proteins—such as the T-cell response to viral NS-3—to enhance its ability to resolve infection.

A constant problem is the knowledge that chimpanzees and humans alike appear to have weak immunity against reinfection. As a result, researchers are hoping to use naked DNA and vector DNA immunizations to broaden the immune response and increase the protective efficacy of the vaccines. At present, however, it seems unlikely that they will be able to achieve a vaccine as effective as those against hepatitis A and B. Still, it will be highly beneficial if they can ameliorate the disease by slowing down or preventing the progression to chronic hepatitis in a significant fraction of subjects.

In response to questions, Dr. Houghton added the following:

- The first population to vaccinate would be high-risk groups such as health care workers, family members of patients, dialysis patients, etc.
- Researchers have not yet identified major differences in the antibody or CTL response of patients who resolve following acute infection compared with those who develop chronic infection. Nor do they understand why they are getting resolution in experimental chimpanzees, although they suspect that the vaccine limits the viral load and spreads sufficiently to allow the host CMI response to deal with the infection.
- The only studies showing resolution have involved HCV subtypes 1-A and 1-B. There seem to be few differences between these two subtypes, but it is impossible to say anything about resolution versus chronicity in the other major strains of HVC.

HUMAN PAPILLOMAVIRUS[4]

Incidence and Burden. Human papillomaviruses (HPVs) are extremely common and widespread. Genital HPV infection is a sexually transmitted disease with an incidence of 5 percent to 40 percent among sexually active women. HPVs are etiologically linked to genital cancers, especially cervical cancer, and infection with a high-risk HPV is by far the most significant risk factor for developing cervical cancer—more than 90 percent of cervical cancers contain HPV DNA. Cervical cancer is approximately the number-six cancer among women in developed countries but its the number-one killer from cancer in developing countries, where Pap smears are not readily available. On a worldwide basis, cervical cancer is the number-two cause of death from cancer in women, after cancer of the breast. It has been estimated that HPV infection is involved in approximately 15 percent of all human cancers.

Pathobiology. HPVs are small, nonenveloped DNA viruses that replicate in the nucleus of the host cell, leading to lesions, warts, and tumors. They are epitheliotropic: replication occurs only in epithelial cells, primarily in the differentiated layers of the epidermis. More than 70 different HPV genotypes have been identified and classified into three large groups according to the region of epithelia they tend to infect:

1. *Cutaneous nongenital HPVs* are commonly seen in dermatological practices and do not appear to have malignant potential. Several million cases are present in the United States at any given time. It is not clear that there would be demand for a prophylactic vaccine, although a therapeutic vaccine might well be important.

2. *Epidermodysplasia verruciformis-specific HPVs* include almost one-half of all known HPV types and are found principally in patients with a predisposition to develop widespread, chronic, nongenital lesions. Some of these patients go on to develop malignancies, but this is a very rare condition.

3. *Mucosal HPVs* include almost 20 different types identified to date. Some are low-risk types associated with nonmalignant disease, particularly HPV-6 and 11. Others are high-risk types that seem to have malignant potential, particularly HPV-16, 18, 31, and 45. In a study of viral DNA in 1,000 cervical cancers from around the world, HPV-16 is by far the most common type, although HPV-18 is also common in Southeast Asia. However, the DNA of multiple HPV types is found in both benign and malignant genital lesions, for which reason a vaccine against genital HPV will need to be polyvalent.

About 50 percent of cervical infections are with high-risk HPVs, but the majority are clinically inapparent and self-limited. Only about 10 percent of the infected women have cytopathological changes on Pap smears, and most of

---

[4] Based on a presentation by Douglas R. Lowy, M.D.

these are early or mild dysplasias. Severe dysplasia is less common and tends to occur in older women, as though there were changes in the cells during persistent infection over a period of years that leads to dysplasia. Presumably this includes virus-specific changes, such as integration of the viral DNA into the host genome, and possibly some cell-specific changes as well.

Viral Gene Products. In cell lines derived from cervical tumors, there is a preferential retention and expression of three oncogenes from the high-risk HPV. Two genes (E6 and E7) in collaboration with each other can establish immortalization of human keratocytes grown in culture: the E6 product binds to and inactivates the p53 tumor-suppressor protein; the E7 product binds to and inactivates the pRB tumor-suppressor protein. These properties are significantly more active in high-risk than in low-risk HPVs. A third transforming gene of HPV is E5, whose product appears to activate the growth-factor receptors; it is not always found in the malignant tumors themselves, but it may play a role in initiating the lesions.

Animal studies suggest that immunization with E6 and E7 does not prevent lesions, but the lesions do regress faster. As a result, trials are now being conducted to evaluate a therapeutic vaccine based on differing combinations of E6 and E7.

Barriers to Vaccine Development. Several problems limit attempts to understand HPV infection and develop a vaccine. Perhaps the most important is the lack of a system to propagate HPV in vitro. Second, researchers have not been able to produce preparative quantities of purified viral capsid proteins. Third, immune parameters have not generally correlated with the benign infection antibodies to E6, E7, E2, and other viral proteins. In addition, there is no animal model of HPV infection—the productive infection is species-specific, although there are several animal systems that might eventually be used as models.

Approaches to Vaccine Development. Most attention has focused on the development of a subunit vaccine. Work at the Laboratory of Cellular Oncology at the National Cancer Institute (NCI) has focused on the two viral structural proteins, major capsid protein L1 and minor capsid protein L2. Researchers found that when they expressed the bovine papillomavirus (BPV) L1 gene in recombinant baculovirus in insect cells, it was sufficient to cause self-assembly of virus-like particles (VLPs)—essentially empty capsid that do not contain the viral genome. When L2 was added to this insect cell system, there was no major differences in immunogenicity, but there was more efficient assembly of VLPs. This self-assembly process can be carried out with HPV, producing VLPs that do not contain the HPV genome. The BPV system now provides the major in vitro test for infection, a conformational test for antibodies to HPV-16 VLPs.

When rabbits are immunized with authentic BPV virions, it induces very high levels of neutralizing antibodies, more than 10^5 titer. VLPs, whether L1 or L1-plus-L2, induce similarly high levels of neutralizing antibodies. When the

VLPs are denatured before immunization, however, they fail to induce the neutralizing antibodies. From this it is possible to conclude that the neutralizing antibodies are directed against conformationally dependent epitopes on L1 that mimic authentic virus. This model seemed most relevant to the development of prophylactic rather than therapeutic vaccine.

In collaboration with the Pasteur Institute, NCI researchers tested this model in a vaccine for cottontail rabbit papilloma virus (CRPV). A total of 39 experimental rabbits were immunized 3 times with VLPs containing CRPV L1 or L1-plus-L2 (in Freund's adjuvant) or L1-plus-L2 (in alum) and then, with 39 controls, challenged with high-dose virus. The results indicated that 90 percent of the controls developed the expected disease, whereas 90 percent of the experimentals developed either no disease or a mild regressing disease that was very self-limited, and only one experimental developed persistent disease. In addition, about 40 percent of the controls developed invasive squamous cell cancer, but none of the experimental animals developed this. Importantly, animals inoculated with bovine L1 and L2 became infected despite high levels of BPV antibodies; the protection against CRPV was type-specific.

Researchers were able to transfer protection passively by transferring serum from immunized to unimmunized animals, thereby confirming that the neutralizing antibodies are the protective mechanism. Other laboratories have demonstrated different techniques for immunizing rabbits, including DNA transfer and the use of vaccinia vectors. The common denominator is the ability to obtain the appropriate conformationally dependent epitopes for viral capsid protein L1.

One drawback of this CRPV model is that it involves a cutaneous infection, whereas the genital HPV infections associated with cervical cancer are mucosal infections. However, an experiment with BPV type 4, which causes oral mucosal disease in cows, showed protection similar to that seen in the CRPV cutaneous system. Another experiment with canine oral papillomavirus also demonstrated very substantial protection from mucosal infection using L1 VLPs that had been expressed in insect cells. In the latter case, researchers were able to wait for as much as a year after immunization before challenge and still obtain very substantial protection, indicating a considerable duration of immunity in this mucosal model. A Rhesus monkey papillomavirus model would be superb, since it would be a mucosal infection and some monkeys develop invasive cervical cancer; however, the virus is not yet available, so this model remains theoretical rather than actual.

Serological Assay. Because there are so many types of mucosal HPVs, the vaccine against genital HPV infection should in principal be polyvalent. Some of the relevant HPVs will probably represent different serotypes. For example, genetic classification according to DNA homology shows that HPV-6 and 11 are closely related; HPV-16 and 31 are closely related; and HPV-18 and 45 are closely related. Whether they represent distinct serotype, however, remains to be established. The serotyping of HPVs is constrained by the unavailability of the appropriate conformationally dependent epitopes for the various types.

NCI researchers have developed an ELISA assay for VLPs of HPV-16, based on reaction to the conformationally dependent epitopes of the L1 protein, but there seems to be some crossreactivity to other high-risk types. That is, women who are infected with HPV-18 and 31 are more likely to be positive on this assay than women infected with the low-risk HPV-6 and 11. The latter show little difference from uninfected women, so the assay does not seem to be detecting antibodies that would be directed against low-risk HPV types. In a prospective study, this assay proved to be about 90 percent accurate in measuring current or past infection with HPV-16, irrespective of cytology, with a maximum false positive of about 3 percent.

This ELISA assay for HPV-16 has been used to look at different groups with various cancers. As expected, there is a highly significant odds ratio for being positive on the ELISA and cervical cancer. However, there is also a significant odds ratio with urethral cancer, vulvar cancer, and possibly, cancer of the esophagus. The association with esophageal cancer is still controversial, in part because most studies fail to find HPV DNA in these cancers. There is well-documented evidence that BPV in conjunction with a carcinogen, is responsible for esophageal cancers in cattle. The viral DNA may be absent from human esophageal cancers because a "hit and run" mechanism is at work.

Hemagglutination Assay. To provide additional information, and to overcome some of the disadvantages of the serological assay, researchers have developed a very sensitive hemagglutination assay using BVP and VLPs. Data published about 20 years ago indicated that incubation with BPV causes agglutination of mouse red blood cells. Researchers found the same response to L1 and L1-plus-L2 VLPs, and that the response is sensitive to differing concentrations and combinations and BPV proteins. Similar results were obtained with other papillomaviruses, including CRPV and several varieties of HPV.

Further research led to the development of a sensitive hemagglutination inhibition (HI) assay, in which the presence of antibodies to papillomavirus will disrupt the viruses and prevent agglutination. The HI assay is type-specific, in that BVP antibodies will prevent hemagglutination in response to VLPs of BVP but not HPV-16, and conversely HPV-16 antibodies will give a negative response for VLPs of HPV-16 but not BVP. This assay has been used to show that rabbits immunized with disrupted VLPs were not protected from CRPV, despite high antibody titers on the ELISA test, while rabbits immunized with intact VLPs were protected. This assay should be useful in measuring natural exposure to papillomaviruses, evaluating immune response after VLP vaccination, and investigating cross-protection from heterologous types after VLP vaccination.

In response to questions from the audience, Dr. Lowy added the following:

• Researchers are studying the role of E7 protease in inducing CTL response—for example, inducing CD8-positive T-cells—but it unclear whether these cells are effective in viral infection or in the treatment of existing human cancer.

• When these studies move into humans for efficacy testing, a logical clinical endpoint would be cytological abnormalities—not cervical cancer. Investigators could also monitor DNA in the cervix.

• There is as yet no data on mucosal routes of administration, although this will be an important issue in the future.

• There is as yet inadequate knowledge of the epitopes of the various papillomavirus subtypes to assess the possibility of making chimeric VLPs containing L1 proteins from multiple serotypes.

• The timetable is uncertain. Some pharmaceutical companies may try to go into Phase I clinical trials in the next couple of years, but it will take a period of time to demonstrate immunological reactivity and safety, and a longer time following women to demonstrate efficacy. Controlled Phase III trials might be completed in more than 5 but less than 10 years.

• The target population for a prophylactic vaccine would be women, hopefully before they become sexually active.

DENGUE HEMORRHAGIC FEVER[5]

Pathobiology. Dengue is a positive-strand RNA virus, like HCV a member of the flavivirus family, and is transmitted by mosquitoes. There are four serotypes, and infection with one serotype results in long-lived immunity against that serotype, as well as sensitization to other serotypes. Dengue virus infection presents as two clinical syndromes: dengue fever (DF) and dengue hemorrhagic fever (DHF). Several days pass between transmission and the appearance of fever. In uncomplicated DF, the fever lasts for 3 or 4 days and then resolves successfully. In a few cases, however, as the fever is resolving, the patient develops capillary leak syndrome, which is a more serious illness commonly called DHF. There is little real hemorrhage but a lot of leakage from the capillaries, and hematocrit rises and body temperature falls. In its most severe form, DHF can result in shock and death. Depending on the speed of diagnosis and treatment, mortality can be anywhere from less than 1 percent to as high as 20 percent. Fortunately, most children respond well to aggressive volume expansion.

Incidence and Burden. Dengue fever (DF) is a frequent childhood infection in tropical and subtropical regions of the world where the mosquito *Aetes aegypti* is prevalent. There are an estimated 100 million cases per year,

---

[5] Based on a presentation by Frances A. Ennis, M.D.

based on the expectation of a 10-percent annual infection rate among children in endemic areas.

The far more severe form of dengue hemorrhagic fever (DHF) has been recognized as a problem in Southeast Asia for the past 40 years. During the 25-year period 1956-1980, there were 3 million cases of DHF in Southeast Asia and 20,000 deaths (0.67 percent). During the first half of the 1980s there were 800,000 cases and 10,000 deaths (1.25 percent). During the second half of the 1980s, there were 900,000 to 1 million cases and 10,000 to 11,000 deaths (1.00 to 1.22 percent).

In the past few years, DHF has been occurring with increasing frequency in other parts of the world, including Cuba and the Caribbean, Central America, and South America—areas that previously had DF but not DHF. The reasons for this are not known. One possibility is a change in the virulence of the various strains of the virus. For example, the dengue type 2 virus that is present in the Caribbean today is different from what was there in the past and more closely resembles the type 2 genotype of Southeast Asia, which may have been transported to the Western Hemisphere.

Epidemiology. However, the current hypothesis, based on epidemiological data, suggests that increased risk of DHF comes from pre-existing infection rather than a more virulent virus. Studies of children aged 1-14 in Thailand indicate that there is an extremely small risk of developing DHF during primary infection with any of the four serotypes. In secondary infection, the vast majority have asymptomatic, self-limited DF, but there is about a 50-fold increased risk of developing the more severe form of DHF. However, DHF is very seldom seen during the first 2 years of life.

This is confirmed by data from Cuba. The island had been free of dengue for generations until an outbreak of dengue type 1 in 1976-1977. The country mobilized in anticipation of an outbreak of DHF, but they observed very little serious illness and no deaths. Then, in 1981, there was an outbreak of dengue type 2 and many cases of DHF, mostly of which occurred in children aged 3 to 12—those who had been sensitized by the preceding type 1 infection. Only one child born between the two outbreaks developed serious disease.

Immunopathogenesis. Recent research has emphasized the immuno-pathogenesis of dengue, and specifically the concept of *antibody-dependent enhancement,* rather than vaccine development per se. The current hypothesis is that, during secondary infection, previously existing crossreactive antibodies are binding the dengue virus and helping it into FC receptor-bearing cells. The receptor hasn't been defined yet, but it seems clear that human monocytes would be the most permissive cell, and that binding with non-neutralizing antibodies will increase the number of infected cells about tenfold. That is, only about 2 percent of human monocytes will normally become infected with dengue virus, but if the virus is bound with crossreactive non-neutralizing antibodies, about 20 percent become infected, and if FC receptors are up-regulated by exposure to interferon-gamma, perhaps 60 percent become infected, with virus yields going up proportionately.

In this case, memory T-cells and CD8 T-cells are present in high numbers because of the recent infection with a crossreactive strain. These T-cells are stimulating their MHC molecules, and as a result they wind up acting at least in part as antigen-presenting cells. They also bear cross-one, cross-two FC receptors on their surface; secondary infection is more efficient because crossreactive antibodies bind to the viral protein and help it enter via the FC receptors. The result is more infected monocytes, which function as virus factories.

Activated T-cells produce cytokines and other products that can affect capillary action, and killed monocyte may also release vasoactive compounds. The target cell for dengue infection appears to be the RE monocyte, and virus antigen is not seen in endothelial cells. Researchers currently believe that endothelial cells are leaking because of cytokine alteration of their function. Hence, research is focusing on the serum, T-cells, and other peripheral monocytes in order to understand the basic mechanism of immunopathogenesis.

Human T-cell Responses to Dengue. The three-dimensional structure of an HLA class II MHC molecule shows a so-called A-2 crypt that holds an endogenous peptide—the antigen. In the case of the dengue virus, CD4 T-cells initially recognize the infection in the form of dengue peptides being presented in HLA class II molecules on the surface of antigen-presenting cells.

Following primary infection with dengue type 1, stimulated peripheral blood monocytes will respond most strongly to the dengue-1 antigen, but there is also a lesser response to the three other serotypes. Analysis shows that about 1 cell in 1,000 will be positive for dengue-1, and about 1 cell in 10,000 will be positive for dengue-2, 3, and 4. To determine the smallest amino acid sequence that CD4 T-cells would recognize, researchers identified and reproduced these crossreactive T-cells using limiting dilution cloning. They then conducted a series of experiments in which the cells were infected with vaccinia virus that expresses the dengue protein. As the protein was truncated, peptide analysis identified the amino acid sequence to which the CD4 T-cell clone responded— in this case, viral nonstructural protein 3 (NS-3).

The results confirm the polymorphism of T-cell response to dengue virus NS-3. As with hepatitis C, dengue NS-3 apparently contains multiple T-cell epitopes with very different specificities. In the case of a subject who had been immunized with dengue-3, all T-cell clones recognized the epitope for dengue-3, but with four degrees of crossreactivity: (1) just dengue-3; (2) dengue-2, 3, and 4, but not 1; (3) dengue-1, 2, and 3, but not 4; and (4) dengue-1 through -4 plus West Nile and yellow fever virus, both of which are also flaviviruses. In another subject immunized with dengue-4, analysis found T-cell clones that reacted to (5) just dengue-4; (6) dengue-2 and 4; and (7) dengue-1, 2, 3, and 4. Within each serotype, there were three or four distinct epitopes on the viral NS-3.

This polymorphism—multiple T-cell epitopes to the viral protein— probably is not unique to dengue. But in dengue it contributes to the T-cell activation level because of the epidemiology of the close circulating viruses.

Comparison of sera from children with DF, DHF, and controls showed significant elevation of soluble CD8 and IL-2 receptor, in those with DHF, evidence of a marked activation of CD8 T-cells and IL-2 receptor-bearing cells. Soluble CD4 was elevated to a lesser degree. Interferon-gamma was elevated in both DF and DHF.

Based on these results, researchers have mounted a prospective study of children recruited from a Thai outpatient clinic. Subjects had fever of 24 to 72 hours duration and no other source of infection. During the first year, 180 children were recruited; 60 were subsequently diagnosed with DF and showed dengue-positive antibody response, and 29 developed DHF. The study is not yet complete, but several interesting findings have emerged. One is that 100 percent of the children with dengue had viremia, while the literature suggests that the positive isolation rate would be 50 percent for DF and 25 percent for DHF. This finding actually makes more sense, in view of the theory that enhancing antibodies were contributing to the increased risk for severe disease. Researchers plan to titrate plasma to see whether the viral burden is greater in children with DHF.

Using T-cell clones from these children, researchers also plan to measure the cytokine production (particularly interferon-gamma) and the selective activation of T-cell receptors. The activation of specific T-cell receptors is of interest in regard to the pathogenesis of many infectious diseases. In previous studies, stimulating with dengue led to the preferential activation of V-beta-17-bearing T-cells, and the majority of dengue-specific T-cell clones also bear the V-beta-17 receptor. It is unclear whether this is an integral part of DHF, but it bears further investigation.

Vaccine Development. Classical studies by Sabin showed long-lived immunity to homologous virus serotype, so the concept of vaccination seems reasonable. The concern is to prevent DHF and not sensitize a population that might later be exposed to a different serotype and find itself at greater risk for more serious disease. For this reason, there is consensus that a successful vaccine must induce immunity to all four serotypes. From a public health point of view, it is also very important to immunize with one dose of a polyvalent vaccine, if at all possible.

A group in Thailand has performed Phase I immunogenicity studies in adults, using live attenuated strains of dengue-1 through 4. They believe that there is adequate immunogenicity in terms of neutralizing antibody response, although enhancing antibody response has not been measured. The group is now beginning studies with combination vaccines, but it is too early to say what the results will be. Polyvalent vaccination appears to be more difficult in children, possibly because of interference between serotypes, and a number of additional studies will be required. Lots of vaccines are being prepared for clinical trials, and there is an expectation that efficacy studies might be conducted by the end of this decade. However, far more information is needed on the safety and antigenicity of the polyvalent vaccine.

Other approaches under investigation might also provide good results, including subunit vaccine, plasma DNA vaccine, and infectious cloned vaccine (e.g., chimeric dengue-4 backbone), and recombinant dengue vaccine containing NS-1 (which is a potent antigen in experimental vaccines against yellow fever). However, there appears to be no practical way to produce neutralizing antibodies without at least some enhancing activity; this will be a safety concern in all dengue vaccines.

Another major concern is the duration of protection. Most cases of DHF occur between ages 3 and 15, at which point children seem to develop an immunity. Hence, dengue vaccines should have a very solid long-term memory, with the ability to induce both B-cell and T-cell responses, as well as good antibody response.

One of the biggest barriers to vaccine development is that there is no suitable animal model for DHF. One team looked at over 100 primate species and couldn't find a model. Primates can be infected, and they develop viremia, but they don't progress to the more serious syndrome of DHF.

In response to questions from the audience, Dr. Ennis added the following:

• Although T-cell activation is V-beta-17 specific, it does not appear to be a super-antigen effect. Instead, host factors such as HLA seem to be contributing to increased risk. HLA typing of the children in Thailand should shed light on this question.

• Antigenic variation doesn't seem to be a major issue. There are four serotypes, but within the serotypes there doesn't seem to be much drift in the antigens or epitopes.

• Immune response to primary infection is serotype-specific, with antibodies appearing after a day or two, about when the virus is cleared. At the beginning of a secondary infection, therefore, the only antibodies that will recognize the new virus will be the crossreactive antibodies. Hence, the triggering of the increased number of infected cells takes place before the antibody response.

• The risk of DHF increases with secondary infection, but it does not appear to increase further when the subject is infected with a third serotype. In fact, risk seems to go down after the second infection, possibly because of cross-neutralization.

• While there is a strong emphasis on developing a quadravalent vaccine, additional studies will be needed to develop a combination vaccine that has 95 percent neutralizing-antibody responses to all four serotypes, instead of 60 percent for one and 95 percent for another.

• Greater knowledge about the polymorphic nature of T-cell response should make it possible to engineer vaccines that contain T-cell epitopes as well as neutralizing epitopes.

CHLAMYDIA TRACHOMATIS[6]

Once considered to be a virus, *Chlamydia* is in fact a bacteria, although distantly related to other familiar bacteria. The genus is composed of three species:

1. *C. psittaci* is a common pathogen on a variety of mammals and birds. It causes psittacosis, or parrot fever, an opportunistic respiratory infection that can be life-threatening when transmitted to humans. However, this disease has been largely controlled by regulation of the trade in exotic birds.

2. *C. pneumoniae* is a new and emerging disease. It is a frequent cause of respiratory infections and associated with pneumonia, especially among young adults in northern Europe. It is also associated with arteriosclerosis, although the relation is not yet known.

3. *C. trachomatis* can be subdivided into three biovariants that cause very different kinds of disease: (a) the *mouse pneumositis* biovariant is not a pathogen of humans; (b) the *lymphogranuloma venereum (LGV)* biovariant, which consists of three serotypes that proliferate in the lymph nodes; and (c) the *trachoma* biovariant, which consists of 15 different serotypes that cause epithelial infections of the eye or of the genital tract.

Incidence and Burden. As an ocular infection, *C. trachomatis* causes trachoma, which remains the leading cause of preventable blindness in the world, affecting some 200 million people. Trachoma is no longer encountered in the United States, but exactly the same strains cause genital infections that have made chlamydia the fastest growing sexually transmitted disease (STD) in this country, with over 5 million new cases per year. (By comparison, there are only about 235 cases of LGV, although it remains an important STD in developing countries.) Most of these 5 million cases present as either nongonococcal urethritis or cervicitis. Significantly, many of these cases are largely asymptomatic, which is a problem both for treatment and for identifying individuals at risk for more serious sequelae.

Among men, chlamydial urethritis is a common cause of epididymitis, but the real focus of attention is on women. In addition to the complications of urethritis and cervicitis, infants born to infected women are also at risk for conjunctivitis and chlamydial pneumonia. Because so many infections are asymptomatic, they often go undiagnosed and develop into more serious problems. One of the most serious is pelvic inflammatory disease, which can lead to chronic pelvic pain, involuntary sterility, or ectopic pregnancy.

Diagnosis, Treatment, and Prevention. Over the past 10 years, researchers have improved substantially the ability of clinicians to diagnose chlamydial

---

[6] Based on a presentation by Richard Stephens, M.D.

infections, moving from self-culture-based assays to culture-independent assays. Nevertheless, even the best molecular assays to date have only a 70 percent sensitivity in high-prevalence populations or symptomatic infections, and less than that in low-prevalence populations or asymptomatic infections. Once diagnosed, chlamydia can be treated with antibiotics and there are as yet no signs of antibiotic resistance, although the infection hasn't really been challenged to date.

Behavior change might be one preventative strategy, but like other STDs, chlamydia is predominantly an infection of teenagers and young adults, with all the problems that entails in terms of recognizing and changing high-risk behavior. There are two biological strategies for preventing the disease: one is the development of a competitive analogue, the other is the development of a vaccine.

Pathobiology. The chlamydiae are nonmotile, obligate intracellular parasites with a distinctive life cycle. The extracellular forms can be detected by direct fluorescent antibody and enzyme immunoassay, but while they are infectious, they are metabolically inactive. The extracellular forms attach to a cell by a mechanism that is not yet understood and, once attached, enter the cell by endocytotic mechanisms. Inside the cell, it remains inside an inclusion—a membrane-bound vacuole that inhibits fusion with lysosomes—throughout its growth cycle.

Chlamydiae can propagate only inside a cell. Once inside, it undergoes changes in its membrane and DNA and begins to differentiate. Researchers believe that it follows one of two pathways: it can multiply and grow like other bacteria, or it can remain in a cryptic state. The latter, which is one of the mechanisms by which this organism persists in the host, is poorly understood. If it multiplies, it will divide by binary fusion some 24 to 72 hours after infection, after which it again differentiates from the vegetative to the elementary or infectious form and is released, by another unknown mechanism, to infect new cells. Importantly, chlamydia does not seem to be able to transmit by cell-to-cell interaction but must leave the cell and thus be exposed to antibodies and other host activity.

Chlamydia is a mucosal pathogen that does not so much kill host cells as cause persistent inflammation. The inflammation causes scarring in both the ocular and genital models, and the scarring accounts for the disease problem—for example, deformation of the eyelashes and blindness. Infection of epithelial cells leads to a potent gamma T-cell response and the excretion of inflammatory cytokines, especially IL-8, which in this case fits the requirements for a mediator for pathogenesis. Other pathogens elicit a similar response early upon uptake, which then fades away; whereas with chlamydia it occurs late in the cycle and endures throughout the infection process.

Adhesion Molecules and Analogues. Researchers believe that the parasite attaches and enters the host cell using a carbohydrate-like ligand that is synthesized on the surface of the chlamydia and somehow mediates entry. This ligand is similar to the heparin sulfate molecule and apparently can be cleaved with an enzyme that is specific to heparin sulfate. When this occurs, the chlamydia decreases or loses attachment and is no longer infectious. When exogenous heparin or heparin sulfate is added, the chlamydia regains its infectivity; indeed, the level of attachment increases by some 50 percent.

Researchers have been able to model this mechanism by coating polystyrene beads with either the natural ligand or heparin sulfate. The beads attach to and enter epithelial cells very efficiently in a manner similar to chlamydia. They also elicit the same pattern of tyrosine polyphospholated host-cell proteins upon uptake, suggesting that they are mimicking the chlamydia pathway. This mechanism may provide a way to target delivery of vaccines to the mucosal surfaces that chlamydia infect.

Understanding of these adhesion molecules also suggests the possibility of a second antimicrobial strategy, that of using analogues to compete with and block the binding activity of chlamydia. Researchers experimented with different forms of heparin and discovered that the N-desulfated, O-sulfated form of the molecule would inhibit binding to the eucaryotic host cells without binding to the chlamydia elementary bodies. This suggests that one could design compounds that would not bind to the organism (which would risk potentiating or rescuing infectivity) and would be potent competitors for the host-cell receptor for this ligand. Such a chlamydia inhibitor might be added to various spermicidal compounds.

Immunology. Epidemiological data, animal models, and early vaccine trials demonstrate serotype-specific immunity to the 15 known serotypes of *C. trachomatis* var. *trachoma.* Immunity is relatively short-lived, typically waning in 6 months to 1 year. It is commonly believed that immunity is related to serotype-specific antigens. Three molecules on the surface of chlamydia are candidates for these targets: (1) the lipopolysaccharide (LPS), (2) the major outer membrane protein (MOMP), and (3) the adhesion-and-invasion ligand (see above).

LPS is genospecific, not serospecific, and neutralization cannot be demonstrated, so it doesn't fit this serovariant-specific model. MOMP, on the other hand, is known to carry serovariant-specific antigens, and antibodies to these molecules neutralize infectivity. Even in polyvalent sera there is a big difference between homologous and heterologous neutralization. Unfortunately, MOMP is the only major surface component that is well understood. There may be other antigens, and this area is worthy of continued investigation.

C. trachomatis has only one gene for MOMP, but the gene and the protein vary across strains. Variation in amino acid sequence occurs in each of four variable sequence (VS) regions called VS1 through VS4; changes are most frequent in VS4 and least frequent in VS3. CD4 T-cell determinants have also been mapped in this protein, including two major ones, one in a conserved region between VS1 and VS2, the other overlapping with VS3. Since there seem to be no antibodies to the VS3 region, however, the serovariant-specific antigens are to be found in VS1 and VS2 or the more broadly reacting antigens of VS4.

Synthetic (linear) peptides from these regions elicit a strong immune response, both independently and in expression vectors such as poliovirus and vaccinia. Relatively little of this response confers on the organism, however, so there is no microbiologic protection. An increasing amount of data suggest that conformational-dependent determinants are important for this target molecule. In VS1, for example, a given 12-amino-acid sequence yields a peptide that is sometimes recognized in linear form but by other serovariants only in circular form. Similar variance occurs in VS2, in which there is good antiserologic response to circular peptides, but not linear.

CD4 and T-cell help is also essential for protection and resolution of infection. A variety of proteins can elicit stimulation for CD4 cells, including MOMP. Animal models also suggest that CD8 cells and cytotoxicity are also important in resolving infection, and possibly in protection. Recent studies have detected CD8-killing of chlamydia-infected epithelial cells in vitro, but it is unknown whether this involves MHC class IA or IB presentation. Research in this area is ongoing.

Issues in Vaccine Development. Unlike some of the viral infections, there are several animal models for chlamydia, including mice, guinea pigs, and monkeys. Murine models include respiratory, systemic, and even genital tract models, including infection with human strains of the pathogen. The guinea pig model is limited to a strain that is a natural pathogen to guinea pigs. Both ocular and genital tract models have been developed in monkeys.

At present, however, there is a need for a better understanding of the cell-mediated immune mechanism, the role of CTLs and antibodies. There also needs to be a clearly differentiated understanding of the role of conformation determinants, the exact nature of the antigenic targets, and how to deliver them. And one of the biggest challenges is to find a way to genetically transform and manipulate these organisms, which currently cannot be grown in the quantities needed to support research.

In response to questions, Dr. Stephens added the following:

• The time frame for developing a vaccine against either MOMP or the adhesion ligand is entirely a function of money. Most of the problems are fairly straightforward; given enough money, the time frame would be quite reasonable.

• Differences in immune response to chlamydia peptides suggest that a small difference in primary sequence may result in a very large difference in the tertiary or quaternary structure of the molecules. In the guinea pig model, protection is totally dependent on conformational determinants. This suggests that researchers need to be more sophisticated in how they look at and present the antigens.

• The hypothesis that heat shock protein 60 (HSP-60) plays a role in the pathogenesis of chlamydia has been called into question by recent experiments showing that immunization with HSP-60 makes no difference in response to infective challenge. In other words, this is not a delayed-type hypersensitivity mechanism, and while HSP-60 may still play a role, it is not responsible for the persistence of inflammation.

• While there may be 15 serovariants, typically 1 or 2 serotypes will be dominant in any given population. Researchers don't understand why, and indeed they can't always differentiate among strains. Nevertheless, in terms of vaccine development, this makes for a much simpler "cocktail", rather than trying to include all 15.

• Studies of antibody passive-immune therapy were conducted before a neu-tralizing assay was available and produced ambiguous results. These studies need to be repeated in light of new understanding of antibody response at mucosal sites.

• Most researchers would agree that the route of administration should be mucosal. It is unclear whether intranasal, rectal, etc., would elicit the best response.

• MOMP is down-regulated by interferon (IFN) gamma, but only in 3 of the 15 serotypes.

TUBERCULOSIS[7]

Incidence and Burden. A third of the world's population is thought to be infected with tuberculosis, and 10 million die from TB each year. In the United States there are an estimated 10 million people infected with TB, and the numbers of infections and deaths has been rising rather than falling—there were more than 50,000 excess deaths between 1985 and 1992. And while a number of effective chemical therapies are available, clinicians are seeing increasing numbers of multiple-drug-resistant strains of TB. The massive epidemiology of this disease demands an effective preventative vaccine.

Problems with Existing Vaccine. Unlike many other infectious diseases, there is already a vaccine for tuberculosis (TB)—the Bacillus Calmette-GuJrin (BCG) vaccine, developed over 70 years ago in France. But while BCG is one of the oldest vaccines, it is also one of the most controversial. Its effectiveness varies considerably, and there is concern over the potential variability among the various strains of the vaccine that have developed over the years. Consequently, there is growing interest in finding a possible replacement for BCG as a vaccine against TB.

BCG is made with attenuated *Mycobacterium bovis,* the other species that, like *M. tuberculosis,* can cause TB. It was developed in the 1920s, but was never cloned and, as it passed through different laboratories throughout the world, a lot

---

[7] Based on a presentation by Daniel Hoft, M.D.

of potential variability has developed among the different strains. Over 3 billion doses have been given worldwide, by multiple routes, and BCG has been shown to be an extremely safe vaccine, even in infants. The original route was oral, but in the past 20 or 30 years the intracutaneous route has become more common.

The efficacy of BCG in producing immunity ranges from 0 percent to 100 percent, depending on trial or study. A number of factors have been postulated to explain this variability. Trial methodology varies considerably and makes it difficult to determine the statistical validity of the results. Different strains of BCG were used in the various trials. Different routes and doses may also have contributed to variability. Crossreactive immunity to environmental mycobacteria may have masked or biased the protective effect of the vaccine. Background rates of TB were sometimes too low to show a significant effect.

A 1994 meta-analysis of the published literature on BCG efficacy found that, overall, BCG was 51-percent protective against pulmonary TB, even more effective against disseminated forms of the disease, and 71 percent protective against death. Comparison of 13 prospective trials and 10 case-controlled studies suggested that neither BCG strain nor age at vaccination was an important variable in terms of efficacy. However, geography was important: the further away from the Equator, the higher the efficacy of BCG vaccination. (This may be related to higher endemic rates of environmental mycobacterial colonization and infection in warmer climates.) Study design was also important: the higher the data validity, the higher the efficacy of BCG.

Special Problems in Developing TB Vaccines. Many of the problems with the current vaccine have to do with the special conditions of TB as a disease, rather than with BCG itself. For example, researchers are greatly hampered by their inability to measure infection rates in vaccine trials with BCG. The best way to identify infection is the purified protein derivative (PPD) delayed hypersensitivity test; unfortunately, BCG induces a positive PPD response. In addition, only 10 percent of people that become infected with *M. tuberculosis* go on to develop disease, and this is often associated with suppression of the immune system. Finally, the long latency of the disease is also a problem; efficacy trials require long-term follow-up, which presents its own difficulties.

It seems obvious that the most important immune response to concentrate on is mycobacteria-specific memory, the only response that could be induced by a vaccine that would persist in vivo and protect against a rechallenge. Much of the in vitro research has not taken this into account. Mycobacteria produce adjuvant-like effects, and it important to have negative lymphocytes as a control or baseline, in order to determine whether an in vitro response is related to memory immune response rather than to an adjuvant or a superantigen-like response that occurs only in vitro.

Four major mycobacteria-specific antigens have been studied as potential vaccine candidates over the past 20 years:

1. *Heat shock proteins* were seemingly dominant in immunoscreening strategies, but many researchers now think that they may be involved in pathology and that it would not be a good idea to use them as a subunit vaccine.

2. *Actively secreted protein component* of mycobacterium may provide the most protective antigens, and this has drawn increasing interest in the past 5 or 10 years.

3. *Isopentenyl pyrophosphate and other pyrophosphates* can stimulate gamma-delta cells, but it is not known whether this immune response can develop a memory.

4. *Mycobacterial lipids* can stimulate the so-called CD4-negative, CD8-double-negative T-cell populations, but again, it is not known whether this immune response can develop a memory. It may have a place in immunotherapy strategies.

Pyrophosphates and lipids will probably prove to be important in therapies where the immune response is being induced in the face of disease.

Interest in actively secreted proteins originated with the finding that live vaccines work better than killed vaccines. It has been shown that culture filtrate proteins, the antigens secreted by mycobacteria in vitro, can induce an immune response in mice and guinea pigs and can protect against experimental challenge. Three of these antigens are: *MPT-57,* which is similar to a heat shock protein; *antigen 85 complex* (Ag85), probably the hottest candidate (see below); and a so-called *less-than-10 kD moiety,* which is also secreted by the mycobacterium. Ag85 complex is currently going into clinical trials, but there has been no good comparison of culture filtrate proteins with BCG.

Animal models provide strong evidence that Th-1 CD4-positive cells are important in protective immunity. These cells produce interleukin 2 (IL-2) and interferon gamma (IFN-gamma), both of which activate macrophages to kill intracellular organisms. These findings have been confirmed in the three human models of protective immunity:

1. People with tuberculosis pleuritis are thought to have an immune response that is controlling the infection, since most of them go on to resolve the disease. Purified lymphocytes from the pleural fluid of these patients produced high levels of IFN-gamma in response to a protein from the cell wall of mycobacterium and to the less-than-10-Kd secreted moiety. This suggests that Th-1 cells are important in this model.

2. People who are PPD-positive but healthy also appear to have protective immunity, since they have not developed disease. Comparison with TB patients showed that these individuals showed a predominant Th-1 response: elevated levels of IL-2 and IFN-gamma, and depressed levels of IL-4. This suggests that it may be important both to induce Th-1 response and to inhibit Th-2 response.

3. People who have been vaccinated with BCG also demonstrate a Th-1-like response. In this case, however, there is a stronger response to whole lysate of mycobacteria (WL) than to culture filtrate (CF), suggesting that BCG induces an immune response to cell-associated antigens rather than to the actively secreted proteins of the CF.

The latter finding may explain why BCG fails to provide as much protection as clinicians might wish. Researchers offer three possible explanations. First, BCG does not induce a predominant immune response against the secreted antigens. Second, there may be other, possibly unidentified antigens that should be considered in developing a vaccine for TB. Third, and consistent with other data, immune response to mycobacterium is highly heterogeneous, making it difficult for a single subunit protein to induce the same levels of immunity that would be induced with multiple antigens or with a whole, attenuated organism.

Routes of Vaccination. Researchers compared the above findings, which were observed following intradermal vaccination, with the immune response following percutaneous vaccination. They found that intradermal vaccination induces statistically increased positive PPD response. Both T-cell proliferative response and T-cell IFN-gamma response to the whole lysate were significantly up-regulated following intradermal vaccination, but not after percutaneous vaccination. These findings are consistent with the finding that, despite the fact that intradermal uses one-tenth as much vaccine, it produces better immune responses.

Since the TB infection is mucosal, however, the vaccine will have to induce good mucosal immunity. Experiments with the mouse model indicate that oral vaccination is a good method of inducing both mucosal and systemic immunity. Internasal vaccination with BCG can also induce immune responses, and this is an important area for future research. It may be important to use a combination of intradermal and oral immunizations in order to induce a Th-1 response systemically, and a Th-2 response locally, within the mucosal surfaces.

Researchers are currently one-third of the way through a double-dose escalation trial using increasing doses of BCG orally versus a placebo; data will be available in 12 to 18 months. In addition, researchers at Colorado State University are doing a study of a mucosal homing molecule that would be expressed after BCG vaccination.

Possible Improvements in TB Vaccines. Among potential subunit vaccines, Ag85 is the best-characterized. It is known to protect guinea pigs, and it is going into clinical trials in humans. Human T-cell epitope mapping studies have been published. Preliminary results using purified Ag85 indicate that it does not stimulate an immune response from BCG. However, there are still no good comparisons of subunit vaccines with BCG itself.

Recombinant BCG vaccines are another possibility. For example, it might be possible to clone high-expression genes for secreted proteins into BCG, thereby inducing better protective immunity. An alternative would be to clone cytokine-expression genes into BCG, thereby potentially inducing higher Th-1 response and lower Th-2 response. A third possibility would be to delete a nonessential antigen from BCG in order to use that antigen, or its absence, as a diagnostic marker; this would be valuable in future trials of protective efficacy for any TB vaccine.

In response to questions from the audience, Dr. Hoft added the following points:

- Efficacy studies show that BCG is more effective in infants than in adults, but this is partly because its easier to detect clinical effects in infants, who have a higher incidence of progressing to disseminated disease. Efficacy is harder to detect in vaccinated adults, who may take 10 or 20 years to progress to disseminated disease.
- Rising rates of TB in adult populations, especially in tropical developing countries, do not point to a major failure in terms of BCG vaccination of adults. At the same time, they point to the need to do better. What is needed is a strategy that concentrates on preventing the spread of infection by detecting and treating asymptomatic as well as symptomatic cases.
- Evidence suggests that Th-2 responses predominate in antibody production, while Th-1 responses induce Ig subsets. The two don't necessarily conflict in the development of protective immunity, but it may be important to learn how to use different schedules of vaccination to induce the two responses in different sites.
- As long as overall rates of infection remain low, the United States will probably not use BCG except for people who are at very high risk for infection with multiple-drug resistant TB.
- There is data on crossreactive immune responses to other mycobacterial species such as M. vaccae. This may have a role as a potential adjuvant in immunotherapy. Further study is needed.
- There are as yet no data on the use of BCG as a carrier for other antigens, but it promises to be a very useful vector. The technique has worked in animals, and MedImmune is currently conducting tests in humans.
- There have at present been no controlled trials of intranasal or oral vaccination with BCG in humans.

HISTOPLASMOSIS AND COCCIDIOIDOMYCOSIS[8]

Pathobiology. *Histoplasma capsulatum* and *Coccidioides immitis* are soil-based dimorphic fungi. In the soil they exist as molds, but they can cause serious disease when inhaled by animals or humans.

---

[8] Based on a presentation by George Deepe, M.D.

In the lungs, histoplasma converts to a yeast phase, a vacuolated intracellular parasite similar to *Leishmania donovani* and *L. mexicana,* that then disseminates into the liver and spleen. It has a predilection for mononuclear phagocytes and grows readily in phagolysosomes. The survival strategy is unclear, but it appears that the organism can alkalinize the phagolysosome to a pH of 6.0 or 6.5, low enough that it can still scavenge iron but high enough to mitigate the effects of acid proteases that are present in the phagolysosome. If the inoculum is sufficiently high with the pulmonary infection, the individual can become moderately to severely ill. In most individuals the infection is self-resolving, often either asymptomatic or with flu-like symptoms. When the immune system is suppressed, however, the organism will disseminate and reactivate to cause progressive disseminated histoplasmosis that, if untreated, can be life-threatening.

When coccidioides enters the lungs it is transformed into spherules that can become quite large, containing up to 1,000 endospores. As with histoplasma, the infection is often self-resolving and asymptomatic, but in an immunocompromised host the organism can disseminate and reactivate, causing Valley fever—progressive disseminated coccidioidomycosis. It shows a predilection for the skin and the meninges, as well as the lungs, and like histoplasma it likes viscera that are rich in mononuclear phagocytes.

Both organisms pose the biggest threat to immunocompromised hosts, in the form of a reactivation disease. Primary infection is followed by a dormant phase that is held in check until a perturbation in the immune system allows the organism to flourish. Except where known, immunosuppressive agents are involved, researchers do not know why otherwise healthy immune systems should break down and allow the organism to replicate.

Incidence and Burden. Incidence can be very high in areas where the pathogen is endemic. During the 1950s, approximately 90 percent of Navy recruits from the Cincinnati area were skin-test positive for histoplasma. The figure may be lower today, yet clinical observations indicate that about 75 percent of the people in Cincinnati who undergo routine chest x-rays have calcifications in their lungs or spleens, and an autopsy series demonstrated that—at least in Cincinnati—most of those calcifications were correlated with the presence of organisms consistent with *Histoplasma capsulatum.* When the National Institute of Occupational Safety and Health (NIOSH), which is located in Cincinnati, tested for the presence of histoplasma in a building being renovated, they found the organism not only in accumulated bat guano inside the building, but also in soil samples from outside the building. After the bat guano was treated with hypochlorite solution, it still tested positive for histoplasma (the usual treatment is formaldehyde).

Immunology. With both histoplasma and coccidioides, cell-mediated immunity is of primary importance. CD4 cells appear to be the primary mediator, although CD8 cells play a smaller role. Humoral immunity has little or no role. In both cases, the transfer of hyperimmune serum results in very little enhancement of phagocytosis by mononuclear phagocytes. One reason is the very rapid intrinsic phagocytosis of the organism—when unopsonized histoplasma are incubated with human mononuclear phagocytes, 80 percent to 90 percent of them are bound to the phagocyte within 5 minutes, and within 10 minutes the same proportion have been ingested.

Other evidence that histoplasma infection leads to cell-mediated immunity include (1) granuloma formation, (2) delayed hypersensitivity, (3) proliferation by peripheral blood mononuclear cells in vitro, (4) greater susceptibility by athymic mice than in their normal littermates, and (5) the ability of T-cells from immunized mice to transfer protection to unimmunized mice. Immunity to coccidioides can also be transferred with T-cells, while T-cell depletion or impairment is associated with poor prognosis. In both cases, however, as in tuberculosis, the result is not so much the killing of the organism as the inhibiting of its growth, since the organism remains dormant for many years following the initial exposure.

In both histoplasmosis and coccidioidymosis, as in tuberculosis, the Th-1 response seems to be most important in controlling infection, at least in the mouse models of these diseases. Resting phagocytes allow the organisms to grow until they are activated by a soluble signal from the T-cells. In mice, that signal seems to be IFN-gamma, but in humans (at least for histoplasma) the signals are IL-3 and the granulocyte and macrophage colony-stimulating factor (GM-CSF). Human mononuclear phagocytes on plastic are activated by neither IFN-gamma nor tumor necrosis factor alpha (TNF-alpha).

Isolating Protective Immunogens for Histoplasma. The literature on histoplasma indicated that a sublethal inoculate of either the conidia (spores) or yeast form of *H. capsulatum* could protect mice from subsequent challenge, and that inactivated conidia or heat-killed yeast could also provide protection. Further analysis showed that a detergent extract of the cell wall and cell membrane from this organism could confer protective immunity, and two antigens were isolated from an extract taken from the virulent strain *H. capsulatum* G217-B, the standard strain used in all animal models.

Researchers were able to demonstrate (1) that one of these extracts, called HIS-62, was recognized by immune sera from mice, (2) that it stimulated proliferation of sensitized lymphocytes in immunized mice, (3) that mouse T-cell clones recognized the crude extract, and finally (4) that vaccination with HIS-62 could confer protective immunity against pulmonary histoplasmosis in three different strains of mice. Upon further analysis, researchers found that the peptide sequence from HIS-62 was highly homologous to heat shock protein 60 (hsp 60)—about 70 percent identity with hsp 60 from *Saccharomyces* (the nearest yeast species), 50 percent identity with hsp 60 from bacteria, and 60 percent to 70 percent identity with mouse or human hsp 60, at the amino acid level. Crossreactivity with anti-GroEL serum confirmed that HIS-62 was a member of the hsp 60 family.

Researchers subsequently isolated the gene that expresses HIS-62 and cloned it into a bacterial expression vector, pET19b. Further tests confirmed that the rHIS-62 induced protective immunity in BALB/c mice against intranasal challenge with a lethal dose of histoplasma. Currently, they are trying to identify the smallest fragment of rHIS-62 that can confer protective immunity, using 4 overlapping fragments of about 250 to 300 amino acids in length. Unfortunately, the hierarchy of proliferation response has been totally different for BALB/c mice immunized with whole *H. capsulatum* (fragment 3 highest, followed by 2, 4, and 1) than for mice immunized with rHIS-62 (fragment 1 highest, followed by 2, 3, and 4). This suggests that the fragments are being recognized and processed differently by the differently immunized mice.

When these proliferation experiments were repeated with Black-6 mice, which differ from BALB/c mice at the MHC locus, the mice immunized with whole organism did not respond to any of the four fragments. For mice immunized with rHIS-62, the hierarchy was fragment 2 highest, followed by 3, 4, and 1. Researchers do not know what the conformation of the antigen is in the organism, but they do know that adjuvants (which were used in these experiments) tend to linearize the antigen; this may explain at least part of the difference in how the fragments are being processed.

On the other hand, when mice were immunized with the four rHIS-62 fragments and challenged intranasally with a sublethal inoculum, fragment 3 produced the best protection in both strains of mice—about a log reduction in colony-forming units in the lungs and livers, and a 30- to 40-percent reduction in the spleens. Thus, there may be no correlation between the degree of stimulation and the degree of protection.

But while whole rHIS-62 had induced protective immunity against a lethal challenge in BALB/c mice, immunization with the fragments provided only 50 percent protection for fragment 4 and no protection at all for 1, 2, or 3. There are two possible explanations. First, hsp 60 has some adjuvant effect, at least in mycobacteria, but the region that induces it may not be on a particular fragment. Second, it may take all of the fragments working together to induce a strong proliferative response. This experiment is being repeated in Black-6 mice against intranasal challenge with a lethal dose of histoplasma. Researchers believe they will be able to demonstrated that fragment 4 of rHIS-62 can induce a protective immune response in mice.

Isolating Protective Immunogens for Coccidioides. Researchers are using a different approach for coccidioides, screening potential antigens with antisera from humans who have recovered from an infection. The genes for these antigens will be introduced into DNA vectors and used to immunize mice in hopes of getting a protective immune response. One of those antigens is the hsp 60 from coccidioides, which has about 90 percent identity with hsp 60 from histoplasma. Researchers have sequenced and cloned this gene and introduced it into a bacterial expression vector, pET21a or b. They have also inserted it into PCNV to see if it can induce genetic vaccination. An interesting question for future research is whether hsp 60 is crossprotective for histoplasma and coccidioides, given the differences in pathogenesis and pathophysiology between the two diseases.

Another potential antigen that has been isolated from the soluble fraction of *C. immitis* is HPPD, an enzyme that is involved in the degradation of aromatic amino acids and the production of pigments. The gene for HPPD is highly conserved from bacteria to humans, and that of coccidioides is about 50 percent identical to the human gene. Researchers have sequenced and cloned the gene and demonstrated that HPPD can evoke a proliferative response in mice immunized with coccidioides. At present, however, there are no data on the protective efficacy of either of these antigens.

Problems in Developing Fungal Vaccines. As with other vaccines, an important question is whom to vaccinate. Clinicians don't know at what age these diseases are acquired. Another important question is when to vaccinate. Because cell-mediated immunity is primary, the timing of interdiction is crucial.

In response to questions from the audience, Dr. Deepe added the following:

• Spherulin, the spherule-based vaccine against coccidioides that was developed 10 or so years ago, does not contain hsp 60. There are questions about its efficacy and side effects, but extensive animal studies have been done and the results of randomized clinical trials were published about 12 months ago.

• One of the differences between the two pathogens is the importance of neutrophils in the histopathology of Coccidioides immitis. By the time there are symptoms and biopsies for histoplasmosis, however, there is no sign of neutrophils.

GROUP A STREPTOCOCCI[9]

Incidence and Burden. Group A streptococcus bacteria cause a wide array of clinical syndromes, ranging from the uncomplicated streptococcal pharyngitis (a very common infection among young children) and streptococcal pyoderma at one extreme, to necrotizing fasciitis, "flesh-eating" pyomyositis, and the newly described streptococcal toxic shock syndrome at the other. The resurgence of serious Group A streptococcal infections has provided a new impetus for the development of vaccines, but the major driving force over the years has been the acute rheumatic fever and chronic rheumatic carditis that can follow Group A infection, causing significant morbidity and mortality.

The past 10 years have seen a significant change in the epidemiology of Group A streptococcal infections in the United States and Europe. In certain U.S. cities, for example, the incidence of rheumatic fever has jumped from 1 per

---

[9] Based on a presentation by James Dale, M.D.

100,000 to 10 or 15 per 100,000. An outbreak of rheumatic fever in Utah has been continuing since the mid-1980s. At the same time, there has been an increase in more serious infections—not just pharyngitis and impetigo without complications, but loss of limbs and even of lives. CDC estimates that there are 15,000 to 20,000 cases of serious streptococcal infection per year in the United States, with mortality of anywhere from 30 to 50 percent. In developing nations, meantime, acute rheumatic fever and life-threatening streptococcal infections continue to be as serious a problem as ever.

Rationale for a Surface M Protein-Based Vaccine. There are several potential antigens for vaccines, but over the years the surface M protein has produces the best evidence for protective immune responses. The surface M protein is a major virulence factor of Group A streptococci, since organisms that are rich in M protein are able to resist phagocytosis in the nonimmune host. Significantly, antibodies to M protein are opsonic.

Given these characteristics, the logical approach would be to extract M proteins from the various serotypes of Group A streptococci and combine them into a vaccine. There are three significant obstacles to this approach:

1. Some of the extracellular products that co-purify with M protein preparations are highly toxic. This obstacle has been overcome by recombinant vaccine technology.

2. There are over 80 serotypes of Group A streptococci, all of which express slightly different M proteins, and it would be extremely difficult to concoct a vaccine containing all 80 M proteins. However, there is evidence that the most serious infections can be prevented by a vaccine containing as few as 14 or 16 different M proteins.

3. Most serious of all, some M proteins contain autoimmune (tissue-crossreactive) epitopes and could theoretically trigger acute rheumatic fever, although there is no direct evidence of their role in the pathogenesis of that disease. For example, antibodies to type 5 M protein bind to human myocardium; antibodies to type 6 bind to neurofibers in human brain tissue; and antibodies to type 18 bind to the surface and chondrocytes of mouse joint bone. Among the other host antigens with which M proteins crossreact are myosin, vimentin, keratin, actin, tropomyosin, phosphorylase, DNA, and a large number of undefined antigens.

The latter obstacle led researchers to undertake 15 years of studies to identify which regions of the M protein evoke opsonic (i.e., protective) antibodies and which regions contain autoimmune or potentially harmful epitopes.

Structural and Functional Domains of M Proteins. A generic M protein, which protrudes from the surface of a Group A streptococcus with the amino terminus outward and the carboxy terminus buried in the cytoplasm, is a highly alpha-helical (coiled coil) molecule whose central rod typically contains internal repeats. However, the exposed amino terminus is nonhelical.

In general, the amino terminus usually contains the epitopes that evoke antibodies with the greatest serotypic specificity and bacteriocidal activity. By contrast, most of the tissue-crossreactive epitopes that have been identified to date occur at a distance from the amino terminus, typically in the A, B, or C repeat regions. Consequently, researchers have attempted to develop a vaccine that incorporates amino terminal fragments of several different M proteins, so that they can evoke opsonic antibodies without evoking tissue-crossreactive antibodies. This approach might be characterized as a "fragment of subunit vaccine." By incorporating these fragments into a single construct, they hope to minimize the total amount of protein injected while representing the largest possible number of serotypes.

Development of Complex, Type-Specific M Protein Vaccines. Using specific PCR primers, researchers amplified the 5-prime regions of the M protein gene from four different serotypes—M24, M5, M6, and M19. They purified the PCR products, ligated them in a hybrid M protein gene, and inserted the gene into an expression vector, in this case a transformed *E. coli.* Schematically, the resulting hybrid protein contained 110 amino acids from M24, 58 from M5, and 35 each from M6 and M19. Recombinant hybrid protein was extracted from the *E. coli,* purified, and used as a vaccine in a series of animal tests.

Three rabbits immunized with the tetravalent protein produced significant levels of antibodies against all four serotypes of native protein. However, the level of relevant (i.e., opsonic) antibodies tended to be higher for the first two fragments (M24 and M5, nearest the amino terminus) and lower for the last two (M6 and M19, nearest the carboxy terminus). Researchers were uncertain whether this difference was a function of the size of the fragments or their position on the hybrid protein. To resolve this uncertainty, researchers added another four fragments toward the carboxy terminus—35 amino acids each from M1, M3, M18, and M2—and injected another set of rabbits with the resulting octavalent protein. Again, the immunized rabbits produced significant levels of antibodies against all of the serotypes, and again the level of opsonic antibodies tended to decline toward the carboxy terminus.

To determine whether multivalent hybrid M protein would be immunogenic when administered locally by the mucosal route, researchers constructed additional hybrid proteins consisting of the entire B subunit of *E. coli* labile toxin (LT-B) ligated to 15 amino acids from type 5 M protein (M5), using a proline- and glycine-rich linker. Mice that were immunized intranasally with the resulting LT-B-M5 vaccine produced opsonic serum antibodies against the M5 component, and this response afforded significant protection when the mice were challenged peritoneally with type 5 streptococci. When this experiment was repeated with a LT-B-tetravalent vaccine, however, one of the components (M19, nearest the carboxy terminus) was not immunogenic at all. These mice also developed secretory immunoglobulin-A (IGA) in their saliva, a sign of mucosal immunity, but the IgA level was not particularly high.

An alternative to this approach concentrates not on the hypervariable amino terminus but instead on epitopes in the so-called C-repeats region, epitopes that are highly conserved from one serotype to another. These conserved epitopes are exposed on the surface of the organism and available for antibody binding. Researchers have shown that antibodies to these C-repeat epitopes can block adherence and colonization, and thus prevent infection, in the mouse model. In this experiment, mice were immunized intranasally with peptide from the C-repeat region of type 5 streptococcus and then challenged with the heterologous type 24 streptococcus. The experimental group showed a higher level of survival and a lower level of colonization compared with controls. While this approach will work, however, it is questionable whether it should be the sole basis for streptococcal vaccines.

There are potential vaccine constructs that might be effective against Type A streptococci. Data on the octavalent vaccine suggest that these high complex hybrid molecules can maintain the conformations that stimulate B-cells to produce the relevant antibodies, and researchers have plans to construct a dodecavalent gene and protein. Linking this multivalent protein to LT-B or another carrier that serves as a mucosal adjuvant would provide for both opsonic and secretory antibodies, or a "cocktail" of monovalent terminal fragments could be mixed together according the epidemiology of the organism. C-repeat fragments linked to a carrier might provide broader, more flexible protection. A strategy that deserves attention in the future is the combination of amino terminal fragments (which evoke opsonic antibodies) and C-repeat epitopes (which evoke IgA that can block colonization); this combination might afford the broadest protective immunity in ultimate vaccine trials.

In response to questions from the audience, Dr. Dale added the following:

- The best candidate at present is the type-specific amino terminal approach. Researchers have had unexpected success with these epitopes, which often evoke a better immune response when buried in the middle of a hybrid molecule than when they are on the end.
- Researchers have not yet tested any of these approaches in humans. A great deal of pure development remains to be done, including the preclinical studies that will be needed to convince FDA that these complex constructs are safe.
- It would be desirable to take a candidate vaccine into limited Phase I trials within 5 years.
- The goal of the vaccine is not just to prevent rheumatic fever and other serious disease, but to prevent streptococcus infection in general. Types 2, 4, and 12 are not particularly rheumatogenic but are highly prevalent; by incorporating them in a multivalent vaccine, it might be possible to have a broad impact on disease.
- The target population for the vaccine is preschool children. If they can be immunized before kindergarten, it might be possible to have an impact on overall incidence.
- In addition to common C-repeats, the so-called M5 family (M5, M6, M18, M19, and others) also has common B-repeats, and these conserved epitopes are opsonic.

- Several companies have expressed interest in becoming partners for further development and preparation for human trials.
- Despite tremendous pressure, Group A streptococcus has not developed antibiotic resistance. Penicillin is still effective in treatment and in prophylaxis.
- There is sometimes a fine line between immunizing epitopes and tissue-crossreactive epitopes. Researchers hope to clarify this issue when the final vaccine construct is tested in animals, especially primates whose immune response genes are most similar to humans.

HELICOBACTER PYLORI[10]

Recent developments indicate that it may soon be possible to use vaccines not only prophylactically, to protect against infection and reinfection with *Helicobacter pylori* (HP), but also therapeutically, using active immunization to clear existing infection and prevent reinfection.

Incidence and Burden. HP is the cause of the vast majority of cases of peptic ulcer, over 90 percent of duodenal ulcers, and perhaps 80 percent of gastric ulcers. Once infected with HP, the lifetime risk of acquiring peptic ulcer disease is about 20 percent, with additional cases of atrophy. The risk of gastric cancer is also significant: overall, the lifetime risk of gastric cancer in the United States is about 1 percent, and 60 percent of these cases are attributable to HP.

The association with cancer is even more important elsewhere in the world. In the United States, seroprevalence is about 50 percent by age 50; in developing countries it approaches 100 percent and the infection is acquired earlier, often in childhood. Early acquisition and decades of chronic inflammation appear to be important in the genesis of gastric cancer. The World Health Organization has classified HP as a definite carcinogen.

Pathobiology. HP is a Gram-negative bacterium that is transmitted by saliva and vomitus; young children are the most active transmitters. Once ingested, the bacterium is well-adapted to penetrate the mucous lining of the stomach and colonize the gastric epithelium. It has a spiral shape designed for boring through this viscous environment, and a polar flagella that provides motility and also plays a role in virulence. HP does not invade the host; instead, it causes an "offshore" or surface infection of the epithelium and sometimes penetrates into the gastric glands. Once established, it is a lifelong persistent infection that is not cleared by host immune response.

The result of chronic infection is inflammation of the gastric epithelium leading ultimately to atrophy and destruction of the gastric glands, lymphoid follicles, and a massive accumulation of T and B cells. Secondary effects of

---

[10] Based on a presentation by Thomas Monath, M.D.

inflammation include gastric ulcer, gastric metaplasia of the duodenal bulb, duodenitis, and ultimately duodenal ulcer. A long-standing infection may lead to intestinal metaplasia and gastric carcinoma. Recently, B-cell lymphomas of the stomach have also been associated with HP.

Issues in Vaccine Development. Because HP is a noninvasive surface infection, vaccines should elicit strong mucosal or secretory IgA immunity against one or more prominent surface proteins of the bacterium. Because HP has several virulence factors, the vaccine should be designed to prevent infection rather than interfere with just one virulence factor. Because the infection persists despite a vigorous immune response by the host, and hosts cured of infection with antibiotics appear to be susceptible to reinfection or recrudescence, natural immunity does not seem to be sufficient to protect against or clear infection; hence the vaccine should elicit a response that is qualitatively or quantitatively different from natural immunity.

In addition, HP antigens may elicit hypersensitivity or autoreactive responses, as was the case with Group A streptococci; for this reason, the vaccine should be based on a well-characterized protein that avoids these reactions. The latter considerations—inadequacy of natural immunity and potential crossreactions—argue against the use of live attenuated vaccines or crude whole-cell preparations.

Finally, HP strains are extremely plastic, showing wide variation at both the genomic and antigenic levels. Consequently, the antigen or antigens used in a vaccine must be highly conserved and must be expressed in vivo, so as to be available as a target for immune response. Several candidate antigens have been investigated, including urease and vacuolating cytotoxin, and the ultimate vaccine may involve a combination of antigens. The balance of the presentation focused on urease.

Urease-Based Prophylactic Vaccine. Urease is an abundant protein on the surface of the bacteria and makes up over 6 percent of its total soluble protein. It is highly conserved across strains of HP and even across different species of *Helicobacter* that can be used in animal models (see below). It is a large molecule (550 kD) with a particulate structure, but natural immunity to HP includes only a weak or inconsistent response to urease. The enzyme functions as a virulence factor: it splits the urea found in gastric secretions into two molecules of ammonia, creating a neutralizing cloud around that bacteria that protects it as it passes through the acid environment of the stomach on its way to the pH-neutral environment under the mucous lining.

The operon that controls urease includes two structural genes, ure-A and ure-B, that code for proteins of about 25 and 60 kD respectively. Six units of each of these proteins make up the intact 550-kD molecule. The rest of the genes in this operon are involved in folding the molecule in such a way as to incorporate a molecule of nickel, the metalloenzyme required for its activity. By cloning the two structural genes and leaving out the rest, researchers were able to generate a recombinant urease that is structurally and antigenically intact but lacks the enzymatic activity that would be harmful to a host. Cloned into *E. coli* and expressed in a high-density fermentation system, this modified operon produces extremely large quantities of this recombinant urease—over 3 grams per liter of culture, when immunization requires microgram or nanogram doses (see below).

Preclinical Results. There are several good animal models in which to test HP vaccines. *H. pilus* is a very similar species that infects mice and cats, and the human pathogen *H. pylori* can also be modified to infect mice. Ferrets are susceptible to a third species. However, the most interesting work has been done with cats, which are highly susceptible to *H. pylori,* naturally infected, and develop gastritis and even ulcer disease that is very similar to humans. Cat immunology is at a relatively advanced state of knowledge, which makes this model even more useful. Finally, researchers are beginning to work with primates as well.

Experience has shown that the most effective schedule for prophylactic vaccination is 4 applications 1 week apart. The animals are then tested for antibodies and challenged with either *H. pilus* or *H. pylori* after an appropriate interval—initially 2 weeks, but now up to 1 year. A total of 2 weeks or longer after challenge, the animals are sacrificed and tested in various ways: spectrophotometry (to measure urease activity in the stomach and hence the presence of bacteria), histology (a silver stain for bacteria), electromicroscopy (for antibodies), and immunocytochemistry (for antibody-secreting cells in the gastric mucosa).

Experiments with *H. pilus* in mice showed that mucosal immunity plays an important role in protective immunity. Experimental animals were immunized with recombinant urease by different routes: oral, oral with bicarbonate, intra-gastric, intragastric with bicarbonate, and subcutaneous. Following challenge, 100 percent of unimmunized controls became infected, while 100 percent of those immunized by the oral route were protected. Intragastric immunization, which bypasses potential induction sites in the oral cavity, was less protective, especially when given without bicarbonate to neutralize gastric acid. Parenteral immunization did not protect at all, although it did induce very high serum IgG antibodies.

Dose-response studies showed this is an incredibly potent immunogen, but that a mucosal adjuvant is required for immunization. When mice were given recombinant urease linked to *E. coli* labile toxin (LT, similar to the LT-B used as an adjuvant in streptococcus vaccines, above) by the oral or intranasal route, doses as low as 50 nanograms provided significant protection. Doses are usually in the microgram range or higher in animal experiments. Without the mucosal adjuvant, however, doses as high as 5 milligrams provided no protection: 100 percent of the animals became infected. Analysis of antibody response indicate that secretory IgA correlates best with protection: animals that were fully or partially protected had IgA in their saliva; those that became infected might have IgG in their serum but had no IgA in their saliva.

Durability of protection is another critical issue, and results to date show very durable immunity after oral immunization with recombinant urease. Animals challenged at various intervals show up to 94 percent protection when challenged 1-year after immunization. Significantly, these animals also have very high concentrations of salivary IgA antibodies one year after immunization. This distinguishes artificial immunity from natural immunity, which in this model is primarily serum IgG. Based on this finding, researchers now theorize that HP may avoid the natural host immune response (at least in part) through an antigen-specific suppression of a Th-2 response (other possible explanations include antigenic variation, molecular mimicry, privileged site of sequestration, and polyclonal stimulation).

Other studies have confirmed that immunized mice produce IgA-class antibodies not only in their saliva but also directly in their stomachs following challenge. Immunocytochemistry reveals a marked increase in the number of IgA-secreting cells in immunized animals and a much lower response in infected controls. In fact, up to 20 percent of the IgA-secreting cells in the gastric mucosa of immunized mice were urease-specific. It was this vigorous local immune response that first suggested the possibility of developing a therapeutic vaccine.

The same results were achieved when these experiments were repeated in the mouse model using *H. pylori* instead of *H. pilus,* and similar studies are now being conducted with *H. pylori* in cats, which may be a better model of the human infection. Domestic cats immunized with urease and LT adjuvant developed salivary IgA responses to urease that peaked at 2 weeks and declined somewhat by 5 weeks. When challenged 8 weeks after immunization and sacrificed 8 weeks after challenge, immunized cats had significantly lower mean numbers of bacteria in the stomach compared with controls, and significant recruitment of urease-specific antibody-secreting cells in the gastric mucosa.

Therapeutic Vaccine. After discovering that immunized animals could become transiently colonized and then clear the infection, researchers designed an experiment to see if they could eradicate an infection by active immunization. Mice were infected, given the typical vaccine course, and then sacrificed after 2 or 8 weeks to determine outcome. Controls were 100-percent infected, but there was a significant decrease in the infection rate in immunized mice. When immunized mice were challenged a second time 4 weeks later, there was significant protection to rechallenge among animals that had cleared their infection.

The next question was how best to use the vaccine therapeutically. Current therapeutic regimes achieve cure rates of up to 90 percent using a combination of antacids and various antibiotics, and vaccine can transiently suppress the infection as well. But neither antibiotics nor vaccine by itself can achieve 100-percent clearance, and bacteria populations tend to drift upward again over time. Working with the mouse model, however, researchers found that the *combination* of amoxicillin, Pepto Bismol, and vaccine was able to achieve 100-percent clearance of the infection and to protect against recrudescence or reinfection.

Current Status of Vaccine. Researchers filed an Investigational New Drug application in 1995. A Phase I safety study indicated that the vaccine was quite safe and well tolerated. Researchers are currently in the middle of an appropriate Phase II study of the safety and immunogenicity of this vaccine, using an appropriate adjuvant.

In response to questions from the audience, Dr. Monath added the following:

• Other groups are investigating other potential immunogens, including vacuolating cytotoxin and other molecules. In the end, some combination of antigens including urease and others may be required to produce a successful vaccine.

• Urease is present on the surface of the bacterium, but researchers don't know how it gets there. They have not discovered the signal sequence. One theory is that as other bacteria are lysed and release cytoplasmic urease, the urease is scavenged by bystander bacteria and collected on their surface.

• HP infection is densest in the antrum of the stomach, but there are also bacteria present in the corpus and even the cardia. There is no clear or well-understood relationship between the site of infection and the subsequent site of ulceration. The mechanism is better understood: infection compromises the protective mucous layer as a result of HP virulence factors—mucinase, ammonia, etc., and this exposes the a region of mucosa to acid.

• HP have been found colonizing dental plaque, as well as the stomach, but there is no evidence that HP replicates in the gut.

NEISSERIA GONORRHOEA[11]

Incidence and Burden. The incidence of gonococcus infections has declined dramatically in Europe, by 80 to 99 percent in most countries and almost to extinction in Sweden. It has also declined by about 40 percent in the United States over the past few years, but the social economics of the disease are such that it is unlikely to disappear from its core regions, which include the inner cities and the rural South. Seroprevalence may be a few percent to 5 percent in these U.S. areas, and gonorrhoea remains a very common disease in much of the rest of the world. In Africa, for example, 5 or 10 percent of many study populations are carrying gonococcus at any one time.

Gonococcus is important not because of its acute symptoms but rather because it causes tubal infertility. In this country, it is probably the number-2 cause of tubal infections, after chlamydia, causing about 100,000 cases per year of salpingitis, ectopic pregnancy, and infertility.

---

[11] Based on a presentation by P. Frederick Sparling, M.D.

More importantly, both gonococcus and chlamydia appear to be important co-factors for HIV transmission. Among African women, for example, gonococcus and chlamydia infections are associated with a fourfold increase in the risk of contracting HIV, and the vaginal secretions of infected HIV-positive women contain an increased amount of virus compared with uninfected HIV-positive women. Recent studies have shown that antibiotic treatment of gonococcal or chlamydial infection dramatically reduces the amount of HIV RNA in semen. In a prospective study, simple syndromic management with antibiotics of minor genital infections, urethritis, and genital ulcer syndrome dramatically decreased HIV transmission.

Gonococcus is developing resistance to antibiotics, however. Clinicians have already lost penicillin and tetracycline, which were the drugs of choice until about 2 years ago. Isolated cases of resistance to ciprofloxacin and chlorinated quinoline have appeared in the United States and will probably spread. If clinicians lose the second- and third-generation cephalosporins, treatment would becomes a very significant problem.

Natural Immunity. Like *Helicobacter pylori*, there is little or no naturally acquired immunity to gonococcus. Infections persist, and reinfections are common. Nevertheless, there are convincing data from the era before antibiotics indicating that a deep and persistent gonococcal infection resulted in an immunological cure. In fact, there are a few articles in the old literature on the use of therapeutic vaccines. Despite the shortcomings of these studies, they do suggest that gonococcus, however elegantly it evades the immune response, cannot completely evade a truly vigorous response, and that this effective immune response could be utilized in a vaccine.

This relative lack of a protective immune response to uncomplicated genital infection is surprising, at first glance, because such infection does result in a very vigorous systemic and mucosal antibody response against a number of gonococcal antigens. The mechanisms by which gonococci escape what might otherwise be an effective immune response include rapid antigenic variation of key surface proteins, masking of surface antigens by sialylation of gonococcal lipooligosaccharide (LOS), production of IgA protease, and stimulation of "blocking" antibodies.

In part because of the lack of a good animal model in which to study immune response, past research has focused on the genetics, molecular biology, and pathophysiology of gonococcus rather than functional or protective immune responses. Researchers have learned a good bit about several of these gonococcal antigens, and this knowledge may provide explanations for the lack of natural immunity, as well as candidate antigens that might become the basis for gonococcal vaccines.

Current Candidate Antigens. Most of the initial research concentrated on different forms of gonococcal pilus, a surface appendate that functions as an adherence ligand, and its main subunit (pilin). Antibodies to pilus block adherence and opsonize phagocytes, but gonococci generate a bewildering antigenic variation in pilus. In a human volunteer study, a pilus subunit vaccine administered intramuscularly resulted in significant protection against urethral challenge by the exact strain from which the vaccine was made, but not against a heterogenous strain. When the U.S. military conducted a field trial of monovalent pilin vaccine in Korea, the vaccine failed completely, and predictably. Attention has therefore shifted to pil-C, a pilus-associated protein that is expressed at the sides and tip of the assembled pilus rod and is crucial for epithelial cell adherence. Pil-C is a relatively minor protein on the cell surface, and little is known about how variable it is or whether antibodies against it are protective. It may nevertheless prove to be a better candidate that pilin.

Another effort has focused on the principal outer membrane protein (Por), which is a more attractive candidate than pirin as a vaccine. Por is the major protein on the surface of the gonococcus; it is expressed constitutively and in thus always plentiful; and it shows relatively little antigenic variability (two major immunochemical classes, and minor variance within classes). Antibodies against Por have been shown to be bacteriocidal and opsonic and to block tissue-culture toxicity. Some antibodies crossreact broadly within one or the other immunotype. All of these properties suggest that a vaccine that stimulated these antibodies would be broadly protective. Several groups have worked on developing vaccines using recombinant porine and peptides based on porine.

One difficulty in developing a Por-based vaccine is that Por occurs on the cell surface in tight clusters with two other molecules, LOS and reduction modifiable protein (Rmp). When sialic acid, a sugar residue, is added to the core sugars in LOS, it physically masks the surface exposure of the critical Por epitopes. Rmp is highly immunogenic, and antibodies to Rmp functionally block the bacteriocidal activity of antibodies to Por. The latter mechanism is confirmed by epidemiological data showing a more or less quantitative relationship between the titer of anti-RMP antibody and the risk of a woman becoming infected through sexual contact with an infected man. This still suggests that a Por vaccine is possible, if it induces sufficiently high titers of antibodies to Por while inducing little or no Rmp antibodies. One proposed strategy is to prepare recombinant protein from an organism in which the Rmp has been genetically knocked out. Several companies are pursuing this strategy, and there may well be Phase I clinical trials of such a Por liposome vaccine within 12 to 18 months.

Another strategy has been to focus on the LOS itself. Certain of the core sugars in this molecule are conserved, and antibodies against them are bacteriocidal and opsonic. Anti-idiotype monoclonal antibodies that mimic these core sugars are also bacteriocidal and opsonic. One such antibody is mAb 2C7, which reacts with an oligosaccharide determinant of LOS. Importantly, this particular epitope is not masked when sialic acid is added to LOS. Screening tests show that this epitope is common and stable during serial passage, and antibodies against it are generated in natural human infection. When mAb 2C7 is used as an immunogen in mice and rabbits, the immune response is broadly bacteriocidal and opsonic. This epitope is clearly of interest for further studies.

Potential Future Candidate Antigens. Four other surface proteins, all of them expressed in vivo under conditions in which the bacteria are starved for nutritional iron, have also attracted attention as potential vaccine candidates. One of them, lactoferrin binding protein 1 (Lbp1) is found in only about 50 percent of gonococci; because it is not uniformly present, it is probably not a serious candidate. The other three molecules are present in virtually every gonococcus, and each has properties that suggest its potential value in a vaccine.

Transferrin binding protein 1 (Tbp1) is an integral outer membrane protein that may form a gated pore through which iron enters the cell. Transferrin binding protein 2 (Tbp2) is a lipoprotein that is loosely tethered to the outer membrane; there are multiples of Tbp2 for each Tbp1. Together they form a functional receptor for binding human transferrin and extracting the iron that the gonococcus must take up in order to grow. (This thesis was tested in human volunteers in early 1996, using mutant gonococcus that do not make Tbp1 and Tbp2, and therefore should not be virulent.)

Tbp1 is a potential vaccine candidate because (1) it is antigenically conserved across gonococci (about 90 percent identity across 3 variants characterized); (2) polyclonal antipeptide sera bind to the conserved surface loops; (3) this binding appears to block transferrin binding, an important cellular function; and (4) unlike Por, sialylation of LOS does not mask the functional exposure of this epitope.

Tbp2 is highly immunogenic in vivo, and it is not masked by sialylation of LOS, but it is strikingly antigenically variable—not a characteristic that would recommend it as a vaccine candidate. However, a consortium of European researchers has done considerable work on Tbp2 in both gonococcus (*N. gonorrhoeae*) and meningococcus (*N. meningitidis*). They have found that meningococcal monoclonal antibodies and polyclonal sera against meningococcal Tbp2 block transferrin binding, are bacteriocidal, and—unexpectedly—are relatively crossreactive among different strains. Sequencing of five different strains of meningococcal Tbp2 revealed that, despite differences throughout the molecules, two regions are highly conserved, both of them in the domain that is necessary for binding transferrin. If these antigenically conserved regions are accessible to antibodies, this would explain why antibodies are more crossreactive than expected. It would also make Tbp2 a candidate for vaccines against both meningococcus and gonococcus.

Finally, iron-repressed protein B (FrpB) is another vaccine candidate. This protein in abundant on the surface of some gonococci and present on all. Its physiological function is unknown, although it appears to be a member of the receptor family. Research on meningococcal FrpB, which is almost identical to the gonococcal protein, shows that antibodies are almost always bacteriocidal and surprisingly crossreactive, given that they fall into 10 different serovariant groups. However, sequencing of two gonococcal genes and one meningococcal gene show that this protein is highly conserved at the amino acid level, even in the surface exposed domains. Further research remains to be done, but this protein might also be included in an "bull's eye" component vaccine.

Human Testing. Several animal models have been attempted, but none has been satisfactory, and this has impeded vaccine development. Because of this, however, researchers have learned a great deal about the genetics, molecular biology, and pathophysiology of the organism—how it works and how it evades the immune response. Many researchers have now decided that the time has come to move to human subjects, the only relevant model, in order to develop a vaccine in an intelligent, rational, and cost-effective manner.

One group has challenged over 80 male human experimental volunteers with gonococci in the past few years, establishing several important points. First of all, it is safe. Second, several proteins appear to be sufficient or facilitative for infection, but no single protein appears to be truly necessary or essential for infection. Third, the core polysaccharides of LOS do appear to be absolutely essential to infection, which is another argument for including antibodies to these surface molecules in a vaccine.

In response to questions from the audience, Dr. Sparling added the following:

• It is possible that there will be Phase I and Phase II trials in the next few years, at least on the pilus- and Por-based vaccines. If these trials don't go well, it will take additional years to develop the information needed to go forward with the other candidate antigens described above.

• Progress is a factor of people and money. The field has been moving relatively slowly because there has been little focus on gonococcus vaccine per se.

• The LOS antigen could be developed as an anti-idiotypic vaccine, but it wouldn't have to be. Another possibility would be to combine that core sugar with another antigen in a complex protein-carbohydrate vaccine.

• The LOS antigen has not yet been tested in humans. It does give a good booster response (IgA and IgM) in mice and rabbits, but this is only a surrogate for opsonic and bacteriocidal activity.

• Work on the other antigens—Tbp1, Tbp2, and FrpB—is still at an early stage of concept development.

• It would be desirable to administer the vaccine orally or intranasally. Shigella might be an attractive vector, but there are other potential vectors, as well as cytokines, to target the vaccine.

• The target population would be, at the least, young people as soon as they've had their first incident of any sexually transmitted disease.

ADJUVANTS[12]

An adjuvant is any agent or substance that enhances an immune response. In most cases, adjuvants do not elicit immunity to themselves, but they can and do influence every aspect of the response to the antigen they accompany: the amount of antibody made, its specificity, which epitopes of a given protein are responded to, the isotype of the response, its avidity, duration, memory, and so on. In a very real sense, they are vital to vaccine development.

General Mechanisms of Adjuvant Action. Most adjuvants induce a protective or neutralizing antibody response, and over the years this has been the focus of most adjuvant research. Fewer adjuvants have been looked at for delayed-type hypersensitivity (DTH) or cellular immune response. And only recently have researchers begun to look at the small number of adjuvants that can induce Class I-restricted CTL responses. This research, going back to 1979, has identified a number of general mechanisms by which adjuvants work. One is the so-called "depot effect"—the antigen persists longer because it has been incorporated in an emulsion and is released slowly over time (e.g., Freund's adjuvant). Another is the selective antigen localization in thymic-dependent areas.

However, the crucial mechanism is probably macrophage activation and the generation of inflammation. Indeed, this is how adjuvants were first discovered early in this century—horses that developed a sterile abscess at the injection site had much higher titers of antibody, so researchers started creating abscesses and injecting antigen into the abscess to boost the response. Freund's adjuvant certainly induces inflammation, which is why it is not used in humans.

Other proposed mechanisms for adjuvant activity include increased uptake and presentation by antibody-presenting cells; processing pathway switching; specific or nonspecific stimulation of various helper T-cells; stimulation of increased cytokine production; B-cell isotype switching; and maturation of precursor cells. The specifics for any given adjuvant can be difficult to work out, because these are fairly complex substances that do several different things at once. In the past few decades, much activity has focussed on refining adjuvants down to a simpler, less toxic substance that can be used with greater safety.

On the molecular level, adjuvants appear to enhance the production of costimulatory cytokines. These include IL-1-beta, IL-6, and tumor necrosis factor (TNF), which are crucial for the initiation of immune response. This in turn upregulates costimulatory molecules such as B7, CD8-28, and various other adhesion molecules on T-cells and B-cells. In the future, it may be possible to formulate new adjuvants that selectively exploit these mechanisms. For example, a recent article indicates that the CTLA-4 ligand on T-cells gives a very inhibitory signal to the T-cell; inhibition of that pathway would probably have very good adjuvant effects.

---

[12] Based on a presentation by Charles Elson, M.D.

Increased local production of cytokines such as GM-CSF, which activates macrophage IL-12 and IFN, will recruit increased numbers of macrophages to the lesion. If a "depot" antigen is sitting there, these larger numbers will mean a greater immune response. In many ways, the action of an adjuvant is to overcome the immune system's basic tone or bias, which is to nonresponse rather than response.

Common Adjuvants. Almost every vaccine experiment in animals involves the use of some form of adjuvant, although it seldom receives prominent attention. The most commonly used adjuvants in experimental animals are Freund's adjuvant, either complete or incomplete; *Bordatella pertussis;* lipopolysaccharide (LPS) or the more refined lipid-A; muramyl dipeptide (MDP, the smallest component of microbacteria that has an adjuvant effect); immunostimulating complexes; glycopolymers; liposomes; and a few others. Some of these adjuvants enhance the Th1 or cellular immune pathway (e.g., Freund's, LPS, MDP); others enhance the Th2 or humoral immune pathway (e.g., alum, pertussis).

Only one adjuvant is currently approved by FDA for use in humans: alum, a mixture of aluminum salts. When injected, shards of crystal in the alum cause inflammation, recruiting macrophages that eat the antigen associated with the crystals, thereby presenting it to the immune system. However, researchers have identified at least six groups of potentially useful agents, most of which are already in human trials:

1. *Monophosphoric lipid-A* (MPL) might be called the active ingredient of LPS, a further refinement that has lower toxicity but retains adjuvant effect. In mice, it stimulates both antibody and cell-mediated immunity. It stimulates macrophage IL-1, TNF, various colony-stimulating factors, and IFN-gamma, and it also up-regulates Class II MHC expression. Like LPS, in enhances nonspecific resistance to bacterial infection and has a global effect on the immune system. One such adjuvant is currently in Phase 3 human trials.

2. *Muramyl dipeptides* (MDPs) include hundreds of derivatives that have been synthesized and tested over the years. Two products are currently in human trials with AIDS vaccines: SAF-1, which contains a blocker polymer (see below); and NF-59, which contains a small amount of lipid. Both products stimulate antibody as well as cell-mediated immunity, costimulating T-cells and up-regulating Class II macrophages. The exact cytokine they are producing is not really clear, but they are candidates for future vaccines.

3. *Immune-stimulating complex* (ISC) was developed by a veterinarian in Europe. It contains cholesterol and safranin (a detergent derived from plants), with which the antigen is mixed, and takes the form of small particles. In animal tests (mice, cats, sheep, cattle, and monkeys), it produces very strong antibody and CMI response, and it is effective for mucosal immunization, which also produces CTL responses. A formulation called QS-21 is in Phase 1 trails in humans.

4. *Glycopolymer* is a polyoximer related to common compounds found in mouthwash, toothpaste, and even food products. It consists of a central segment of hydrophobic polyoxyl propylene polymer, with a hydrophilic polyoxyl ethylene at each end; the lengths of these segments are critical to the activity of the molecules. They enhance antibody, IgG1 and IgG2a, and cell-mediated responses. They appear to have a depot effect and have been shown to be effective as an adjuvant with peptides, proteins, and polysaccharides in oil and water emulsions. Currently available as an animal preparation under the name Titer-Max, it is fairly expensive but may be cheaper in broader human use. It is currently in Phase 1 trials.

5. *Cytokines* are a logical target of research: if adjuvants stimulate cytokines, why not use the cytokines themselves? GM-CSF is a leading candidate because both stimulate the production of macrophages in bone marrow and activate the macrophages; it will soon be approved for use in cancer gene therapy. *IL-12* preferentially stimulates the Th1 pathway in mice and might be attractive, but there are toxicity problems. IFN-gamma, IL-4, and anti-IL-4 might also be useful to preferentially activate or block certain response pathways, depending on the antigen.

Human Testing. One of the biggest hurdles in the development of new adjuvants is the difficulty of testing them in humans. Under FDA rules, new adjuvants can only be tested in cancer patients (where the standards of harm and side effects are lowered). Cancer vaccines aren't really that similar to infectious disease vaccines, and adjuvants that fail in a cancer vaccine might still be excellent adjuvants for other applications. Moreover, no single adjuvant is going to be universally effective; many different adjuvants, each with their own particular application, might be needed.

Mucosal Immunization. Most pathogens invade or colonize the mucosal surfaces, and parenteral immunization does not protect mucosal surfaces. On the other hand, the majority of lymphoid cells in the body are at mucosal surfaces, particularly in the gut, which has more lymphoid cells than all other lymphoid organs put together. The lymphoid follicles in the gastrointestinal tract and the nose are important entry or inductive sites for mucosal immune responses. Cells that are induced in one site are transported to other mucosal surfaces, making it possible to immunize the respiratory epithelium (for example) by immunizing the gut or the nose. This has led to considerable interest in nasal immunization.

Unfortunately, there are at present no adjuvants for mucosal immunization that are approved for human use, nothing in human trials, and very little even in early stages of development. Experimentally, however, both cholera toxin (CT) and *E. coli* heat labile toxin (two molecules with similar three-dimensional structures) have been shown to have adjuvant effects at mucosal surfaces.

For example, when mice are fed keyhole limpet hemocyanin (KLH) there is no response in the gut, but when CT is mixed with the KLH there is an IgA response to KLH. This finding has been repeated with a wide spectrum on antigens, including not only proteins (e.g., KLH) but also polysaccharides, whole bacteria (e.g., *H. pylori*), whole viruses (e.g., influenza, Sendai, measles), and even whole protozoa (e.g., *Toxoplasma gondii*). Unlike LPS, CT and the antigen have to be administered together by the mucosal route, and in mice this usually requires microgranules. But all the properties of CT as an immunogen seem to rub off on the accompanying antigen, notably a prolonged memory response. Researchers have also succeeded in attaching peptide antigens directly to the CT molecule, with similar results.

Adjuvant Action of Cholera Toxin. CT has stimulatory effects on macrophages for IL-6 production, about a 30-fold increase. LPS has a somewhat greater effect, but the two together have even greater effect than either alone. On the other hand, CT does not stimulate TNF production, and it inhibits the stimulatory effect of LPS on TNF production.

Researchers have also achieved interesting effects by varying the sequence in which antigen-presenting cells are stimulated. Using bone marrow macrophages grown in vitro with M-CSF, for example, they found that both IFN and CT stimulate IL-6, and the combination stimulates better than either alone. But when the macrophages are "primed" with IFN for as little as 30 minutes before CT is introduced, there is an enormous increase in IL-6 production. This finding suggests that the sequence in which the immune system is stimulated may be more important than the mixture of stimulants.

Researchers are finding similar effects on production of the costimulatory molecule B7: CT alone stimulates 1.7 percent to 10.3 percent of cells to express B7, while CT and IFN together stimulate 40 percent (as measured by flow cytometry). Further analysis shows that B7 comes in two varieties, B7-1 (thought to preferentially stimulate the Th1 pathway) and B7-2 (thought to stimulate the Th2 pathway). B7-1 remains fairly constant regardless of stimulus, while B7-2 increases from 4 percent to 20 percent with CT, to 20 percent with IFN, to 56 percent with CT and IFN together. In short, CT appears to have a preferential, up-regulation effect on B7-2, the molecule that appears to be responsible for the costimulatory effect of CT and IFN. CT produces these effects down to the nanogram range, so it is a potent, very-low-dose effect of CT.

In vivo, the net effect of cholera toxin is to enhance T-cell priming, probably through its effects on macrophages. A single injection of CT plus KLH produces enhanced proliferation in response to KLH from multiple tissues, with cells producing a variety of cytokines for both the Th1 and Th2 pathways. CT also increases precursor cell frequency from 1:23,000 to 1:900. The net effect of all these biologic effects is strong stimulation.

There is a single dominant epitope for T cells on the CT molecule, a peptide designated CTV-89-100. Experiments with this peptide in mice have shown that when the animal is tolerized to CT as an antigen, CT loses its adjuvant effect—both the T-cell and B-cell responses were blocked. Other experiments have shown that the adjuvant effect is also blocked unless both the A subunit and B subunit of the CT molecule are present.

Prospects for Future Adjuvants. Adjuvants will be required for most of the emerging vaccine candidates, and it is likely that different adjuvants will be required for different antigens, particularly to shape the immune response in the most beneficial direction. At present, however, there is no detailed understanding of how the adjuvant mechanism operates at the molecular level; this understanding is needed in the future. Almost no work is being done on adjuvants for mucosal vaccines, and this should be a particular priority.

At present, the number of candidate vaccines greatly exceeds the number of candidate adjuvants, and this imbalance will only increase as genomes are sequenced for increasing numbers of pathogens. In this situation, the lack of new adjuvants may become the principal limiting factor in the development of human vaccines in general and mucosal vaccines in particular. Another limiting factor, however, will be the necessity of testing new vaccines on cancer patients; after all, is their immune system so normal?

In response to questions from the audience, Dr. Elson added the following:

• Researchers have not yet repeated the CT experiments in mice at lower doses, but in all likelihood when it no longer works as an adjuvant it will also loses it effect on T-cells. The mouse experiments were done in the B6 mouse, which has the best response to CTV-89-100.

• In countries where cholera is endemic, the IgA system is fully developed by age 1 or 2, whereas in the United States you would not see adult levels of IgA until the teenage years.

• CT-vibrio vaccine (CTV) appears to be a stronger immunogen than CT itself, in humans if not in mice, and it may also prove to be a better adjuvant in humans. It represents one way to avoid the potential toxicity of CT.

• Another way to avoid toxicity is to use multiple emulsions to sequester the toxin from the epithelium and deliver it instead to the lymphoid follicles of the intestine. This technique has been tested in mice and does not produce fluid secretion. It is much faster than developing correct microencapsulation, which also requires that the antigen be denatured. In addition, multiple emulsions seem to require smaller amounts of antigen and can contain several antigens at once.

• Mucosal immune memory for antigens presented with CT extends for up to 1 year.

• The adjuvanticity of CT seems to be tied to its immunogenicity; mutants that lack adjuvant activity also aren't immunized to themselves. It might to identify a single-amino-acid mutation that lacks toxicity but retains adjuvant activity; but it is not clear how this would be accomplished.

• A tremendous amount of very basic work remains to be done before this knowledge could be used to produce vaccines for use by providers. University research can handle some of the questions, but commercial partners will be needed for development.

ANTIGEN DELIVERY SYSTEMS[13]

To dramatize the importance of mucosal antigen delivery systems, three important concepts bear repeating:

1. *Most infectious diseases or agents enter through the mucosal tissues.* In terms of incidence and burden, this includes a billion cases of diarrhea at any given time. *Bacteria* such as salmonella, Shigella, vibrio, etc., spread at roughly one-half million cases per hour, just among children, 500 of whom will die. *Viruses* such as hemophilus, pneumococcus, and measles infect some 14,000 case per hour. *AIDS* infects 340 people per hour, 80 percent of 90 percent of them through a mucosal surface.

2. *The entire immune system is stimulated by what we eat and by what compromises our mucosal surfaces.* There are roughly 10^{14} bacteria living in the human gut. Each person ingests about one metric ton of solids and liquids per year. About 10 milligrams of undigested protein are "injected" into the circulation every day. Some 70 percent of all lymphoid cells are associated with mucosal tissues, and the gut has more macrophages than the liver.

3. *There is a common immune system.* The concept of systemic immunization, first recognized by Erlich in 1891, involves the stimulation of cells from inductive sites (e.g., Peyer's patches in the intestine) to remote sites (e.g., nasal passages, salivary glands, even the genital tract). In both monkeys and mice, for example, intranasal immunization produces a greater antibody response in the genital tract than any other route. The instrument of this response is the M-cell, which can internalize both particulate and soluble antigens.

Research on Antigen Delivery Systems. The central problem with mucosal application of antigens is the small quantity of antigen that is absorbed, due to degradation by enzymes, mucous coatings, etc. Typical absorption rates for proteins are only 1:100,000. Taking antigen with food can reduce degradation somewhat, as can encapsulation—protecting the antigen from the stomach in order to deliver it to a desired segment of the intestine.

A few groups in Europe and the United States are using liposomes to deliver antigens. In the mouth, this can reduce the formation of plaque and the incidence of dental caries. However, liposomes are relatively unstable in the internal environment. Others are working with mucosal adhesives, microspheres, CT and CPB conjugates, and live pathogen delivery systems.

The goal of this research could be called the "dream vaccine"—something safe and stable that might be produced locally, could be administered orally in one dose to provide both systemic and mucosal immunity, possibly to several

---

[13] Based on a presentation by Jeri Mestecky, M.D.

different pathogens at the same time. At present, 60 percent of the cost of vaccine delivery is spent on refrigeration, and another large fraction on syringes and health professionals. Some of these vaccines would make it possible to immunize thousands or even millions of people in a single day without doctors, needles, or pain.

Mucosal Adhesives. Other researchers are developing new mucosal adhesives, which increase absorption by extending the period of time during which antigen is exposed to the mucosal surface. Substances such as carboxymethyl-cellulose adhere very nicely to the mucosal surfaces and could be used to deliver antigen to those tissues. Investigators in Iceland have tested mucosal adhesives containing influenza virus in the nasal cavity of animals and even humans. It produced stronger and longer-lasting immune response than the injectable vaccine.

Microspheres. Microspheres are already in common use for the delivery of drugs and are being developed for the delivery of hormones and insulin. Because M-cells preferentially internalize particles, it should be possible to use them to introduce soluble antigen to the macrophage. A company in Korea has applied to develop a hepatitis-B vaccine using microspheres that has the considerable advantage of requiring only one injection. (Compliance is a problem with the current vaccine, which requires 3 injections: only 60 percent of patients return for the second shot, and 40 percent for the third.) The spheres themselves are totally biodegradable and nontoxic; varying the composition regulates the rate (and hence the location) at which individual microspheres dissolve.

Injectable microspheres can be up to 50 microns and still be effective, and in the gut these larger spheres collect in the Peyer's patch, where they induce a mucosal immune response (circulatory IgG). They must be less than 10 microns to be absorbed by the intestine. These smaller microspheres can later be found in the mesentery lymph nodes and spleen, as well as in circulation. In some cases (e.g., SIV) they can also induce T-cell-mediated immunity in cytotoxic T-cells, although this is not seen with other antigens (e.g., influenza and polio virus). The reasons for this difference should be addressed in future research.

Obviously, the prospect of a vaccine that could be eaten and would induce both mucosal and system immunity is very attractive. Because microspheres protect against degradation by gastric acid in the stomach, 100 percent of the antigen reaches the gut. At present, however, less than 1 percent of ingested microspheres are internalized. The rate of absorption might be increased through surface modifications or coadministration with CT or CPB, which has increased absorption in animals.

Other development problems also remain. In numerous animal experiments, antigen in microspheres induced much high titers of specific antigen that raw antigen. However, several vaccines that work in animals haven't worked in humans. In some cases, the organic solvents used in preparing the microspheres can denature the antigen unless it is relatively stable. And improvements may be needed in the reproducibility of microsphere preparation.

Live Virus and Bacteria. Another delivery system that is attracting attention is the use of recombinant technology to create yeast viruses and bacteria that express antigen. This has already been done with hepatitis B, removing DNA from the pathogen and introducing it into a vector that then produces the immunizing antigen. Some potential vectors can be administered intranasally, orally, and/or rectally. It may also be possible to induce more than one antigen in a single vector, and the cost of producing these vaccines is fairly low.

Among the bacteria being explored as vectors are *E. coli,* BCG (attenuated *Mycobacterium bovis*), *Shigella,* and lactobacilli. These microbial vectors are immunogenic by themselves, and consequently they cannot be used for a second immunization. Lactobacilli show particular promise because children are usually colonized at an early age, so the immune response is minimal. There is some risk of contaminating the environment with recombinant bacteria.

Viruses may have many advantages, including better control over the conformation and glycosylation of the expressed antigen. Promising vectors include poliovirus, influenza, canarypox, and rhinovirus. Both influenza and canarypox have been used to express HIV antigens in human experiments.

These vectors have disadvantages that must be overcome. For example, the dominant response is always to the vector rather than the antigen. The major problem for immunology, however, is that the level of expression of the desired antigen is extremely low; this might be overcome by inserting multiple copies of the gene. In addition, bacterial vectors do not always produce antigen with the proper secondary and tertiary structure.

Plants. Several groups are looking at plants as possible delivery systems. The tobacco plant in particular is called "the white mouse of botany" because its genes are well known and easy to manipulate using the tobacco mosaic virus, which can infect 400 other plants. Researchers in England have already succeeded in producing hepatitis B antigens in tobacco leaves. Other plants that are being considered as delivery systems include potato, beet, rice, lettuce, tomato, and bananas. Bananas would be particularly attractive in tropical areas, but the intended antigen is produced at low levels—100 micrograms of hepatitis B protein per banana, rather than the 10 milligrams researchers had hoped for.

Plants can also be used to produce specific antigens, including secretory IgA containing the secretory element. This has been done by introducing genes for the heavy chains of IgA into tobacco, and could conceivably be done with edible plants as well. The result could be an edible delivery system for highly specific secretory IgA antibodies against rotavirus, salmonella, etc., as well as antigens. This could become one of the vaccines of the future.

DNA Immunization. DNA vaccines are covered in greater detail in the following summary. However, this is a difficult route of immunization because of generally poor reproducibility and low uptake of DNA. It may be possible to increase uptake using microspheres or other systems. It is unclear at present whether DNA introduced through the Peyer's patch will lead to the synthesis of desired antigens, as it does when injected into muscle or skin.

Barriers to Vaccine Development. Tolerance is a major problem with some of these delivery systems. In addition to reducing the immune response, this can also lead to systemic unresponsiveness or even collapse at the T-cell level, the B-cell level, and even the antibody level. This can be addressed by changing the form or delivery of the antigen—globulin given in large oral doses induces tolerance, but globulin in microspheres continues to produce a good immune response. Frequency and timing of exposure also plays a role. Studies of humans immunized with keyhole limpet hemocyanin (KLH) demonstrated that oral administration "primes" the systemic response and reduces both hypersensitivity and tolerance. The nasal route appears to be more effective than eating the antigen.

Other Applications. These delivery systems might be used to introduce proteins that would treat or protect against autoimmune diseases such as rheumatoid arthritis and multiple sclerosis. Another possible application might be in the control of fertility—researchers working with rats have found that the sperm antigen SP-10, introduced orally, produces specific secretory antibodies against sperm in the female genital tract. The result is a temporary infertility mediated by specific IgA, temporary because IgA immune response is not long-lasting.

In response to questions from the audience, Dr. Mestecky added the following:

- "Immune tolerance" is the wrong name for what happens in oral adminisration. "Mucosal deviation" might be better, since it changes the response rather than causing total unresponsiveness.
- The intranasal route induced better tolerance that the oral route with the same antigen in mice. This work involved animal models of arthritis.
- Antigens produced by plants may not be as "naked" as desired. Antigens like HIV, SIV, and GP-120 and 160 are generally heavily glycosylated, but glycosylation in plants is different from that in mammalian cells.
- Since the immune response to the vector is a limiting factor, systems that are inert might be preferable to live vectors.
- Parenteral immunization is relatively ineffective in inducing mucosal immunity. Studies with a variety of antigens demonstrated that it is almost never possible to boost the secretory IgA response by systemic immunization. Similarly, IgG in the genital tract is not derived from the circulation; systemic IgG cannot prevent the pathogen from crossing the mucosal membrane.

Systemic, intranasal, and internal immunization produce very different patterns of potential homing receptors on the surface of B-cells. Researchers have not looked at receptors on T-cells yet.

DNA VACCINES[14]

Unlike other vaccines, which deliver the antigen itself in some form, a DNA vaccine delivers only the genes that encode for the antigen of interest. In this sense, it is nonreplicating bacterial plasma in a fairly generic expression vector that is expressed by mammalian (and ultimately primate) muscle tissue. These are not yet clinical entities, since none have been approved as yet for use in humans. However, researchers have had success with bacterial and viral antigens in a number of animal experiments, and work is beginning in England on cancer antigens as well.

Research in this area began with a paper published in 1990, detailing a process for transfecting genes into cells in vitro. When reporter genes were put into expression vectors and injected intramuscularly, the tissue expressed the protein encoded in the gene. It is still not known why muscle tissue expressed protein better that other cell and tissues types. Researchers estimate that no more than 1,000 cells actually take up the DNA and express the protein. This technique did not appear promising for gene therapy, but since there was amplification of the immune system, it might be a good way to generate antigen in situ.

Researchers had been looking for a way to deliver antigens to the cytoplasm of the cell, where their epitopes would evoke class I restricted cytotoxic T-lymphocyte responses. Because every individual's MHC molecules are different, this would allow different HLA haplotypes to select their own epitopes, instead of concocting a "cocktail" of different types to cover an entire population. Muscle cells aren't usually thought of as antigen-presenting cells, but the DNA vaccine approach did provide a way to have the antigen produced endogenously by a host cell.

Viral DNA Vaccines. For a protection experiment based on cytotoxic T-cell response, researchers extracted the gene-encoding nucleate protein from influenza virus. This internal protein is highly conserved between different strains of the virus. Mice were immunized with the gene taken from an H1-N1 strain from 1934, and then challenged with a very different H3-NT strain called Compound 68. The results showed that there was a cell-mediated response, and that it was protective. Antibodies were generated as well, but since they were antibodies to an internal protein this response was not protective.

Researchers have since improved on both the vector and the expression of the target protein. In recent tests, 100 percent of immunized animals survive, while 90 percent of controls die. Controls receive either saline immunization or "control DNA" that does not encode for the nucleate protein. Two years after immunization, there is still cytotoxic T-lymphocyte activity that is specific for peptide target cells and influenza-infected cells. Since this is a class I restricted

---

[14] Based on a presentation by Margaret Liu, M.D.

peptide, this is a CD8 response. Protection does not appear to persist as long as the CTL response.

Another group has done similar experiments with aged mice. They were able to get CTLs with the same precursor frequencies in the aged mice as in younger mice, with good antibodies and good small-dose protection. This is an important issue in diseases like influenza, where the elderly are the population at greatest risk.

To determine whether is would also be possible to get efficacious B-cell and antibody responses, as well as CTL response, researchers repeated the experiment using the gene encoding for influenza hemagglutin, a surface glycoprotein that is the antigen against which the major neutralizing antibody is directed. (These proteins change frequently, which is why the current influenza vaccine must be reformulated every year.) The result was a very good level of functional antibodies, with titers comparable to live infection and probably high enough to be protective in humans. These antibody levels have been sustained for 20 months, although duration might not be as great in humans. Researchers are uncertain whether antigen is still being expressed after this interval; one study suggests that the DNA persists and expresses for up to 24 months.

One unexpected finding was that the DNA vaccine encoding for hemaglutin induced antibodies with a different profile from those induced by commercial vaccines containing inactivated influenza, notably a greater predominance of IgG2a. The latter is thought to be important in providing protection from influenza. Doses as low as 1 microgram, given twice 3 weeks apart, provide 100 percent survival in mice and little or no morbidity as measured by weight loss and grooming behavior. Further tests indicate that DNA vaccines also stimulated greater lymphocyte proliferation from splenocytes and higher levels of IL-2 and IFN-gamma on restimulation. This and the absence of IL-4 point to a Th1-like helper response.

HIV DNA Vaccines. It is increasingly accepted that the same kind of Th1-like helper response and CTLs are major factors in preventing HIV infection, or at least prolonging the phase of latent disease. This is supported by recent findings that high-risk individuals who remain seronegative have good Th blood-type responses, and that those with the less virulent HIV-2 are at decreased risk for HIV-1.

Initial work on HIV envelope proteins focused on surface antigens such as B3, GP-120, and GP-160, looking for a neutralizing epitope and trying to make it recombinant. It has become increasingly clear that the antibody response is more complicated, and that memorization in particular involves dimeric dimers of GP-160 that form conformational epitopes. Accordingly, effort has shifted from peptide vaccines to ways of making intact oligomeric GP-160. DNA vaccines offer the advantage that the protein is synthesized in situ, with normal glycosylation.

Researchers gave African green monkeys two injections of a DNA vaccine based on a truncated GP-160-like construct. Animals developed relatively high antibody titers that show diverse neutralizing responses, which is desirable given the diversity of HIV types. However, antibodies are not at levels that would be protective against SIV challenge. Researchers hope to improve antibody titers in the future.

To look for CTL responses, researchers also vaccinated monkeys with a DNA vaccine based on envelope proteins with known CTL epitopes. The animals developed good CTL response, with precursor frequencies as high as animals that have been infected with SIV. This may not be high enough to challenge at present, but researchers are encouraged by the combination of antibody and CTL response. Future work may focus on conserved envelope protein such as GAG and POL.

Similar results were obtained in mice immunized with DNA GP-120 vaccine. When splenocytes were restimulated in vitro with GP-120, they proliferated and produced a lot of IFN-gamma and IL-4—again characteristic of a Th1-type response. Lymphocytes from other sites—mesenteric, iliac, inguinal, and peripheral blood—also proliferated in response to antigen, even 6 months after vaccination in the quadriceps. This kind of long-lived response, with both cytokines and helper CTLs, would be particularly desirable in an HIV vaccine.

TB DNA Vaccines. TB remains a major health problem, with perhaps one-third of the world's population infected, and it is a growing problem with multidrug resistance in the United States. An effective vaccine would be important at least until new antibiotics are available. Researchers prepared a vaccine containing the DNA coding for antigen Ag-85, one of the secreted antigens of TB, and were able to induce CTLs. These lymphocytes were not antigen-restimulated, however, but rather were ConA- and IL-2-restimulated. Vaccinated animals also produced IFN-gamma and GM-CSF, the latter also being important for protective response.

In preliminary challenge studies, immunization with DNA Ag-85 protected just as well as BCG against intravenous and inhalation challenges. This may not be a very good vaccine—yet—but it is working as well as the vaccine that many people are getting now. The next step may be to add genes for additional antigens.

Researchers had thought that one of the advantages of DNA vaccines would be mammalian post-translational modifications in the antigen. In the case of TB, however, this was not necessarily desirable. Fortunately, it was fairly easy to remake the vectors—cleaving Ag-85 and altering the leader sequence, glycosylation points, etc., to get the desired form. Nevertheless, researchers still weren't sure whether they were getting true oligomerization of the resulting envelope proteins.

HPV DNA Vaccine. L1, the major capsid protein of human papillomavirus, forms pentimers that come together to form the capsid. The neutralizing antibody is directed at conformational epitopes, so the protein must have the correct structure and oligomerization to act as antigen. This protein is targeted to the nucleus, where new viruses are assembled and then excreted from the cell. For these reasons, it wasn't clear that the DNA vaccine would work.

Researchers prepared DNA vaccine using the L1 protein from rabbit papilloma virus and immunized rabbits. Following a single immunization, animals made a good titer of antibody that has persisted out to 32 weeks, although this doesn't predict what will happen in humans. The animals are challenged by scarifying the skin and applying virus, resulting in a wart. This is not how infection occurs in humans, but it does allow measurement of neutralizing antibodies. Animals immunized with L1 DNA were all protected from getting warts, so at least in this model it was possible to get neutralizing antibodies to a protein that forms a conformational epitope.

Herpes DNA Vaccine. HSV is an interesting case because there is a good animal model for mucosal challenge. Researchers would like to develop a mucosal delivery mechanism for DNA vaccine, since the current procedure does not produce mucosal antibodies.

In the first study, mice were vaccinated with DNA encoding for the surface glycoprotein GC and challenged intraparenterally with a lethal dose. About 90 percent of controls died, while animals immunized with as little as 800 nanograms of vaccine were protected to some extent.

In a second study, guinea pigs were immunized and then challenged intravaginally. This is thought to resemble closely what happens in humans. The results showed that immunizing the animals with one or two doses of DNA vaccine provided very good protection from the lesions that occur in the group injected with saline solution.

Other Approaches. The DNA vaccine technology is relatively simple: just put a gene into a vector and immunize with it. But in less than 3 years since the first study was published, the technique has been proven effective against a broad range of targets, including parasites as well as viruses, microbacteria, and cancer. One group has used the technique to construct "expression libraries," in which an organism's genome is broken into perhaps 2,000 fragments and then used to immunize experimental animals that are subsequently challenged. A decoding process identifies which antigens elicited protective immune responses. The process is slow and animal-intensive, and there may be problems with antigenic competition or partial conformations, but this approach does offer potential application for vaccine discovery efforts for antigens.

Issues in DNA Vaccine Development. Three sets of key issues raise questions about the ultimate importance of DNA vaccine technology: (1) safety, (2) human efficacy, and (3) process and stability. The stability issue in particular poses the danger of overselling the potential of the technology.

There is a need for a full safety profile. Some of the key points raised by regulatory personnel concerned subintegration: i.e., does insertional mutagenesis occur, are pathogenic anti-DNA antibodies generated, and does tolerance occur? To date there is no evidence of any of these problems. Researchers have performed a very sensitive PCR-based assay on tissue from 13 different organs and found no evidence of the inserted DNA. Mutations are less likely in double-stranded DNA than in single strands. Tolerance is a more difficult issue, but researchers are monitoring it. One advantage of this approach is that there is no danger of viral disease, since the vaccine does not contain replicating virus.

On the question of efficacy, native protein is made endogenously, with the appropriate mammalian post-translational modifications, and it induces neutralizing antibody even across conformational epitopes. There are cytotoxic T-lymphocytes and cross-strain protection. The muscle cells, while they may not be antigen-presenting cells, definitely do transfer antigen, and there is good helper T-cell response.

On the question of production, it is (or will be) a generic technology. Once the manufacturing process is in place, producing different vaccines will be no different than producing different flavors of ice cream. The process is the same, and so is the host strain. The technology will also be useful as a laboratory tool for producing and screening antibodies.

In response to questions from the audience, Dr. Liu added the following:

• It would appear that the DNA itself is modulating the Th1-like response. Recombinant nucleate proteins induce antibodies to recombinant nucleate proteins, but when you add plasma DNA—even if it doesn't encode for anything— you get a Th1-like response with predominance of IgG2A. In a sense, the DNA acts as an adjuvant.

• Researchers don't know whether the muscle cells that are generating antigen will be attacked and lysed by antigen-specific CTLs. For one thing, they are multinucleated; for another, they are very large. In any event, very few muscle cells are transfected: the number of plasmic copies drops from 2,000 initially to about 1,500 at 4 weeks and 500 at 18 weeks.

• Researchers have tried various routes of immunization. Subcutaneous injection produces good antibody response but no CTL or helper T-cell response. They have also applied DNA directly to mucosal tissues; the result was IgG antibody response without IgA, and no CTL response. Nevertheless, their goal is to move toward mucosal delivery if only because of the ease of delivery.

• Researchers have not yet investigated the class II response in detail.

• Histologic studies of transfected muscle cells reveal no inflammatory myopathies. The needle track remains visible and is infiltrated with lymphocytes, but the response was much less marked than the response to an antibiotic that is injected intramuscularly and known to be a mild irritant.

• Researchers still don't understand the exact mechanism by which antigen expressed in muscle cells induces antibodies. Clearly it makes it out of the cell, but that could be due to (1) transfer by the myoblasts or (2) transfection of antigen-presenting cells that happen to be in the muscle tissue. They plan to pursue this question using experiments in which transfected myoblasts are transplanted to bone marrow chimeras.

- The DNA plasma in the vaccine is not integrated, because the gene itself does not replicate, even though there is expression of the antigen that it encodes for.
- The TB studies have looked at three major forms of Ag-85—A, B, and C—and at different variations of these forms (with and without leaders, etc.). They are just now beginning to work with ESET6, the other major secreted antigen that is believed to provide some protection.
- It is very difficult to say how soon there might be a vaccine for humans. Work seems to be on track in terms of addressing safety concerns. The biggest unknown is whether they will be allowed to test an IND in healthy humans instead of cancer and HIV patients as is currently the case. A great deal depends on the regulatory agency.
- The influenza vaccine is the most advanced candidate, even though it may not be the best choice for a DNA vaccine because of antigenic drift. And there are influenza vaccines already, but no vaccines for herpes, HIV, etc.
- Studies have not been conducted with newborn mice, because of their very small size. Studies have used mice from 3 weeks to aged. There might be some advantage to using this technology for something like a measles vaccine to cover the period of 6 to 12 months, before maternal antibodies decline. But this will not be the first population that a commercial laboratory would focus on because of regulatory problems.
- Tolerance is unlikely to be a problem unless expression is boosted considerably, or unless the dosage is increased significantly. However, more needs to be known about the phenomenon of tolerance induction.
- From a safety point of view, it might be desirable to transfect a more differentiated but shorter-lasting cell, such as a dendritic cell, rather than a muscle cell. Researchers will probably continue to explore this question.

PREVENTIVE VACCINE FOR DIABETES[15]

Clinicians have noticed that when insulin replacement therapy is begun, it often appears to reverse the disease process. This led to experiments in which non-obese diabetic (NOD) mice were given daily prophylactic doses of insulin at the outset of the inflammatory lesion in the pancreatic islets. The results showed that diabetes is not only preventable, but also reversible. Photomicrographs of the pancreas of an NOD mouse showed some islets that were completely free of lymphocytic infiltration, while others were full of lymphocytes.

This raises the question of mechanism, and one possibility is that of beta cell rest: if the animal receives insulin every day, the islets don't need to produce it, and the suppressed cells don't produce autoantigens that are reactive to the immune system. In this case, insulin itself seems to be acting in some speci-

---

[15] Based on a presentation by Noel Maclaren, M.D.

fic immunological way. Based on this experience in NOD mice, the researchers have organized a Diabetes Prevention Trial Type 1, which is ongoing. They have also conducted further experiments in antigen-specific immunotherapy in the NOD mouse.

The strategy in general is to tolerize against the harmful Th-1 immune cells, and if possible transform the response from a harmful Th-1 to an ostensibly harmless Th-2. This can be accomplished by immunizing with various antigens and adjuvants, either orally or intravenously. Three possible autoantigens have the greatest relevance for human diabetes:

    1. Glutamic acid decarboxylase (GAD), usually GAD-65 rather than a higher molecular weight isoform;

    2. Transmembrane tyrosine phosphatases, one called IA2 and the other IA2-beta; and

    3. Insulin and insulin receptors.

Experiments with IA-2 and IA-2-beta are ongoing; results are available for experiments with GAD and insulin.

Oral Antigen Therapy Experiment. In one experiment, NOD mice were fed doses of 1.0 milligram (mg) of insulin or 0.5 mg of GAD (from pig brain) per day. Over time, most of the controls developed diabetes, while insulin and GAD both provided significant but not absolute protection. Feeding the two antigens together seems to have some additive effect, particularly in maintaining protection. At about 12 weeks of age, when diabetes begins to occur in the NOD mouse colony, the insulitis score (based on level of inflammation observed by microscope) is much lower in mice fed GAD, insulin, or both.

This anergy or suppression of T-cell response is antigen-specific: feeding insulin suppresses insulin responses; feeding GAD suppresses GAD responses; and feeding together suppresses both, but there is no bystander suppression. Most of the antibodies in the NOD mouse are of the IgG-B2 variety, and oral feeding doesn't suppress the animal's ability to make antibodies, or switch the subtype of antibodies made.

Two cytokines of interest are induced: tumor necrosis factor beta (TNF-beta) and interferon gamma (IFN-gamma). Feeding regimes did not change TNF-beta levels, but controls had much higher levels of IFN-gamma in islet infiltrates, most of it from Th-1 CD4 cells. This is evidence of down-regulation of Th-1 response in animals fed insulin and/or GAD. In the Peyer's patch, too, researchers found an inhibition of elaboration of messenger RNA for IFN-gamma, as well as increases in interleukin four (IL-4) and possibly IL-10, evidence of down-regulation of Th-1 response and possibly of up-regulation of Th-2.

Intravenous Antigen Therapy Experiments. Large amounts of IV insulin will kill the mice, so researchers used biologically inactive forms, including

A chain, B chain, desoxyinsulin, and pro-insulin, as well as human GAD. In this case, only GAD was effective in providing protection.

Subcutaneous Immunization Experiments. Researchers immunized animals at 4, 8, and 12 weeks. Controls received incomplete Freund's adjuvant (IFA) with a diluent, which had been shown to give no protection. (Mycobacterium antigen in a complete Freund's does give marked but nonspecific protection.) Experimentals received A chain, B chain, or whole insulin with IFA. The A chain provided insignificant protection, but animals immunized with B chain developed marked protection that was transferrable to irradiated animals. The protective epitope turns out to be amino acids 9 through 23 on the B chain of the insulin molecule. Similar experiments are now under way with GAD peptides and various whole GAD molecules.

Since oily adjuvants such as IFA cannot be used in humans, researchers have investigated other adjuvants that might be approvable. Alum plus B chain proved to be effective, although alum by itself may have some effect as well. Diphtheria, tetanus toxoids, and pertussis vaccine (DTP), a common childhood vaccine that contains alum, also proved to be a good adjuvant, at least in mice. Clearly, however, DTP itself causes a nonspecific stimulation that biases the animal to a Th-2-type peripheral phenotype. Analysis of cytokines produced in DTP-treated animals shows an increase in IL-4 and a big increase in IL-10, but not the same decrease in IFN-gamma that was seen following oral administration.

This process is not anergy but instead an immune response. Responses to GAD are not decreased but actually enhanced. Researchers believe that this is an IL-4-driven response. Regardless of regime, including DTP by itself, the treated animals had increased responses to GAD. Consequently, this is an active process.

Conclusions. Oral administration of autoantigens may be leading to tolerance. Intravenous administration of insulin is relatively ineffective in delaying diabetes. Subcutaneous administration in IFA proved to be the easiest route and to have the longest-lasting effect. Alum and DTP are effective substitutes for IFA as an adjuvant. The process seems to involve, at least in part, switching from a destructive Th-1 to a protective Th-2 response. These findings could now be subjected to human trials, if the B chain epitope is similarly reproduced in humans.

Other groups have reported that the T-cells of NOD mice have a high density of receptors for insulin, and that transfer of these cells to irradiated mice uniformly transferred diabetes as well. It is possible that immunization against the B chain of insulin deviates these cells from homing on the pancreatic islets that express insulin. Researchers have already constructed a viral vaccine designed to immunize against the B chain of insulin experiments are ongoing, and they look forward to subjecting it to provisional human feasibility studies.

In response to questions from the audience, Dr. McLaren added the following:

• Researchers repeated the oral experiments using pig brain GAD and eventually baculoviral-expressed GAD to remove questions about specificity of response. However, they also found that—while there isn't an additive effect—the best results are obtained by giving both antigens.

• Researchers are now looking at costimulation and using antibodies such as neutralizing IL-4 and neutralizing IL-10.

• Transfer of protection depends on both CD4 and CD8 cells, but mainly CD4.

• Researchers have not looked at the question of prior maternal sensitization, but they have found that age at time of immunization is important.

• These experiments used human insulin, but insulin is a highly conserved molecule. Human and pig insulin differ by only one amino acid, human and mouse by only three amino acids. Human and pig brain GAD are somewhat less conserved, perhaps 70 percent homologous. The possibility of foreign protein response makes it difficult to factor in the results.

CYTOKINE MODIFICATION OF AUTOREACTIVITY[16]

There are two general theories with regard to autoimmune disease:

1. The antigen is the primary effector of the immune response, but a pathogenic response leads to disease; and
2. Disease is a problem of immune regulation.

It is well known that Th-1 and Th-2 cells counterregulate each other. Th-1 cells are thought to promote autoimmune disease, but their action can be counterregulated by Th-2 cytokines, particularly IL-10 and IL-4 and, to a lesser extent, tumor growth factor beta (TGF-beta).

Working with NOD mice, which are a good model for human diabetes, researchers first tried to determine whether IL-10—whose primary role is to down-regulate IFN-gamma (the prototypic Th-1 cytokine)—could regulate this autoimmune response. This was done by eliciting the cytokine locally, in the pancreatic islets of a transgenic (BALB/c) mouse, using the insulin promoter. This attracted inflammatory lymphocytes, but this response did not induce diabetes in a nonsusceptible mouse.

IL-10. The next step was to see whether IL-10, which down-regulates IFN-gamma, is capable of regulating the disease in the NOD mouse. Researchers introduced the genetic loci onto the BALB/c background by backcrossing to F1s, then backcrossed again to N2s, at which point they expected to

---

[16] Based on a presentation by Nora Sarvetnick, M.D.

see a 10 percent incidence of diabetes. Instead, they found a 94 percent incidence of diabetes in MHC-susceptible animals and no diabetes in IL-10-negative, MHC-susceptible animals. Mice with BALB/c MHC did not develop diabetes.

In other words, the effect of IL-10 was completely the opposite of what they had expected—not only did it accelerate the disease process, it also seemed to overcome the requirement for a lot of susceptibility information. (There are numerous susceptibility alleles in the NOD mouse, and more are being mapped all the time.) It seemed that IL-10 was actually a very strong potentiator of disease, at least in this and other transgenic mouse models. To see whether or not IL-10 plays a role in the natural disease, researchers have conducted depletion experiments with neutralizing (anti-IL-10) antibodies. In one experiment, NOD mice that were treated with anti-IL-10 from a young age developed far less insulitis than controls. In another experiment, irradiated NOD mice were injected with sensitized lymphocytes from diabetic mice and then treated with anti-IL-10, but the neutralizing antibody had no effect in this transfer model, which involved older (9-week old) mice.

Researchers interpret these results to indicate that IL-10 is required early on in the natural disease, but that it is dispensable later on. NOD disease differs from other autoimmune diseases in its diversity—many new antigens are still being identified, and a corresponding variety of T cells mediate and regulate the disease. Hence, the progression of the disease seems to involve three stages:

1. Presentation (seeing the antigen or antigens);
2. Diversification (sensitizing lots of T cells to islet antigens); and
3. Effector phase (leading to destruction).

Researchers hypothesize that IL-10 acts in the diversification process, specifically through its ability to activate B cells and (through them) to diversify the immune response. Researchers are conducting further experiments to test this hypothesis, using anti-IL-10-treated NOD mice, but focussing on responses to peptides of GAD. The two immunodominant determinants, GAD 34 and GAD 35, respond similarly in the presence or absence of anti-IL-10, but the neutralizing antibody inhibits the spreading of the cryptic determinants, GAD 23 and GAD 17. Since there are high ratios of B cells in the islet infiltrates, this response may be critical to the clinical manifestation in the natural NOD disease, and possibly in the human disease as well.

IL-4. Unlike, IL-10, IL-4 totally blocks the disease. This colony of NOD mice has an 85-percent incidence of diabetes, usually developing the disease between 16 and 24 weeks. Targeted IL-4 to the pancreatic islets reduced the incidence of diabetes to zero, for over a year. To determine whether this reflects a state of tolerance, researchers transplanted NOD islets into transgenic mice that express IL-4 and looked for signs of rejection. The graft was accepted, indicating tolerance of an unknown mechanism.

When researchers reversed the transplant, however—putting islets expressing IL-4 into diabetic mice—the grafts were rejected. The beta cells in the transplanted islets were destroyed, while the alpha cells remained stupidly in the graft. This suggests that, once autoreactivity develops, you cannot stop committed or primed cells from killing the islet.

On the other hand, when researchers transplanted splenocytes from NOD diabetic mice into an NOD IL-4 transgenic recipient, they again saw protection, while disease was transferred when splenocytes were transplanted to NOD controls. Researchers recognize that these are contradictory results and suggest that the difference has to do with the "audience." That is, circulating cells have a much higher proportion of primed, or memory cells, whereas the spleen contains both primed and unprimed, memory and naive cells; the presence of at least some naive cells in the tissue being transferred allows for some regulation. Researchers are currently testing this hypothesis.

These results suggest that the immune system must see antigen in order to produce tolerance, but only if it is seen in the presence of IL-4. If the antigen is seen alone, the result is destruction, and seeing it a second time in the presence of IL-4 doesn't seem to give any kind of regulation. They also suggest that the T-cells enter the islet naive, and that priming occurs within the islet. This in turn suggests that therapy could be accomplished locally if it were possible to "speak" to the cells as they entered the islet. This could be done more elegantly if it were possible to merely add the proper determinants, but this will require a better understanding of natural Th-2 determinants, conditions for priming, site of priming, cytokines, etc.

In response to questions from the audience, Dr. Sarvetnick added the following:

- The IL-4 in these experiments was murine IL-4, so this could not be the reason for the rejection.
- An IL-4-producing islet from a BALB/c donor is not rejected when transplanted into a BALB/c recipient, only by an NOD recipient.
- The results with TGF-beta are far less interesting—essentially a fibrosis of the pancreas without any sign of blocking diabetes, at least in their lab. Other researchers have found some signs of inhibition.
- Researchers have not looked at the pattern of B-cell development or how it is altered in transgenic mice, except with regard to IFN-gamma. B7-1 and B7-2 are in the infiltrates in the NOD mouse, but they have not looked at whether that is down-regulated. It would be a good experiment.
- Slides of the islets of transgenic mice show lymphocytes surrounding but not infiltrating the islets. This suggests that the protective effect of IL-4 may come from altering the receptors or adhesion molecules on lymphocytes.
- Researchers have not looked at endothelial markers extensively.

- Researchers believe that the homing patterns of primed Th-1 cells are different from those of primed Th-2 cells. In addition, Th-2 cells seem to turn over very rapidly—there is circumstantial evidence of Th-2 cells homing away from the islet and dying in the adjacent lymphoid aggregate.

- Cytotoxic T lymphocytes (CTLs) appear to be involved in the initial insult, but not enough to cause disease or killing. Experiments with NOD Class I knockouts showed that both CD8 and CD4 cells are required. Results suggest that IL-10 can attract CD8 cells and enhance CD8 CTL activity in-vitro. However, researchers found relatively few CD8 cells in the infiltrate compared to CD4s and B-cells. Breeding a Class I knockout onto an NOD mouse would apparently require nine backcrosses.

Noel Rose of Johns Hopkins University described a new model he and his coworkers have developed showing the role of IFN-gamma in inducing autoimmune thyroiditis. This involves transgenic mice that express IFN-gamma in response to thyroglobulin promoter. The results are dramatic: the mice develop severe thyroiditis, their thyroids are almost completely infiltrated and destroyed, and they become profoundly hypothyroid, with very low levels of circulating T4. All of this is caused by local expression of IFN-gamma in the thyroid. The mice in question were C57 blacks, a susceptible strain.

T-CELL SUBSET CHOICE ON THE
OUTCOME OF AUTOIMMUNE DISEASE[17]

Transgenic T-cell models allow researchers to ask questions that cannot be asked in clinical disease, primarily because they limit the dramatic diversity of diabetes. In both humans and NOD mice, diabetes involves a plethora of antiens and T-cells and cytokines. Researchers try to constrain these variables in such a way as to gain some insight on the total disease.

When a naive T-cell first enters the islet or encounters antigen, it becomes a Th-0 or initially activated cell that can produce both IL-4 and IFN-gamma, as well as a host of other lymphokines. IFN-gamma will stimulate macrophages to make IL-12, which will drive the Th-0 cell towards the Th-1 phenotype. IL-4, on the other hand—either autocrine or paracrine (from a cell not yet defined, possibly a mast cell or CD1-restricted CD4-positive T-cell)—will drive the Th-0 cell towards the Th-2 phenotype. These are the two very distinct arms of the immune system. IL-4 feeds back and down-regulates IL-12 responsiveness, and IL-12 down-regulates IL-4 responsiveness—a very nice polarizing system. Other researchers have shown that T-complement (Tc-1 and Tc-2) cells are very analogous to the Th-1 and Th-2 phenotypes, with the same signature lymphokines.

---

[17] Based on a presentation by Jonathan Katz, M.D.

Other Disease Models. Researchers have found interesting dichotomies involving these same pathways and lymphokine profiles; in *nematode infections,* for example, giving IL-4, results in lower fecundity of eggs in the gut and more rapid shedding of the eggs, with a curative effect. In *leprosy,* the tuberculoid form of the disease produces more IFN-gamma; and IL-2, while the lepromatous form produces higher antigen levels and more CD8 cells, IL-4, and IL-10. In *listeriosis,* the pathogen induces macrophages to release IL-12 that drives the response down the Th-1 pathway.

Experiments have show that genetic influences may establish "default pathways" in certain individuals or strains—predispositions that researchers will need to consider when developing vaccine strategies. In response to the *leishmaniasis* pathogen, for example, B10.D2 mice produce an initial burst of IL-4, followed by rising levels of IL-12 and ultimately a Th-1 response with rising levels of IFN-gamma; while BALB/c mice produce a sustained level of IL-4 with rising levels of IL-12 and ultimately a Th-2 response with low levels of IFN-gamma. In this case, it appears that the polarizing variable is not the IL-12 per se but the IFN-unresponsiveness of the BALB/c mouse compared with the B10.D2 mouse. Further experiments confirmed that the difference between the two responses lay in a constitutive part of the IL-12 beta chain; a surface component (which is inducible by IL-12) allows the IL-12 molecule to bind to the Th-1 cell surface, actually competing with the signalling pathway that tells the Th-1 cell to produce IFN-gamma.

Diabetes. Type 1 diabetes accounts for about 7 percent of all diabetics in the United States, some 1.4 million individuals. Since this is a T-cell-dependent disease, the relevant questions are (1) what kind of T-cells transfer the disease and (2) how these T-cells develop. Sequencing the T-cell receptor of a Class II-restricted, CD4-positive clone revealed nothing that would mark it as a diabetogenic T-cell. Researchers developed a transgenic mouse model in which to observe T-cell development in the thymus and periphery, and in which to learn how to control that development. The transgenic was crossed onto the C-alpha knockout background, because they lacked a neutralizing antibody for the endogenous alpha chain.

The result is a line of "hypertransgenic" mice with CD4-positive T-cells that differ from the original phenotype only in the expression of the V-beta-4 T-cell receptor. These mice, as well as the regular transgenic mice, develop destructive insulitis at about 120 days, with infiltration of the beta granules and loss of insulin production. The next question is what type of cells are important in transferring disease.

In an earlier experiment, islet-specific T-cells were generated and then forced their development towards either Th-1 or Th-2. When transferred into the mice, diabetes developed only in the Th-1 recipients. This experiment had no control for antigen specificity or receptor affinity and avidity, which play a role in determining Th-1 vs. Th-2 responses. However, researchers could use the transgenic mouse, which had only one particular T-cell receptor, to control for this diversity. This "mixing" experiment is described below.

Researchers removed peripheral T-cells from the spleens and the mesenteric and inguinal lymph nodes of transgenic mice and polarized them by stimulating with concanavalin A (conA) in the presence of recombinant IL-2, IFN-gamma, and anti-IL-4 (to generate Th-1) or in the presence of recombinant IL-4 and anti-IFN-gamma (to generate Th-2). The resulting T-cells had a high level of expression of D-beta-4 TCR, up-regulated the proper activation markers (CD44 and CD25), and down-regulated CD62L (also called L-select). After stimulating with islet cells and culturing for about a week, researchers transferred the cells into perinatal (5 to 7 days old) NOD mice and waited 14 to 28 days to see if insulitis and diabetes developed.

The results indicated that within 3 or 4 days after transfer, there is infiltration of the islets by both Th-1 and Th-2 cells, with resulting peri-insulitis and insulitis. However, only the Th-1 recipients go on to develop diabetes. This suggests that, at some point in the future, it may be possible to regulate diabetes by forcing a Th-2 response, even when that cell carries the TCR for the as-yet-unknown antigen in the beta granules of the islets. Unfortunately, other experiments indicate that Th-2 does not provide this same protection when Th-1 is also present, even in small amounts.

Researchers are now conducting further experiments to test the hypothesis suggested above, namely that the real differentiation event is the loss of the beta chain of the IL-12 receptor. If it were possible to insert this receptor early on, it should be possible to generate a Th-0 cell that responds to IL-12 and makes IFN-gamma while still producing IL-4. It may be that the Th-2 cells produced in the mixing experiment have the IL-12 receptor and revert to Th-0 in an IL-12-producing environment, thereby preventing the desired suppression. Hence, researchers are trying to produce very heavily polarized Th-1 and Th-2 cells with no high-level expression of the receptor to see if this pattern will hold. Other possibilities for negative regulation of T-cell development include blocking the CD40 ligands or blocking the CD28 and B7 pathway, which may be important in the development of Th-1-type cells. Another is a soluble IL-12 receptor that might also switch the balance, even if the default is toward a Th-1 response.

In response to questions from the audience, Dr. Katz added the following:

• It may be possible in the future to overcome genetic predispositions by choosing the correct immunogenic peptide, with correct affinity, to induce a strong Th-1 or Th-2 response. At present, however, researchers don't know the antigens and peptides, and can't answer questions about affinity.

• The antigen in question copurifies with beta granule fraction by normal fractionation.

• Researchers are conducting experiments to see whether they can activate a Th-2 population by immunization while blocking Th-1 cells, but they have no data as yet.

- Knockouts and backcrossing with various mouse strains can be problematic, because many of the traits of interest are in the same cluster of genes.
- It is now assumed that the effector cell in diabetes is the CD-4-positive ultra-T-cell.
- Th-2 transfers also result in massive eosinophil infiltration. The Th-2 cells themselves persist for 5 to 7 weeks at the longest, and dye experiments to trace their fate show that, like a lot of transferred cells, they end up in the liver and get stuck there. It is unclear why; researchers are currently conduting more detailed histology.

ANTIGEN-INDUCED PROGRAMMED T-CELL DEATH AS A NEW APPROACH TO IMMUNE THERAPY[18]

Another new class of vaccines has an intended effect the opposite of all currently available vaccines—that is, to extinguish rather than activate an immune response—by means of eliminating the catalytic cell of immune responses—the T-cell—by using antigen to specifically program those T-cells to die. Such vaccines could play an important role in the treatment of disease in which T-cells play an important role in pathogenesis, including autoimmune diseases, graft rejection, allergies, and some others. Such vaccines would use the inherent specificity of the immune system itself to treat immunological diseases.

Researchers were prompted to propose this class of vaccines in response to the surprising observation that T-cells could be specifically programmed to die by antigen. More surprisingly, the agent that primed them for receptor-driven death was IL-2 T-cell growth factor: when cells that are cycling IL-2 are exposed to a peptide antigen on the antigen-presenting cells, a large fraction of them undergo programmed death. Almost any TCR ligand will have this effect; the original observation involve 2C11, an antibody against the CD3-epsilon chain of the TCR. That this was apoptosis was indicated by the fact that IL-2 or 2C11 alone did not disrupt genomic DNA, whereas IL-2 followed by 2C11 resulted in DNA fragmentation suggesting cleavage between nucleosomes, one of the hallmarks of programmed cell death.

The usual in vitro protocol for producing this effect involves (1) exposing the T-cells to conA, a nonspecific TCR ligand that up-regulates the high-affinity IL-2 receptor; (2) bathing the cells in various doses of IL-2; (3) restimulating the cells with various doses of antigen; and (4) recovering viable cells from the culture. The results are from a strain of mouse that is transgenic for a T-cell receptor that recognizes a peptide of myelin basic protein (MBP), by virtue of which these mice are susceptible to a disease called experimental allergic encephalomyelitis (EAE, see below). As expected, T-cells proliferate in

---

[18] Based on a presentation by Michael J. Leonardo, M.D.

response to increasing doses of IL-2, but when restimulated by increasing doses of antigen there is a substantial decline in the number of viable cells. The exception is at low doses of IL-2, and even here proliferation drops off in response to higher doses of antigen, which induce endogenous IL-2 that supplements the existing level in the culture.

This finding—that the things that stimulate T-cells (i.e., antigen receptor occupancy and IL-2) can also program them to die—creates a paradox. After infection with a replicating pathogen, one might hope that T-cell response would increase along with the pathogen challenge. Researchers now believe that this is negative feedback regulation: the system appears to recognize that a strong immune response represents a potentially dangerous alteration in normal physiology, and therefore modulates the response in a very specific way that is tied to the particular antigen and the amount of stimulation received. There are, in fact, many examples of noncytopathic (parasitic) viruses in which the immune response is the detrimental component of the disease, rather than the replication of the microorganism itself. It is also known from clinical trials that several of the T-cell-derived cytokines are very toxic in the high doses that would result from an unregulated response to heavy antigen load.

Researchers tested this hypothesis by repeatedly challenging BALB/c mice with a superantigen, staphylococcal enterotoxin B (SEB), that is similar to toxic shock toxin. They administered large amounts of SEB to initiate immune response, followed by smaller doses on days 3 and 5 to maintain a large population of cycling cells, while also giving the animals regular doses of an antibody that would block the IL-2 receptor and thus prevent IL-2 responses. They sacrificed the animals at day 8, harvested the lymph nodes, and measured the populations of V-beta-8 T-cells (which specifically respond to SEB) and V-beta-6 T-cells (which do not). The results showed that the fraction of V-beta-8 cells dropped from 22 percent to 7.5 percent—a deletion of 60 to 70 percent of specifically responding T-cells through exposure to the very superantigen that caused them to undergo mitogenesis.

Evidence of Active Programmed T-Cell Death. This finding, which has been reproduced by other groups and with peptide antigens, fits a feedback regulation model that researchers call "propriocidal regulation," a name borrowed from neural feedback regulatory loops. Activated T-cells both produce and respond to IL-2, and when cycling or proliferating T-cells are rechallenged by high doses of antigen a fraction of them will be shunted into an active programmed death pathway. This is not a mechanism to mop up T-cells at the end of an immune response, when the antigen is cleared—it occurs during the immune response and is a means of regulating that response when antigen is still present.

On the molecular level, active programmed death requires strong engagement of the T-cell receptor, which stimulates high-level production of death-inducing cytokines, including tumor necrosis factor (TNF) and Fas ligand. These cytokines engage specific receptors on the cell surface, engaging intracellular mechanisms that produce apoptotic proteins. Through several steps that have not yet been characterized, this leads to the activation of a cystine protease that is related to IL-1-beta-converting enzyme (ICE) into an active tetramer that can cleave a number of molecules.

Genetic evidence for this pathway can be seen in mice that are homozygously deficient for the IL-2 receptor; such animals have a severe disregulation of peripheral T-cell homeostasis and are unable to eliminate mature T-cells as they are supposed to do. The SEB experiment described above demonstrated that animals lacking the IL-2 receptor are unable to delete V-beta-8 cells from their mature repertoire. Other experiments have shown that deficiencies in the TNF receptor will also prevent mature T-cell death. And the immunology community has known for some time that mice as well as children with mutations in the Fas molecule will develop lymphoproliferative autoimmune disease very early in life.

Controlled Use of Programmed T-Cell Death in Autoimmune Therapy. To determine whether the active programmed cell death pathway could be used in a controlled way, to eliminate T-cells that were causing T-cell disease, researchers used an animal model—experimental allergic encephalomyelitis (EAE)—in laboratory mice. EAE was first observed in patients who were vaccinated against rabies but developed a disease that looked a lot like multiple sclerosis (MS). It is a murine autoimmune disease in which CD4 cells react against various protein components of the myelin sheath, causing demyelinization and inflammation that leads to various neurological deficits, including paralysis and sensory defects. Certain forms of EAE are relapsing conditions very similar to human MS.

The protocol follows the paradigm of the SEB experiment described above to see if readministration of large doses of antigen at defined times would program a fraction of the activated T-cells for death and thereby prevent the autoimmune sequelae. The clinical results demonstrated that repeated doses of 400 micrograms of antigen, coadministered with 30,000 units of IL-2, can dramatically suppress the severity of the disease compared with untreated mice. In fact, two of the five animals in the experimental group showed no signs of disease and were indistinguishable from their litter mates.

Since pretreatment is unlikely in a clinical setting, researchers also delayed the administration of therapy for 9 days (until the first symptoms of disease) and then 17 days (until the first signs of chronic disease, namely the first wave of paralysis). Administering MBP alone at day 9 dramatically reduced the severity of disease, and even at day 17, when the disease was fully established, the treatment produced statistically significant improvement. Even after 40 days, following the second wave of paralysis, treatment produced statistically significant improvement in clinical scores, although it did not reverse the damage to the spinal cords. After several months, the treatment has proved to be very long-lasting, and most of the animals do not suffer relapses.

This does not seem to be a classic suppressive-type mechanism, however, since readministering encephalogenic T-cells causes re-exacerbation of the disease. The data supports the idea that the treatment effect comes from eliminating the offending T-cells. Histology revealed that untreated animals show severe disruption of myelin architecture and inflammatory cell infiltrate in the subarachnoid space, while treated animals show little or no disruption of the normal architecture.

Researchers also wondered whether there is a fundamental immunoregulatory problem that might prohibit apoptosis and thus lead to autoimmune disease. The current state of knowledge may not be sufficient to rule this out. However, researchers have repeated the MBP experiment with T-cells from a number of human MS patients and found that they could indeed induce dramatic apoptosis in vitro. They are now initiating studies to look at other antigens.

Conclusions. Researchers now believe that there is a sound scientific basis for a new class of vaccines that will target T-cells for programmed cell death using specific antigen. They are encouraged by preclinical studies that show that this is effective and safe. They are moving on to study this question in nonhuman primates, establishing a marmoset model of EAE. They urge IOM to consider this type of vaccine in their priorities.

In response to questions from the audience, Dr. Leonardo added the following:

- Activated T-cells may represent a reservoir of antigen; when they undergo apoptosis, they release the antigen, recruiting inflammatory cells and leading to relapses.
- Evidence suggests that T-cells are in fact killed, not just switched off or pushed away from their target tissues (e.g., the brain).
- Costimulatory molecules and interactions (e.g., B7-CD28, CTL-A4-IgE) seem to have little effect on the killing phase, or indeed any time after the immune response is initiated. Once the cell is primed, it appears that antigen itself is sufficient to kill it; in fact, a strong TCR ligand alone is enough to kill the cell.
- It appears that different molecular parts of the TCR are important for activation and death. For example, the epsilon chain is capable of stimulating IL-2 production, but the zeta chain is particularly important for programming the cell to die through Fas or TNF. However, researchers do not yet know how to manipulate these differences.
- This appears to be a high-affinity phenomenon, in which the most avid cells would be most quickly deleted, but while low-level stimulation does not eliminate, researchers have not looked into the exact affinity requirements. [Dr. Berzofsky volunteered that high doses of antigen with high epitope densities will selectively produce apoptosis in high-affinity CTLs, but will actually stimulate low-affinity CTLs; he and his coworkers have not looked at CD4 CTLs in this regard.]

INDUCTION, PROPAGATION, AND IMMUNOREGULATION OF AUTOIMMUNE DISEASES OF THE CENTRAL NERVOUS SYSTEM[19]

Possible Mechanisms of Pathogenesis of MS. There are two schools of thought about the etiology of MS. Most people believe that there is a loss of immune regulation, leading to an autoimmune response against neural antigens. This theory is modeled by the murine EAE model described above. However, many epidemiological studies suggest that there is an infectious or environmental component, possibly a virus, that triggers this response. The model for this theory is Tyler's murine encephalomyelitis (TMEV).

If the putative virus is directly cytopathic to oligodendrocytes in the myelin, there would be a primary demyelination, but this doesn't appear to be happening in either MS or TMEV. On the other hand, the virus might induce demyelination—directly or indirectly—as a result of the immune response against the putative infection. One possible mechanism for this process might be called "bystander demyelination": provided the infection persists in the target organ, it can induce Th-1 responses and activate macrophages that somehow, through a process of "molecular mimicry," begin to crossreact with the self-antigenic determinant, leading to a cascade of inflammatory events.

In an alternative mechanism that might be called "epitope spreading," the virus causes the initial damage—either directly by targeting the oligodendrocytes, or indirectly by inducing a chronic inflammatory response in the target organ—and exposes self-antigenic proteins to the immune system, but the chronic stage of the disease is mediated at least in part by responses against the autoantigens that were released by the virus infection.

Murine Models of Virus-Induced MS. Researchers use different mouse models for the two forms of human MS. Both employ the SJL strain of mouse. Experimental allergic encephalomyelitis (EAE) can be induced with myelin basic protein (MBP) or proteolipid protein MOG (another myelin antigen), or by transferring T-cells specific for those epitopes; it develops into a relapsing-remitting form of autoimmune disease. In contrast, TMEV expresses a chronic progressive disease pattern that mimics the other, more serious form of human MS.

The progression of induction in these diseases at the Th-1 level is described below. A particular peptide is recognized in conjunction with MHC Class II and—provided the appropriate costimulatory signals are sent through the CD28 molecule—it induces the proliferation and activation of potential immunopathogenic T-cells. These primed T-cells leave the peripheral lymphoid tissue and penetrate the blood-brain barrier. When they again encounter the same epitope on APCs, they release chemokines and cytokines that activate and recruit mononu-

---

[19] Based on a presentation by Stephen Miller, M.D.

clear cells—microglial cells of the astrocytes, in the case of the central nervous system—which in turn produce the oxygen radicals, nitric oxide, etc., that destroy self-tissue.

Over the past 15 years, several groups of researchers have used immune tolerance as a tool for investigating the specificity of immune response in these two models of MS. This line of research began with the serendipitous observation that Th-1-type or delayed-type hypersensitivity responses could be inhibited by injecting naive animals with a population of MHC Class II-bearing APCs that had been incubated with a particular antigen or peptide in the presence of a crosslinking reagent called ethylene carbodiamide (ECDI). Further experiments revealed that this procedure altered the APC in such a way as to block the costimulatory signal 2, leading not to activation but to anergy and/or deletion of the antigen-specific T-cells.

Potential for Peptide Immunotherapy in Relapsing Autoimmune Disease. Building on these findings, researchers discovered that if it was possible to induce EAE by injecting mice with MBP-specific T-cells at day 0, it was also possible to effectively turn off that response by tolerizing the animals anywhere from 7 days prior to 5 days after injection—i.e., prior to initial clinical tissue damage—either with whole MBP (in a mouse spinal cord homogenate or MSCH) or with its immunodominant epitope (in the 84-104 region of the MBP molecule). If they delayed tolerance until after the acute phase of disease, however, it delayed the disease but the animals tolerized with 84-104 eventually relapsed at the same rate as controls, while the crude MSCH (containing not only MBP but every other potential neuroantigen) did a very effective job of inhibiting any further relapses.

The reason for these findings, researchers suspected, was that the initial phase of disease is directed primarily against the immunodominant epitope, but that tissue damage during the acute phase activates responses against endogenous epitopes, a process others have called *epitope* or *determinant spreading*. In a more defined experiment, they induced disease with the immunodominant epitope of PLP (amino acids 139-151) and then measured specificity of the responses that followed. The results show that, following the acute phase, there is a clear and consistent response against the secondary 178-191 epitope, a response that was not seen before the acute phase. Researchers also found that 139-151-specific T-cells could be reactivated with the noncrossreactive 178-191 epitope and would then transfer disease to naive animals, suggesting that—although 139-151 is the first self-response to arise—178-191 is primarily responsible for disease relapse. And indeed, tolerizing the animals with either 178 alone or 178 plus 139 protected the animals against further relapses, good evidence that the secondary epitopes have a major role in mediating relapses in this model.

This points to a major problem in using peptide vaccines and peptide therapies: the target keeps changing as time goes on. Other researchers have attempted to circumvent this problem by targeting the B7.1 and B7.2 molecules themselves, and hence inhibiting costimulation. They found that infusing anti-

B7.2 antibodies following the acute phase had no effect on relapses, either regulatory or enhancing, and that intact anti-B7.1 antibody actually exacerbated the disease. However, the Fab fragment of anti-B7.1 did protect animals from relapse, apparently by blockading the B7.1 molecule. Other studies have shown that the B7.1 molecule is dramatically up-regulated in the target organ during the preclinical stages of EAE, suggesting that it has a role in breaking down central nervous system (CNS) mononuclear cells into either F480 macrophages, B220 B-cells, or CD3 T-cells.

Potential for Peptide Immunotherapy in Progressive Autoimmune Disease. Researchers believe that tissue damage in TMEV is at least initiated because the virus is trophic for the CNS, where it lives in APC-like cells and can persist for long periods of time. Tolerizing animals with MSCH, as described above for MBP-induced EAE, has no effect at all on the development of TMEV-induced demyelinating disease. However, inducing tolerance against viral epitopes prior to infection does a very good job of shutting off the initiation of this disease. In fact, there are no neuroantigen-specific responses against MBP or PLP epitopes in the first 30 to 40 days after immunization, when the disease is already evident. By day 87, however, there is evidence of a response directed against the dominant 139-151 epitope of PLP, a response that first appears somewhere between days 42 and 52. And by day 164, there are responses not only against 139-151 but also against the secondary 178-191 epitope, the MOG epitope, and a third 56-70 epitope of PLP.

These findings strongly suggest that the tissue damage in the chronic, progressive TMEV model is initiated by virus-specific T-cells that target virus in the CNS and induce the initial inflammatory response. As tissue damage progresses, however, more and more self-epitopes seem to get recruited into this response. It is not yet clear whether these self-responses are playing a role in the chronic pathogenesis, or whether its course can be changed with peptide therapy; researchers are currently conducting reactivation, serial transfer, and tolerizing experiments—similar to those for EAE described above—to answer these questions.

For example, researchers are particularly interested in whether the initial self-response arises because of mimicry between 139-151 and some epitope in the virus, or because of the elaboration of myelin epitopes caused by the chronic inflammatory response. They identified three immunodominant epitopes of TMEV (lying on the VP1, VP2, and VP3 of the capsid) and developed T-cell clones and hybridomas specific for each. However, none of these hybridomas crossreacted with any of the neuroantigens or myelin epitopes that get recruited in the disease, nor do naive animals primed with neural epitopes develop any crossreactivity with the viral epitopes. This argues against molecular mimicry as an explanation of the disease, as does the fact that the response against self-antigens doesn't arise until after tissue damage has occurred, whereas the response to viral antigens arises within 2 or 3 weeks after infection, before the initial expression of disease.

Conclusions. T-cell responses in MS and other Th1-mediated autoimmune diseases appear to evolve dynamically during the course of both relapsing-remitting and chronic-progressive types of disease. Autoimmune reactivity in MS may in part be a secondary consequence of chronic CNS damage initiated by some putative persisting virus. Over the past 15 to 20 years, perhaps 15 or 20 different viruses have been associated with MS, but none has stood the test of time. One of the most recent is herpes virus type 6, which has been reported to be associated with oligodendrocytes in some cases of MS.

The dynamic nature of the T-cell repertoire has important implications for treatment modalities that employ antigen-specific strategies. Because the target changes as the disease progresses, for example, researchers hope to target the B7.1 molecule and costimulation generally, in order to inhibit disease progression without prior knowledge of the epitopes or T-cell receptors that are involved.

The model that emerges. The inducing epitope may be either a self-antigen or a viral antigen, provided the virus persists in the target organ. A Th1-type response leads to inflammation and tissue destruction that produces myelin debris, which stimulates T-cells expressed against endogenous myelin epitopes. Examples of such viruses in humans include Theiler's virus, encephalomyocarditis virus (EMCV), and Coxsackie virus, all of which have been shown to persist in tissues and to be associated with autoimmune sequelae. With EMCV and Coxsackie the sequelae depends on the strain of virus, and the latter may be involved with human diabetes.

In response to questions from the audience, Dr. Miller added the following:

- Researchers still know relatively little about what induces the remissions that follow the acute phase: a Th1-to-Th2 switch, antigen-induced programmed cell death, or some combination of processes. However, the persistence of some of the primed T-cells argues against propriocidal cell death as the sole explanation.

- In Coxsackie B3-induced myocarditis, the inflammation produced by viral infection releases myosin, which is the antigen in the autoimmune phase. However, researchers have blocked the secondary autoimmune response by giving susceptible mice IL-1 receptor antagonist. They have also induced autoimmune myocarditis in normally nonsusceptible mice by administering IL-1. Hence it would appear that inflammation, and especially the cytokines induced by the viral infection, are critical in activating the true autoimmune process.

- TMEV can be a lytic virus. It lives in some APCs, but primarily in F480 macrophages, where it undergoes defective replication, producing more viral antigen than infectious viral particles. The virus can persist in mice up to 18 months after infection. Because it lives in APCs, it may interfere with endogenous IL-12 and IFN-gamma production to maintain a milieu that doesn't lead to remission, but instead encourages inflammation to continue.

PEPTIDE-MEDIATED REGULATION OF AUTOIMMUNITY[20]

Unlike Jenner and Pasteur, who were trying to *initiate* a strong immune response in order to get rid of a pathogen, the problem in autoimmune diseases is to *turn off* a strong immune response against an autoantigen. And while there are many differences among autoimmune diseases, and a welter of potential autoantigens, it is nevertheless worth asking if there may not be some more generic form of treatment that would work for many or all of these conditions. It may be hard to envision a single antigen or a single T-cell receptor that could be used in a range of immunotherapies, but if there were a sufficient understanding of the mechanisms of the immune response, it might be possible to develop strategies that would deliver regulatory products—cytokines or other products—to the sites of inflammation.

Regulatory Peptides. Peptides or proteins delivered in nonaggregated form, in the absence of strong adjuvants, lead to a form of immune unresponsiveness that can be adapted for immunotherapeutic intervention. In at least three different animal models of autoimmune disease (EAE, diabetes, and type 2 collagen-induced arthritis), whether spontaneous or induced, it is possible to use peptides of major dominant autoantigens in a "tolerogenic" fashion to turn off the disease. This presentation focused on EAE, which had been discussed by several other speakers (see above).

The first step in developing vaccine strategies is to test the obvious sites of potential intervention in preclinical models, to ensure that the vaccine will not make the disease worse. This would be the worst possible outcome—to take a patient with a mild case of MS or arthritis and put them in a wheelchair. In the case of EAE, this intervention might come at two different stages in the development of the disease: (1) prior to the initiation of symptoms, and (2) during remission following the onset of disease.

Peptide Immunotherapy. In the first case, mice were given synthetic peptides of immunodominant determinants of myelin protein in a tolerizing regime to block the initiation of symptoms. Earlier studies had shown that mice tolerized prior to time zero with peptides of myelin sheath do not develop disease in response to MBP. More recent work has shown that a "cocktail" of peptides is more effective than either the major immunodominant (AC1-11) or secondary immunodominant (AC35-47). Even AC1-11 is a rather weak antigen, however, with very poor MHC binding. Researchers have determined that peptide substitution—using a tyrosine at the fourth position of the acetylated 11

---

[20] Based on a presentation by Garrison Fathman, M.D.

N-terminal amino acids of MBP—produces a more efficient MHC binder, enhanced immune phenomena, and a more efficient immunotherapeutic.

More importantly, substituted peptides also worked at a later and more clinically relevant stage of the disease, i.e., during remission after the onset of clinical symptoms. When researchers took mice that had progressed to stage 2 of EAE and tolerized them with the 4-tyrosine-substituted peptide, the mice did not get worse; in fact, they got better and stayed better for a long time. The peptide did not cause a relapse, and seemed to block a relapse—in short, it appeared to induce remission in clinically ill animals. Obviously, this result suggests a more realistic and clinically relevant way to administer the vaccine, namely when patients present with clinical disease. This model would be particularly important in diseases marked by a similar exacerbation-and-remission cycle, including rheumatoid arthritis, systemic lupus erythematosus, and MS.

To address concerns about the "innocent bystander" effects that this approach might cause, researchers tolerized mice with a single determinant of MBP and then induced them with spinal cord homogenate containing the entire gamut of proteins from the myelin sheath. The mice were protected. And in a related experiment, separate T-cell clones recognizing determinants A and B of myelin were transferred to naive mice, but when they were then tolerized with a single determinant, it turned off both clones. Something other than the apoptosis or anergy of that single T-cell clone was occurring. Whatever the mechanism, however, the results were dramatic: sick mice looked and acted normal after 24 hours, and their large inflammatory lesions had disappeared.

Researchers speculate that the peptide was not just killing cells but also turning off the inflammatory milieu through some unknown counter-regulatory mechanism. This has important implications for vaccine development strategies: instead of identifying the autoantigens, and hence the regulatory peptide, it might be possible to understand the counterinflammatory mechanisms and thereby bypass peptide immunotherapy entirely. One candidate involves not only the recognition of the antigen but also the regulation of T-cells themselves. Research currently underway suggests that this T-cell immunoregulatory circuit is very active in the exacerbating-remitting characteristics of EAE and may have a role to play in immunotherapy.

The idea would be to enhance this regulatory role, possibly by using peptides of T-cell receptors, but at present researchers do not know which T-cell receptors to pursue. In the clonal transfer experiment cited above, peptide A administered when disease has progressed to stage 2 will turn the disease off; but if anti-IL-4 is administered at the same time, it completely blocks the therapeutic effect of the peptide. This suggests, but by no means proves, that regulatory cytokines might be a central focus in efforts to bypass peptide vaccination immunotherapy and treat autoimmune diseases more directly.

T-Cell Hybridoma Cytokine Regulation. Researchers have investigated this question in a line of retroviral gene products that make it possible to transduce or infect cells with selected genes. For example, researchers "tag" retroviruses with green fluorescent protein to tell which cells are infected, or insert LAK-Z to target the retroviruses. In one study, researchers used this technique to produce a T-cell hybridoma that was prototypically Th1-like and had a receptor for MBP (i.e., was encephalogenic or at least had the capacity to traffic to the CNS) and then transduced it with gene sets for the expression of either IL-4, IL-10, or LAK-Z (as a control). When researchers administered transduced hybridoma T-cells to mice that had been immunized with MBP but had not yet developed EAE, the targeted IL-4 hybridoma appeared to delay the onset and decrease the incidence of disease. In a second experiment, the hybridoma was given a receptor for myoglobin, and hence targeted muscle rather than nerve tissue; in this case the systemic application of IL-4 was not protective, while the targeted CNS-localizing hybridoma was protective.

These results again suggest, but by no means prove, that immunodominant peptides may have a role in inducing immune unresponsiveness. If that role is generic, it might make possible therapeutic strategies that are relevant to multiple autoimmune disorders. An earlier presentation pointed out that the expression of IL-4 under the right insulin promoter seemed to block the development of NOD diabetes. There is some indication in the literature that IL-4 may also be a down-regulatory product in rheumatoid arthritis.

Retrovirus Transduction. Retrovirus transduction may provide a tool for targeted specificity, restoring regulatory cytokines to sites of inflammation. Other studies have suggested different strategies for targeting retrovirus, specifically to activated T-cells and lesions of autoimmunity, where they restore expression of the cytokine of choice. In the future—when funding becomes available—researchers would like to pursue this approach using a retrovirus that is targeted to OX40, a TNF-family receptor that is expressed on the surface of activated T-cells in lesions of EAE. OX40 is also expressed in rheumatoid arthritis and possibly in diabetes as well, although researchers have not yet looked for it in NOD mice. The plan is to add to the retroviral coat a chimeric protein that includes not only the usual gp120 but also some structure (e.g., a single-chain variable region of an antibody) targeting the OX40 ligand of the OX40 receptor. This would target the retrovirus on activated T-cells in sites of inflammation, where the expression of regulatory cytokines would turn off the inflammation. If it proves feasible, this approach promises to provide an alternative mechanism for the delivery of regulatory products that bypasses the vaccine approach altogether.

In response to questions from the audience, Dr. Fathman added the following:

• Evidence from some studies, including those using IL-4 knockout mice, suggests that there may be multiple compensatory mechanisms in the immune response, mechanisms that could regulate inflammation in the absence of IL-4. At present, however, the significant finding is that IL-4 has the capacity to turn off the inflammatory events in three separate preclinical animal models of autoimmune disease.

• The alternative strategy of transferring huge numbers of fully activated Th1-type T-cells may simply overwhelm the immune system, when the goal is simply to restore homeostasis. More importantly, very few of the transferred T-cells would find their way to the CNS joints or beta cells. The transgene approach doesn't allow for the restoration of homeostasis; for that, one needs immunoregulation.

• An alternative approach is to develop preventive immunization that is harmless enough to use in genetically predisposed individuals. This approach has been used in thyroiditis, where the etiologic autoantigen is well known and studied. There is a long list of potential autoantigens in other diseases, however, and much remains to be learned about them.

• Human studies have been limited. Chimpanzees with MS responded well to an extract of myelin sheath containing MBP and other peptides. Human trials of MBP were conducted in the 1970s, but the subcutaneous route proved to be disastrously wrong, and several patients died of fulminating encephalomyelitis. There will be Phase I clinical trials this fall using immunodominant determinants of myelin protein, as described above.

• Researchers do not know if the retrovirus will persist after homeostasis is restored.

• There have been anecdotal reports of patients whose autoimmune diseases were cured when they received autologous bone marrow transplants for other reasons, such as cancer therapy, but this approach is far too radical to use pre-ventively—for example, in prediabetic children that aren't yet sick. An alternative that may be much simpler is stem cell rescue: if the patient becomes heterozygous, this protects against diabetes, although it may allow other diseases to be induced. This approach has been successful in animal models, but humans will have to wait until the next century—at least 25 years—for well-thought-out strategies involving bone marrow transplantation or stem cell reconstitution to (1) induce chimerism and heterozygosity or (2) induce homozygosity for nonpermissive alleles.

• Researchers got protection with IL-10, as well, and TGF-beta may be a good regulatory cytokine as well. They pursued IL-4 initially because they got the best results with it in early tests. Researchers will eventually look at a wider range of regulatory and counterregulatory inflammatory cytokines, alone and in combinations.

• The genetics of human diabetes is similar to that of the NOD mouse. MHC typing reveals five genomic intervals related to the disease, none of which has been targeted. In NOD mice, there is a clear B-chain epitope on the MHC that, when used to immunize naive animals, does not cause inflammation. If this epitope is sufficiently conserved to be relevant to human disease, it will not cause harm there either. However, the targets include antigen processing and presentation, as well as MHC. Researchers know nothing about processing at present.

STIMULATION AND COSTIMULATION[21]

Full activation of a T-cell requires two different signals. The first, *antigen-specific signal,* comes when the T-cell receptor recognizes a peptide-MHC complex on the surface of an antigen-presenting cell (APC). This first signal causes events and reactions that can be quantified, such as the expression of the growth factor receptor or IL-2 receptor or the release of certain cytokine molecules. However, full activation of the T-cell requires a second, *costimulatory signal* involving a different ligand and receptor. Indeed, the antigen-specific signal by itself is a negative regulator of the system and can be used to induce tolerance, as shown in several of the preceding presentations.

At a more complex level, the costimulatory signal appears to be particularly important in activating the CD4 helper cells, which—in either the Th-1 or Th-2 form—plays a critical role in activating other cells of the immune system. And while the signal it transits to the B-lymphocyte may be antigen-nonspecific (e.g., cytyokines such as IL-4), the activation of the helper T-cell is antigen-specific. In this sense, both of the signals received by the B-cell are antigen-specific.

Molecular Signaling in Costimulation. A range of ligands and receptors have been shown to play various roles in costimulatory signals. Perhaps the best-known are the B7 family, which are expressed on the APC in two well-characterized forms, B7.1 and B7.2 (a third form has been proposed). These molecules interact with the CD28 and/or CTLA4 molecules, which are normally expressed on the surface of the responding T-cell. When B7 molecules engage CD28, they turn the T-cell on; when they engage CTLA4, they turn the cell off, thereby providing a feedback loop.

In their resting state, the APC expresses a low level of B7 on its surface, and the T-cell expresses a large amount of the CD28 receptor, and a low but detectable amount of CTLA4. The CTLA4 acts as a buffer, preventing nonspecific activation, because it has about a tenfold-higher affinity for the B7 ligands and, under the limiting conditions of B7, it preferentially occupies these receptors and gives negative signals to the cell. Activation up-regulates B7 on the surface of the APC (first B7.2, later B7.1), rapidly saturating the few CTLA4 receptors on the T-cell and then occupying CD28 molecules, sending positive signals and initiating costimulation. Between 24 and 48 hours later, there is a gradual shift from B7.2 to B7.1 on the APC, inducing an increase in CTLA4 molecules that compete for B7 molecules, send increasing negative signals, and turn off the T-cell—or at least this pathway.

Molecular Response to Costimulation. When CD28 is stimulated in vitro, the predominant effect in tissue culture is a 30- to 100-fold increase in the production of the T-cell growth hormone IL-2, relative to the amount produced

[21] Based on a presentation by Ronald Schwartz, M.D.

in the absence of costimulation. Two different mechanisms have been proposed for this dramatic effect:

1. *Increased transactivation of the IL-2 gene.* The initial signal transduction events are not clear, but it appears that the CD28 cytoplasmic tail will bind to PI-3 kinase after tyrosine phosphorylation. There is also one controversial report of acidic sphingomyelinase activity, leading (probably through several steps) to the activation of Jun N-terminal kinase.

2. *Stability of the IL-2 message.* This mechanism for augmenting IL-2 production has been well studied in the mouse and human systems. Early studies postulated that sequences in the 3-prime-1 translated region were important for message stability, but other studies are underway to identify additional critical factors.

Message stability has an effect on the duration as well as the intensity of the response. When the T-cell was stimulated with signal 1 alone (e.g., anti-TCR), the increase in IL-2 message peaks at 4 hours and then falls off fairly rapidly. When the T-cell also received signal 2 (e.g., anti-CD28), the IL-2 message was more prolonged, and there was about a 35-fold difference in the amount of IL-2 produced. Because of this, some researchers believe that message stability rather than transactivation is the dominant effect.

Studies with Knockout Mice. Researchers have also studied costimulation in vivo using CD28 and CTLA4 knockout mice. When they knocked out the CTLA4 gene, which provides the negative feedback loop, they observed massive lymphoproliferation and death at about 3 weeks as lymphocytes infiltrate and destroy multiple organs. These were the effects that might be expected in the absence of a negative feedback. There was some indication that it was actually cardiac problems that killed the mice.

When researchers knocked out the gene for CD28, however, the data were more ambiguous. IgG antibody responses were impaired, but there were normal cytotoxic responses to L, C, and V viruses. Subsequent studies showed impaired cytotoxic responses to VSV viruses, and a measurable but minor impairment of CD4 proliferative responses. These differences were not as dramatic as would be expected, were CD28 the key molecule in costimulation. This has led to further studies in search of the "missing component."

Other Costimulatory Molecules. Given that the CD28-B7 mechanism does not appear to be the whole story, researchers' attention will probably turn to additional biochemical mechanisms for costimulation. Among the ligands and receptors listed in Table 3 (above), the cell adhesion molecules such as LFA-1 and ICAMs are important because they allow the cells to come together, and adding antibodies to LFA-1 will block the initiation of T-cell response. The LFA-3-CD2 combination also appears to augment TCR signalling. Other outliers have been known for years, including heat-stable antigen (HSA) and the invariant chain (Ii-c.s.).

Several groups are currently studying the TNF super-family (IL-1, etc.), which includes several members that can send both positive and negative signals to cells. IL-1 was the first costimulatory molecule to be defined, and there is good evidence that it participates in initiating events in the immune response. The best-characterized of the family is the CD40-ligand interaction—antibodies that block this interaction will also impair immune responses, and researchers are now waiting for the combination studies and knockout studies that will demonstrate whether this is the "missing component." IL-12 helps initiate Th-1 responses, and GM-CSF helps initiate macrophages. Even chemokines have been reported to give costimulation. In short, there are entire families of molecules that could potentially be manipulated in a vaccine strategy.

Cytokine-Induced Apoptosis and Anergy. TNF and fas can also induce apoptosis. But activation in the absence of costimulation sends a negative signal to the T-cell, driving it into a nonresponsive state. The T-cell does not die, although it does function less well than it did before it was given signal 1 alone, and the term "anergy" was borrowed from B-cell research to describe this state. If the anergic T-cell is restimulated by a normal APC with full costimulation, it generally fails to divide and proliferate, primarily because it fails to produce IL-2, the T-cell growth factor. Production of some additional cytokines such as IL-3 and GM-CSF are down by intermediate amounts, but others such as IFN-gamma don't seem to be affected.

Only when researchers developed a mouse that produced Th-0 cells, which produce both IL-4 and IFN-gamma, were they able to investigate these effects. They found that anergy didn't significantly decrease the production of either IL-4 *or* IFN-gamma, but at the same time the cell was blocked from proliferating in response to IL-4. IL-4 can be a growth factor in the same way as IL-2, but in this case the lack of response wasn't related to shutting off production.

Researchers concluded from this that the cell has a special kind of regulation that stops proliferation—in short, T-cell anergy (at least in vitro) is really a state of growth arrest, possibly involved through a differentiation process. If it occurs very early, however—i.e., after the cell down-regulates IL-2, but before, has had a chance to turn on its IFN-gamma and IL-4 genes—it can also be a mechanism of tolerance, because it prevents cells from expanding and differentiating.

Molecular Basis for Cytokine-Induced Anergy. Researchers are gaining a clearer understanding of the mechanisms that block signal transduction and prevent IL-2 production (for example) in anergized cells. Early studies demonstrated that the intracellular calcium pathway was completely intact. Other studies showed that transactivation through AP-1 was inhibited, and most recently that the problem is in the activation of ras. In particular, they showed that the Shc, Grb2, and SOS activations were normal, but that downstream events from ras such as RAF and the ERK kinases can activate the Jun kinases and thereby block AP-1. There are a variety of other ways to regulate ras, including exchange factors like SOS and VAB as well as GTG-ase activity and another pathway activated by protein kinase C (PKC). As researchers zero in on these molecular mechanisms, they will eventually have a full understanding of this process.

At bottom, then, anergy can be characterized as *negative regulation induced by T-cell receptor occupancy in the absence of costimulation.* Signal 1 alone actually induces an inhibitor that operates on the ras pathway, blocking ras activation. Because this happens at the same time that the signals activating the IL-2 gene, the initial response is to produce IL-2. But the inhibitor persists after the initial response dies down, and when the cell is restimulated it behaves like a negative feedback loop, preventing subsequent activation.

When signals 1 and 2 are both received, on the other hand, there is a far greater production of IL-2, followed by proliferation of the cell. At first researchers thought that cell division alone was enough to dilute out the inhibitor; it now appears that signal transduction through the IL-2 receptor, particularly the gamma chain, can antagonize the induction of anergy, presumably by inhibiting the production of the inhibitor. The biochemical basis of this mechanism has not yet been worked out. In this case, it would appear that costimulation antagonizes the anergic effect in two ways: (1) by augmenting IL-2 production, and (2) by inhibiting inhibitor production.

Finally, recent studies have demonstrated that, even in the presence of normal costimulation, it is possible to modify the peptides in certain MHC complexes by making certain amino acid substitutions that probably decrease the affinity of interaction with the TCR. These so-called "partial agonists" are also capable of inducing anergy, apparently by interfering with the transduction of signal 1 and preventing the downstream event, namely the production of IL-2. This result demonstrates that it is possible to achieve anergy through two different biochemical mechanisms—lack of costimulation, and partial signal transduction.

T-Cell Receptors and Apoptosis. Programmed cell death was described above. However, the resting T-cell has on its surface the CD95 molecule, which is fas. When the cell is activated through antigen stimulation and costimulation, one result is the production of additional fas ligands on the surface. These ligands form a trimeric complex that can interact with the receptor on the same cell, or those on other cells. Researchers hypothesize that this interaction may be what signals the cell to undergo apoptosis. This would explain why interfering with the CD28 system had no effect on apoptosis.

Another team of researchers investigated the roles of antigen-specific and costimulatory receptors by looking at T-cells stimulated with anti-CD3 and measuring the effect of anti-CD28, as reflected in the production of Bcl-2 family members, which are important in protecting the cell against apoptosis. They found that the combination of the two signals resulted in very high levels of Bcl-x. In this case, the antagonist to CD28 was solubilized CTLA4 receptor (with its greater affinity for B7) that has been fused with immunoglobulin for stability. In vitro, this fusion protein (CTLA4-Ig) blocked the costimulatory pathway, Bcl-x production was negligible, and the cells died.

Immunotherapeutic Applications. The NZD mouse is an animal model for lupus. When the animal is treated with the solubilized CTLA4 receptor, which blocks costimulation through CD28-B7 interactions, autoantibody production is reduced and the life of the animal is prolonged. CTLA4-Ig had an ameliorative effect even when given late in the disease. In young NOD mice, on the other hand, CTLA4-Ig reduced the incidence of diabetes but not insulitis, and it had no effect in mice over 10 weeks of age. These partial effects may be related to the fact that CD28-B7 is not the only costimulatory pathway, but further research will be needed.

In tumor immunity, the APC must activate cytotoxic T-cells in order to eliminate tumor cells. Normally, this is done by stimulating T-helper cells, using both signals and producing IL-2 to encourage T-cell proliferation (as in A). In some cases, a precytotoxic T-cell can respond to antigen in the absence of costimulation, but this leads to anergy or apoptosis through the mechanisms described above (as in B). However, a number of studies have shown that when various costimulatory ligands are introduced into the tumor (e.g., B7, as in C), it is possible to enhance CD8 cytotoxicity in the absence of CD4 help, and even in the absence of costimulation by the tumor itself, so long as the peptide ligand is recognized. This strategy has worked in limited situations.

Another group has followed a slightly different track. Because CD28 turns on the costimulatory signal, but also leads to a negative feedback loop when the CTLA4 molecule is stimulated, they developed a monoclonal antibody against CTLA4 (as opposed to CTLA4-Ig, which is a soluble form of the molecule itself). By preventing the negative feedback signal, once the T-cell response has been activated naturally, this strategy results in a tremendous augmentation of T-cell cytotoxic responses that can eliminate certain tumors that wouldn't be eliminated under other conditions.

In response to questions from the audience, Dr. Schwartz added the following:

- IL-2 drives the T-cells into S phase. However, the immune response is not the physiological effect of IL-2, but rather what IL-2 does to the biology of the cell. It's nothing special, just cell cycling.

- Chemokines are part of a nonadaptive immune response in which their major role is to call in T-cells. Neutrophils in particular are the second line of defense, after the skin and mucosal tissue, and the earliest kind of hematopoietic cells to respond to inflammation, trying to destroy whatever organism or invader it finds. Chemokines are released both by the neutrophils and by local tissue. In a generalized sense, they too represent a kind of costimulation, and some investigators are beginning to think that the entire inflammatory process should be considered in up-regulating specific molecules to talk to T-lymphocytes.

VIRAL THERAPEUTIC VACCINES—HEPATITIS B[22]

Peptide-Mediated Vaccines. Researchers sought to develop therapeutic vaccines to treat tumors and chronic viral infections, focusing initially on chronic hepatitis B virus (HBV) infection. In such an infection, large amounts of antigen are present in host tissues but are presented by inappropriate cells. Their approach was to introduce antigen in a more efficacious form by using peptides as the source of antigen.

One advantage of this peptide-mediated approach is the ability to target the type of immunity by selecting peptides with either Class I- or Class II-restricted epitopes. It also avoids the confounding effects of producing a lot of antibody, which might have negative effects on cellular immunity. More importantly, it offers the possibility of using peptides that are conserved across various viral isolates, especially in RNA viruses such as hepatitis C and HIV, in which epitope drift is considerable. Finally, it should be possible to select epitopes that might not be tolerized in the host.

The disadvantage of peptides is that they are MHC-restricted, and for this reason a single peptide can only be expected to mount immune responses in a limited number of individuals in the population. As a result, there is a quantitative problem of how many epitopes are required to mount an effective immune response.

The strategy adopted by the researchers—identifying the epitopes that are most capable of inducing CTL responses—required them first to identify the binding motifs responsible for peptide-MHC interaction, then to investigate their immunogenicity, both in vitro and in vivo.

Peptide-MHC Binding Motifs. Researchers began with the most common alleles of human leukocyte antigen group A (HLA-A) and studied their MHC binding motifs. They discovered that some alleles have very similar motifs, such as A3 and A11, which favor hydrophobic residues in position 2 and lysine at the C terminal position. When they examined the binding activity of different peptides, roughly half of the peptides they tested bound significantly to both A3 and A11.

This led to the concept of "super-motifs," which has been further investigated by several groups. The results show that a combination of peptides that share three of these super-motifs will provide coverage for a very large percentage of all human populations. In this case, the A2 proteins are hydrophobics in the B and F pockets; A3 is hydrophobic and basic; and B7 binds almost any peptide in the F pocket. This finding greatly reduces the number of peptides that must be isolated in order to immunize an outbred population.

The binding motif does not fully define the binding affinity of the peptide, however. Indeed, researchers have observed 10,000-fold differences in binding affinities among peptides that are identical at their anchor positions but differ at

---

[22] Based on a presentation by Howard Grey, M.D.

other positions. Researchers analyzed the importance of each nonanchor residue by comparing a very large set of peptides. They found that charged residues (positive or negative) are deleterious to binding, whereas aromatic residues are generally favorable. This allows researchers to predict with high efficiency the binding capacity of peptides that bear a given motif. In general, a peptide bearing one of the favored residues has about a 25-percent chance of binding, but when it contains one favored residue and none of the deleterious residues the chances of high-affinity binding increase to approximately 80 percent.

Binding Affinity and Immunogenicity. Based on the literature, about 90 percent of normal T-cell epitopes bind to the restriction element with high affinity, defined as a KD of 50 nanomolar. Peptides that are naturally processed by MHC also tend to fall into this high-affinity category. High-affinity peptides from transgenic mice also tended to be preferred immunogens. When researchers repeated this analysis for known epitopes of viral and tumor antigens, however, they found that 90 percent of viral epitopes are high-affinity binders for MHC, while less than half of tumor epitopes are high-affinity binders. Because tolerance tends to favor high-affinity, immunodominant peptides, a possible vaccine in situations of significant tolerance would be to shift to subdominant, lower-affinity peptides as potential immunogens.

In order to vaccinate with these peptides, researchers decided to include a "helper epitope" along with the classical CTL epitope. To this they added palmitic acids, which according to the literature enhance the immunogenicity of peptides. The data showed that the lipidated helper-CTL epitopes was a very efficient immunogen, and that it is equally efficient to a similar construct without the lipid but using IFA as an adjuvant.

Peptide-Mediated HBV Vaccine. Based on these findings, researchers proceeded to construct a CTL vaccine for hepatitis B. The rationale for such a vaccine was that CTL responsiveness was known to be associated with (1) clearance of acute HBV infection, (2) spontaneous clearance of chronic HBV infection, and (3) successful IFN-alpha therapy.

The vaccine used in preliminary studies consisted of an immunodominant epitope derived from the HBV core (18-27), combined with a helper epitope from tetanus toxin (830-843, which is relatively MNH-unrestricted), plus lipids. Phase I clinical data showed a clear immune response (measured in CTL activity) in normal subjects at a dosage of 500 micrograms of antigen, administered with a single booster shot. Higher and lower doses produced corresponding responses.

Preliminary Phase II clinical data show similar responses in about one dozen patients with chronic HBV infection who were given two injections of lipidated peptide as antigen. The "ALT flare" refers to liver damage with release of transaminase enzymes, which would be expected to follow the induction of CTL and is in fact an important indicator of CTL response. A similar flare can be observed in patients treated with IFN-alpha who clear the virus. DNA levels were also measured, often decreasing by anywhere from 50 percent to complete clearance. These results are very early, but they do show that—even in the face of chronic antigen load and viral infection—introducing the antigen in a suitably immunogenic form can lead to an immune response to the virus.

While the tetanus toxin (TT) peptide in this vaccine is relatively MHC-unrestricted, there are nevertheless several MHC haplotypes to which it will not bind, in which cases it is not immunogenic. Examples include DR4 and some of the DR2 splits. Researchers had already developed several peptides that were known to bind to most DR alleles, but when they tried to immunize peripheral blood in vitro with a "pan-DR" peptide, they got very little response compared with TT. The reason had to do with the topography of this particular peptide: the MHC contact residues were on a polyalanine background that gave the TCR very little to recognize except the short methyl groups on the side chain of alanine. Researchers substituted lysine and tryptophan for alanine in three positions, giving the TCR more interesting side chains to recognize, and the resulting peptide induces a better proliferative response in vitro than did TT.

Like TT, pan-DR represents a helper epitope that may be very useful in conjunction with CTL epitopes to augment the immune response. It also shows considerable usefulness in helping antibody responses, and it might be an interesting peptide to add to some of the prophylactic vaccines that are currently used to generate carbohydrate antigen antibodies.

In response to questions from the audience, Dr. Grey added the following:

• Peripheral blood is admittedly a poor compartment in which to observe CTL response, and these in vitro results may not be predictive.

• Normal subjects in the Phase I study were subsequently given traditional surface antigen vaccine and responded normally—decreasing EA, DMA, and surface antigen levels, indicating that the vaccine is in fact affecting viral expression.

• Once they are linked to helper epitopes, the peptides no longer bind directly to the MHC Class I molecules on the APCs. However, they are being processed somewhere—intra- or extracellularly—and the linkage does not destroy their ability to prime CD8 cells. Perhaps phagocytic cells are taking up these lipopeptide adjuvants.

• The original DR peptides were originally developed as MHC blockers in autoimmune disease. They worked well in vitro, but in vivo they have an extremely short half-life and quickly fall below the concentration needed to demonstrate MHC blockade.

• HIV peptide vaccine studies have shown that the CTL epitope and helper or adjuvant must be covalently linked—a mixture doesn't work. Processing appears to extracellular, and the small size of the peptides may allow them to bypass the Class I processing pathway.

• These short peptides pulsed onto dendritic cells have effective properties in vitro, which Dr. Berzofsky will address in the following presentation (see below). Briefly, part of the function of CD4 help in inducing CD8 CTLs is in regulating stimulated molecules and APCs. If the peptides are presented on dendritic cells, it might be possible to induce CTLs in a CD4-independent mechanism.

• There is concern that inducing CTL may increase the severity of cell loss, but studies in HBV-transgenic mice indicate that passive transfer of large amounts of CTL clones does not lead to massive liver damage. There might be a patchy necrosis, in addition to a cytokine-mediated decrease in viral DNA due to IFN-gamma and TNF, but CTL does not appear to kill liver cells, even when 100 percent of those cells express antigen.

CD8 CTL TO MUTATED ONCOPROTEINS AND FUSION PROTEINS[23]

Mutant Proteins and Peptides as Target Antigens. Whatever the inciting carcinogenic event, most types of cancer involve either the inactivation of tumor suppressor genes or the activation of oncogenes. Often, but not always, that involves point mutations or translocations that potentially create neoantigenic determinants that might serve as tumor antigens and thereby serve as the targets of vaccines. Since these mutations or translocations would occur only in the tumor cell, they could provide unique markers that distinguish the tumor cell from normal host tissues to make a specific vaccine.

The problem with this approach, from the point of view of conventional tumor vaccine work, is that most tumor antigens have been described using antibodies, which can only recognize proteins on the surface of tumor cells. The products of these oncogenes and tumor suppressor genes are generally intracellular proteins, often nuclear proteins, that are not expressed on the surface of the cell. However, this limitation does not apply to CD8 cytotoxic T-lymphocytes (CTLs), which is able to "see" any protein synthesized in the cell. This is because those proteins, or some subset of them, are degraded into peptide fragments that are actively transported into the endoplasmic reticulum, where they bind to newly formed Class I MHC molecules and are transported to the cell surface, at which point the peptide fragments can be recognized by CD8 CTLs.

In this way, nucleo- and cytoplasmic proteins can operate as tumor antigens for CTLs. Among the many mutant proteins, researchers have thus far focused on p53 and ras, both of which occur in many of the most common types of cancer. This presentation focuses on p53; a later presentation focuses on ras (see below).

Mutant p53 Tumor Vaccine. The strategy followed was to make a short synthetic peptide spanning the site of a point mutation, and then immunize with

---

[23] Based on a presentation by Jay Berzofsky, M.D.

the peptide to raise CD8 CTLs against the peptide. This approach was based on earlier work with HIV peptides in mice, using peptide-pulsed spleen cells; however, researchers found that they could also use peripheral blood mononuclear cells (PBMCs). Both contain about 1 or 2 percent dendritic cells. Peptide can bind to the MHC Class I molecules on these dendritic cells without going through the intracellular processing pathway. When the cells are washed, irradiated, and reinjected intravenously, they induced CD8 CTLs and specific lysis.

The key cell in this process is the dendritic cell. Researchers found that immunizing with 100,000 purified dendritic cells produced as much or more specific lysis as 8 million peptide-pulsed spleen cells. This is consistent with the ratio of one or two dendritic cells per 100 spleen cells.

Previous experiments had shown that HIV peptide 18, part of the V3 loop of the envelope protein, was a major target for CTLs in BALB/c mice. Other researchers had successfully demonstrated that this same peptide-pulsed spleen cell immunization technique could protect against a mouse tumor that was expressing HIV gp160 (made tumorigenic by cotransfecting with ras). Based on this, investigators decided to use the same approach with peptides corresponding to mutations of p53, specifically a mutation called T1272, that came from a human lung carcinoma.

Researchers immunized BALB/c mice with peptides corresponding to this mutation and were able to induce CTLs that would kill targets. Using various truncated peptides, they mapped the minimal epitope to a tenmer that contained the point mutation (a cystine to tyrosine). Interestingly, this epitope avoids the differences between human p53 and mouse p53, and the induced CTLs are specific only for the mutation difference—they do not kill controls or targets pulsed with wild-type peptide.

In other words, the cystine-to-tyrosine mutation created a new antigenic determinant that was not present in natural p53. This peptide is presented by KFD, whose binding motif involves a tyrosine at position 2. Since natural p53 doesn't bind to KFD, and isn't recognized by the CTLs, there should be no danger of inducing autoimmune disease if the subject were a human with cancer.

The key question was whether endogenously expressed mutant p53 would be processed and presented in such a way, and in sufficient quantity, to be killed by the induced CTLs. Researchers transfected mouse tumor cells with mutant p53 and found that they were killed, whereas untransfected cells were killed only if peptide was added to the culture. In addition, the level of mutant p53 expressed by the transfected cells was at the low end of what is found in natural human and murine tumors. This indicated that the tumor antigen was not produced by overexpression of p53 and would in fact work at the levels found in natural tumors.

Researchers concluded from these findings that endogenously expressed mutant tumor suppressor oncogene product p53 can serve as a target antigen for CD8 CTLs, and that such CTLs can be induced by peptide immunization. They chose this method of immunization in part to avoid the need to attach a helper epitope (see presentation by Ronald Schwartz, above). Adjuvants containing helper epitopes can be very important, but when peptides are pulsed into dendritic cells, helper epitopes seem to be less critical. Consequently, researchers would be able to immunize numerous patients, each with a different mutation of p53 requiring a unique peptide—challenge enough—without also having to attach a helper epitope to each unique peptide.

Tumor Immunotherapeutic Experiments. To test the ability of the mutant peptide vaccine to treat a mouse with an established tumor, researchers injected tumor cells, waited 8 days until they could see or palpate tumor nodules that were 2 to 4 millimeters in diameter, and then immunized with peptide-pulsed dendritic cells either (1) a single time or (2) repeatedly every 4 or 5 days. The single immunization did not change the rate of growth of established tumors, but multiple immunizations significantly inhibited tumor growth. This protection lasts as long as immunizations continued; when immunization stopped, the tumors eventually began growing again. The animals were not cured, but the tumors were suppressed as long as researchers kept boosting their immunity.

Based on these results, researchers have started a clinical trial with human subjects. They performed a biopsy of the patient's tumor to determine if there was a mutation of p53 or ras, synthesized the corresponding peptide, pulsed it onto autologous PBMCs, and then reinfused the cells into the patient to immunize. This trial is still at an early stage, and it would be premature to report any results, but in most cases the patients had bulky tumors and extensive prior treatment with chemotherapy, which has left them with very poor immune systems (e.g., many are unable to make a CTL response to flu). However, researchers have shown the safety of this approach, and a few patients with less severe disease they have seen hints of either cytokine or CTL responses. This clinical trial is now moving into a new stage involving patients with less tumor bulk, or no tumor bulk, in whom investigators expect to see a better response because the immune system is more intact. This new stage may also immunize with larger numbers of cells, or with purified dendritic cells.

Fusion Proteins as Target Antigens. A similar approach has been tried in a different disease system found in Ewing's sarcoma and alveolar rhabdomyosarcoma (AR). These two pediatric sarcomas involve chromosomal translocations that create fusion proteins. For example, in about 90 percent of AR patients, there is a fusion between the PAX3 and FKHR genes, both of which are transcriptional regulators. In a chromosomal translocation between chromosomes 2 and 13, the DNA-binding domains of PAX3 are juxtaposed with the activation domain of FORCO, creating an aberrant transcription factor that is believed to be causative in this sarcoma. However, this break point also creates a potential neoantigenic determinant.

Researchers therefore asked whether there was a similar type of fusion in Ewing's sarcoma, which involves translocations between chromosomes 11 and

22. In contrast to the single break point of AR, they found several different break points that can occur between the EWS chain and the FLI1 gene. But while several peptides might be needed, depending on the patient, the same principle does apply: the translocation events generate new tumor-specific antigens capable of binding to MHC molecules and eliciting T-cell responses.

Fortunately, the sequences of the peptides surrounding the break points contain a number of different binding motifs for both human and mouse Class I and Class II MHC molecules. Researchers do not yet have binding data and cannot be sure all of these motifs will actually lead to binding, but (1) all of these peptides span the break point, and (2) none of them are present in normal cells. Hence they have the same properties as point mutations: these MHC-binding motifs are unique to the tumor.

Researchers tested these results by immunizing mice with peptide-pulsed spleen cells and found that they could induce CTLs that would kill a tumor cell, in this case CT26, an H2D-positive BALB/c mouse colon carcinoma cell. Very importantly, a transfected cell that endogenously expressed the whole PAX3-FORCO fusion protein were also killed. This demonstrated that, as with mutant p53, endogenously expressed whole fusion protein is appropriately processed and presented on Class I molecules to be seen by CD8 CTLs.

Fusion Protein Protective Vaccines. Researchers "mock immunized" two groups of mice (A and B) as controls and immunized two other groups (C and D) with PAX3-FKHR peptide. They then injected all four groups with tumor cells from lung metastases—A and C with wild-type cells, but B and D with tumor cells that had been transfected to express fusion protein, called F8. Autopsy showed no difference in the number of number of nodules in the lungs of groups A and C, which received wild-type tumor cells. However, there was statistically significant protection in group D—immunized mice had substantially fewer nodules than unimmunized mice in group B. This experiment wasn't perfect—transfected cells didn't grow as well as wild-type in vivo, many mice in both arms had micrometastases that couldn't be counted, and the results need to be repeated—but these preliminary results are encouraging.

In another experiment, researchers injected tumor cells first, allowing them to establish micrometastases, and then—24 hours later—adoptively transferred cells from immunized mice into the infected mice. Again, there was no protection against wild-type tumor cells, but there was a substantial reduction in the number of tumor modules in mice that received both transfected tumor cells and immunized CTLs. The results were not quite statistically significant, and there was the same problem with micrometastases, but researchers were encouraged by the trend, and by the fact that two of the animals had no detectable nodules whatsoever.

Conclusions. Researchers concluded from these experiments that the characteristic T-11-22 translocation of Ewing's sarcoma and T-13 translocation of AR generate fusion proteins that act as neoantigens. Sequence analysis of these fusion proteins suggests the presence of MHC Class I and II binding motifs for both mouse and human. Immunization of experimental animals with synthetic peptides corresponding to the fusion break point results in generation of specific CTL responses. Immunized animals have reduced tumor burden following tumor challenge, compared with controls. Adoptive transfer of bulk spleen cells from immunized animals mediated partial reduction in tumor burden in animals with established disease. These preliminary results need to be repeated with additional controls, and that work is in progress. Researchers are now planning a clinical trial in patients with these pediatric sarcomas.

Tumor Immunogenicity. These strategies would be unnecessary if the tumor itself were more immunogenic. At least five possible explanations have been offered for the failure of the tumor to elicit a CTL immune response:

1. *Failure of the mutant epitope in the oncogene product or fusion protein to be presented by an individual's MHC alleles.* Research cannot overcome this problem, but it is not the only way to induce an immune response.

2. *The tumor down-regulates the MHC allele responsible for presentation.* Research has shown that it takes a much higher density of MHC-peptide complexes to induce an immune response than it does to be the target of a CTL immune response. In this case, even if MHC is expressed at a level insufficient to induce an immune response, it is still possible to induce an immune response on professional APCs that will induce CTLs to kill the tumor.

3. *The tumor processes antigen inefficiently, and hence at insufficient levels to induce immune response.*

4. *Loss of costimulatory molecules.* Several groups have shown that tumor cells transfected for the B7 costimulatory molecule become immunogenic and induce CD8 CTLs that will kill the tumor. That is, costimulation is necessary for the afferent (inducing) but not the efferent (killing) limb of the immune response.

5. *Tumor cells may be tolerogenic.* They present signal 1 without signal 2, and so instead of prolonging memory they kill the CTLs induced by immunization. Evidence for this is seen in the need to immunize repeatedly to suppress the tumor. Even this may have a beneficial effect in terms of the longevity of the patient.

In response to questions from the audience, Dr. Berzofsky added the following:

- Investigators have intentionally avoided the nonmutated portions of p53, etc., because they don't want to induce autoimmune responses. Because mutant p53 is overexpressed (due to prolonged survival rather than increased synthesis), this risk is particularly great.
- Tumor genotype will become an important component of designing specific tumor vaccines. In the case of ras, there is a handful of common mutations, and the peptide is probably already synthesized. There are hundreds of different

mutations of p53, however, and a new peptide must be synthesized for almost every new patient. For this approach to work, clinicians will need to have on the shelf a repertoire of at least the most common peptides.

• Researchers know the binding motifs for only a handful of human MHC molecules. Preliminary binding studies suggest that there is a match between the mutation and the patient's HLA allele in about 35 percent of cases. However, even 35 percent of cancer patients is more than can be treated at present.

• Because different types of cancer will have different biologies and different escape routes (see above), strategies that fail with one cancer may still succeed with others.

• Phase I trials were aimed at safety rather than efficacy, and there have been clinical remissions to date, but a few patients have unexpected stability.

• Tumor immunotherapy may prove to be most useful as a "cancer adjuvant," for patients who have already had the bulk of their disease removed by surgery or other therapy, but remain at high risk of recurrence from micrometastases.

• More than 100 common mutations of p53 have been observed in lung, breast, and other cancers. The necessary "repertoire" of mutant p53 peptides is the correspondingly large. This may not be, most cost-effective approach, but it is a first step. It may eventually be possible to make a DNA vaccine of these constructs.

• Patients in clinical studies are immunized with autologous peptide-pulsed PBMCs, a 2-hour process. If researchers move to purified dendritic cells, grown in GM-CSF or IL-4, quality control is better but several days are required for incubation, and the patient must be available for up to a week at a time.

• The current route of immunization is intravenous. This is not the best way to make antibodies, but experiments in mice have shown that the intravenous route induces CTLs more effectively than either subcutaneous or intraperitoneal when working with either spleen or dendritic cells.

CTL SCREENING FOR TUMOR ANTIGENS[24]

Researchers attempted to characterize tumor antigens that are recognized by CTLs, in hopes of targeting the immune system for these antigens. Using mixed lymphocyte-tumor cell culture, they obtained CTL clones that lyse autologous /tumor cells. Most of this work has been done with melanoma, which proved to be easier to work with that other tumor types that are now under investigation (e.g., sarcoma, lung, blood, renal, and head and neck carcinoma).

Investigators used a genetic approach to isolate genes coding for the proeins from which tumor antigens are derived. There are three categories of human tumor antigens:

---

[24] Based on a presentation by Pierre van der Bruggen, M.D.

1. antigens encoded by genes expressed in different tumor types but not in most normal tissue;

2. antigens encoded by genes expressed in both tumors and normal tissues (e.g., melanoma and normal melanocytes); and

3. antigens derived from abnormal proteins such as mutated proteins and fusion proteins (see preceding presentation).

Tumor Antigens (MAGE, BAGE, GAGE, RAGE). The first gene they isolated was called melanoma antigen 1 (MAGE-1), a previously unknown gene whose sequence is the same in DNA from melanoma cells and blood lymphocytes of the same patient. MAGE-1 belongs to a family of genes that are expressed in melanoma and other tumors; the coding regions in a terminal segment include about 300 amino acids for the putative proteins.

All of the MAGE genes are located in the long arm of chromosome X. Other teams have recently identified a related cluster of genes in the short arm that present strong homology with the MAGE family. Homology is even stronger with a cluster of genes isolated in the mouse genome. Researchers do not currently know the function of the MAGE genes; they will attempt to develop knockout mice in which to study the function of the proteins they encode.

Researchers used a specific PCR approach to detect the expression of the MAGE genes, and they found that they are expressed in a wide range of tumor types. They are not expressed in renal carcinoma, nor in leukemia and lymphoma; MAGE-2 and MAGE-3 are more frequently expressed than MAGE-1; and they tend to be expressed in a higher percentage of metastases and infiltrating tumors. The latter have a relatively bad prognosis, but the higher expression of MAGE genes is probably related not to higher metabolic potential but rather to the methylation status of the gene promoter.

The transcription factors capable of activating the MAGE-1 promoter are present in most if not all cells, including those that don't express MAGE-1. The MAGE-1 promoter region contains two major elements that have ETS binding sites. It also contains a number of methylation sites (vertical bars) and HPA2 restriction sites (H), where it will be cut and digested if it is undermethylated. PCR analysis of DNA from different tumors demonstrated an inverse correlation between expression of MAGE-1 and overall degree of DNA methylation. In general, however, MAGE genes are not expressed in normal tissues, with two exceptions: testes (male germ cell lines undergo genome-wide demethylation), an placenta (primarily MAGE-4).

Two additional gene families have been found to encode for antigens that were recognized on the melanoma of the same patient. Designated BAGE and GAGE, they are expressed over the same range of tumor types, although at lower levels than MAGE-1 through 3. They are not expressed in leukemia or lymphoma, renal carcinoma, or colorectal carcinoma; and like MAGE they are not expressed in normal tissues, except the testes.

All three families of genes have been found to encode for antigens that are expressed specifically by tumors, presented by different HLAs, and recognized by different CTLs:

• MAGE-1 protein has two such epitopes, located at different regions of the protein; one is presented by HLA-1, the other by HLA-C16, and researchers have identified CTLs expressing at least three different T-cell receptors. MAGE-3 also encodes for one antigen presented on HLA-1, a second presented on HLA-B44, and four others that are expressed on HLA-2.

• BAGE seems to belong to a family of several genes. The protein it encodes is very short, with the immunogenic peptide located at the amino terminus. The peptide is presented to CTL by HLA-C16, so again different CTLs with different TCRs are able to recognize the peptide-HLA combination.

• GAGE also belongs to a family of several genes. Researchers have isolated six cDNAs; GAGE-1 and GAGE-2 encode a peptide presented by HLA-C6, while the others encode peptides presented by HLA-A29.

The only normal tissues in which these genes express themselves are the testes and placenta. However, it appears unlikely that immunization against one or more of these antigens will cause harmful side effects due to expression in the testes. First of all, expression was found only in germ line cells, spermatocytes and spermatogonia, and since these cells do not express MHC molecules, gene expression should not result in antigen expression. Secondly, the PGFB-type fas ligand is present normally in testes and would not contribute to destructive inflammatory reactions. Third, experiments with mouse p815 tumor antigen (also expressed in the testes) produce strong CTL response in male mice, with no signs of inflammation and no loss of fertility.

Finally, other investigators have isolated an antigen from a renal carcinoma gene, designated RAGE. The protein is very short and the antigen is presented by HLA-B7. Researchers have been able to obtain a CTL response that recognizes HLA-B7 renal tumors but not B7 normal tissues. RAGE is not expressed in normal tissues except the retina, which (like the testes) do not express MHC molecules—an immunologically privileged site. However, RAGE is expressed in only 2 percent of renal cell carcinomas.

Antigens of Both Tumors and Normal Tissue. CTL responses are readily generated against several different antigens encoded on normal melanocytes as well as on melanoma. This finding was unexpected several years ago, but several genes encoding such antigens have been identified, including tyrosinase, Pmel17-gp100, Melan-A-MART-1, and TRP-1-gp75. Most of the antigenic peptides are presented by HLA-2, although other peptide combinations have been found. The pattern of CTL precursors against these antigens is very different from that observed with the MAGE-like antigens.

In fact, most melanoma patients have CTL precursors that can be readily restimulated in vitro by autologous tumor cells. This implies that immunization should be possible, and should increase the levels of such CTLs. On the other hand, most of these patients have progressive disease, and that suggests that these CTL precursors are not very effective. There is also concern for side effects—not vitiligo (due to destruction of normal melanocytes), which can occur without unacceptable consequences, but rather in the pigmented cells in the choroid layer of the retina, where the expression of fas ligand and TGJ-beta could contribute to inflammatory reactions. Nevertheless, several groups are going forward with plans for carefully devised clinical trials of immunotherapy against these antigens.

Antigens of Mutated Protein. Point mutations can also generate antigens on melanoma that are recognized by CTLs. One of the most interesting is a protein that normally binds to p16 in the regulation of the cell cycle. The mutation prevents this binding, thereby increasing entry into the S phase of the cell cycle. This mutation is both antigenic and oncogenic.

Another mutation antigen was isolated in renal carcinoma using CTL clones that recognize renal tumors but not autologous Epstein-Barr virus-transformed B-lymphocytes. The gene was identified by transfecting cos cells in combination with HLA-A21, because the lysis of this clone was inhibited by anti-HLA-A2 antibodies. Surprisingly, the cDNA alone could confer recognition, and the sequence was the sequence of HLA-A21 molecule that was mutated at position 117.

Experimental Results. Identification of tumor antigens has three advantages: (1) the patients are easily identified; (2) the antigens can be engineered for optimal immunization; and (3) there are several modes of immunization. Of those that have been tried thus far, one of the most impressive is adenoviral injection.

One experiment used mouse tumor antigen p815-A, a known epitope presented to CTL by LD molecules. Researchers inserted the sequence encoding for this peptide into the genome of an E3,E1-deletion mutant of adenovirus serotype 5. The location of the insertion was just after the promoter, which is a strong promoter active in a wide range of mammalian cells. Varying amounts of the plaque-forming units of adeno.P1A were injected intradermally in the ears of experimental mice, while other animals received equal numbers of control adenovirus. After 14 days, researchers removed spleen cells and stimulated them in vitro in the presence of L1210 cells transfected with either P1A or P1A and B7.1. Experimental animals that received higher concentrations produced a strong CTL response, especially if the stimulated cells were also transfected with B7.1. Results were similar when IL-2 was used in place of B7.1. Otherwise, however, results were less impressive: there was a CTL response, but never enough to protect against challenge with living p815 tumor cells, and prior infection with MD adenovirus prevented CTL responses to p815.

Prospects for Human Immunotherapy. Given the frequency of expression of different tumor antigen genes and the frequency of different HLA alleles in the human population, up to 82 percent of melanoma patients might theoretically be eligible for immunotherapy. In practice, because some tumors express different tumor antigens, about 60 percent of melanoma patients could be eligible, and lower percentages of patients with other tumor types.

In a preliminary study, patients received three different dosages (30, 100, or 300 micrograms) of MAGE-1 peptide, without adjuvant, subcutaneously, at monthly intervals. After three injections, there was little or no toxicity, no tumor response, and no CTL response. In a second study, patients received either 100 or 300 micrograms of MAGE-3 peptide, again subcutaneously and at monthly intervals. There was no toxicity, but significant tumor response and at least one possible case of CTL response. One melanoma patient showed considerable response by the day of the third injection, but unfortunately died a month later of a brain metastasis. A second patient with 100 metastases around a skin graft showed significant regression after three injections and one year later is tumor-free. A third patient, designated AVL3, had primary melanomas removed in 1990, but in April 1995 had several metastases in the lung; by October 1995 the patient was disease-free, although the tumor subsequently relapsed.

In response to questions from the audience, Dr. van der Bruggen added the following:

• Human patients show tumor response but no CTL response, either spleen or peripheral blood; experimental mice show CTL responses but no regression of tumors.

• Researchers have not had the opportunity to look for tumor-infiltrating lymphocytes, nor have they looked for antibodies against MAGE-1 and MAGE-3, although this is planned.

• Researchers cannot explain why regressions are observed only after the third injection. One member of the audience speculated that CTLs have fairly short memory, and since the tumor itself may not be a good source of antigen, multiple injections are needed to maintain a high level of CTLs.

• It may be possible to elicit a CD4 restricted response (e.g., to tumor lysate) as a supplement to the initial CD8 response.

IMMUNITY TO ONCOGENIC SELF-PROTEINS[25]

Immunity to Mutated Ras. Researchers asked whether or not oncogenic proteins can be targeted for vaccine and T-cell therapy. They first examine mutated ras as a prototype. Ras is activated by point mutations that are common in diverse tumors. Ras is present in about 15 percent of all human tumors, including 50 percent of colon cancer and 95 percent of pancreas cancer.

Animal experiments demonstrated that ras can function as a tumor-specific antigen, eliciting both helper T-cell and CTL responses that can decrease the growth of tumor in vitro and in vivo. Researchers have also found existent immune responses in a few patients with pancreatic and colon cancers. Most are antibody responses to normal ras, but a small number have a very restricted antibody response to the mutated protein. Other patients have a very specific T-cell response to the mutated segment of ras, but there is a problem in trying to focus immune attack against a single epitope. More importantly, oncogenic proteins that are activated by mutation have increased function, and proteins that have increased function don't have to be present in abundant amounts.

Immunity to HER-2/neu. Rather than looking at immune responses to proteins that weren't abundant, researchers asked whether or not it was possible to focus an immune attack against an oncogenic protein that is present in large amounts. Their prototype was HER-2/neu, a very large nonmutated protein that is expressed in very low amounts in some normal tissues, but is amplified in about 25 percent of breast cancer patients. When amplified, it is overexpressed and substantially more abundant. The structure of HER-2/neu includes a very large extracellular domain, so large that there are potentially epitopes for every individual.

Initial experiments revealed that 15 percent or 16 percent of breast cancer patients have existent antibody responses to HER-2/neu, including 42 percent of patients with documented overexpression of the protein. In the latter case, the immune response is assumed to be elicited by virtue of the fact that the protein is overexpressed. Unfortunately, some normal patients also have a response, between 2 percent and 5 percent based on screening of blood donors. Experience has shown that by setting the cutoff level high enough—in this case, a titer of less than 1:500—it is possible to exclude virtually all responses in normal individuals while retaining a much more specific response for breast cancer patients.

In many cases, the responses are extremely low, between 1:100 and 1:500, but five patients out of 96 had very substantial antibody responses, with titers of greater than 1:12,000. As it happened, these same five patients also had stage I or stage II breast cancer, as opposed to more advanced disease. In general,

---

[25] Based on a presentation by Martin Cheever, M.D.

antibody titer tended to be highest in patients with early breast cancer, and to decrease with more advanced disease. However, HER-2/neu was overexpressed in about 25 percent of patients with advanced breast cancer, where it was associated with more aggressive disease. Researchers speculate that the existent immunity occurs early on in the course of disease and prevents the progression of some patients.

Researchers have shown that the antibody response is to the whole protein and to both the intracellular and extracellular domains. This appears to be due to cell breakdown, which releases previously sequestered segments of the protein. The extracellular domain functions as a growth factor receptor, so that when it is amplified and overexpressed, the signalling through this protein is part and parcel of the aggressiveness of the disease. Some monoclonal antibodies to HER-2/neu have agonistic effects, some have antagonistic effects; hence, antibodies to the extracellular domain might either inhibit or stimulate the growth of breast cancer cells.

Researchers studied the patients with the highest antibody titer in greater detail. In several of these patients, the IgG antibody binds to the same tumor cells that overexpress HER-2/neu. Using epitope mapping, they have discovered a segment of the extracellular domain that is rich in cystine and thus a potential binding site. The researchers are now investigating whether this is a functional antibody.

Some patients with an IgG antibody response also showed a proliferative T-cell response to HER-2/neu. The patient with the highest antibody response also had the greatest T-cell response, to both whole protein and to peptides from the intra- and extracellular domains. Other patients showed proliferative response to peptides but not whole protein. Researchers have not yet mapped all of the epitopes involved.

Animal Models. To learn how to immunize with the HER-2/neu protein, researchers needed to develop an animal model. In the mouse, the neu sequence is not evident and has not been closed. Rat neu protein is quite homologous to human HER-2/neu, but when researchers immunized rats with purified neu protein in complete Freund's adjuvant, they could find neither proliferative T-cell response nor antibody response.

Earlier researchers had developed a vaccinia virus vector that expressed the extracellular domain of rat neu protein. While this vector was immunogenic in mice, however, it too failed to elicit a response in rats. Those researchers had concluded that the failure to elicit a response was due to tolerance to self. However, subsequent screening has identified patients with existent immune response, proving that is possible to overcome tolerance to HER-2/neu.

Researchers therefore began to focus on immunizing to fragments of the protein. They found that immunizing rats with groups of intracellular domain neu peptides resulted in peptide-specific T-cell and antibody responses, and that the T-cells that responded to peptide also responded to whole protein. They were also able to immunize to peptides from the extracellular domain, but the response was much weaker. This may be due to a biological principle—i.e., tolerance of extracellular domain is more stringent because it is a shed protein that is more available to the thymus for induction of tolerance—or it may be because researchers merely picked the wrong peptides to work with.

Sequencing shows that the peptides to which rats were immunized are identical in the human protein (rat neu and human HER-2/neu are about 89 percent homologous at the amino acid level). Hence, the antibodies that will immunoprecipitate the rat protein will also immunoprecipitate the human protein. These are also peptides to which at least some human patients have responded.

Researchers now plan to go forward with a vaccine trial in which humans patients will be immunized with peptides identified as immunogenic in rats. The adjuvant used in the rat studies was complete Freund's, which is too toxic for standard use in humans, so they plan to use GM-CSF as an adjuvant. Instead of growing dendritic cells in vitro with GM-CSF, the cytokine is injected intradermally with the peptide. Animal tests have shown that it is possible to generate immune response to intra- and extracellular domain peptides with GM-CSF as the adjuvant, and indeed that the DTH assay is much stronger that when using complete Freund's adjuvant. Researchers have submitted to an IRB a protocol to immunize patients with breast and ovarian cancers with peptides. FDA has signed off, and the protocol should begin within months. Data should be available before 2000 on whether these peptides are toxic and/or efficacious in vivo.

Autoimmune Cancer Therapy. Generating an immune response to self-protein does not resolve the issue of whether it is possible to induce an aggressive autoimmune response as a form of cancer therapy. To answer this question, researchers focused on the prostate—once the prostate becomes malignant, it is often removed, at which point any prostate tissue left in the body is by definition malignant. If it were possible to induce a rapidly destructive, aggressive autoimmune prostatitis, it would have therapeutic benefit.

There are several problems in this use of autoimmune prostatitis; not the least is immunological tolerance to self-proteins. There is no information available on which prostate-specific proteins are immunogenic; nor have experiments confirmed that autoimmunity can destroy normal prostate tissue. In addition, most autoimmune disease is relapsing and often resolves spontaneously, while this strategy requires a rapid and aggressive autoimmunity that can eradicate the organ. (Parenthetically, there is a general lack of attention to CTLs in the field of autoimmunity, possibly because autoimmunity isn't mediated by CTLs, or possibly because CTLs are too difficult to deal with.)

Researchers first tried to immunize to prostatic acid phosphatase (PAP), a common and well-characterized marker for human prostate tumor for which the sequence of a rodent model is also known. PAP is a glycoprotein secreted exclusively by prostate epithelial cells. It is expressed by all normal prostate tissue and by most prostate cancers. And while portions of the molecule are similar to acid phosphatases from other tissues, other portions are prostate-specific. All of these factors made it an appealing target.

As with HER-2/neu, purified rat PAP with complete Freund's adjuvant induced neither helper T-cell nor antibody response. Peptides induced helper T-cell responses in female rats, which had little or no protein in their systems, and in two cases the response was peptide-specific. But rat peptides failed to induce any response in male rats. Trying another approach, researchers first immunized male rats to homologous human PAP peptides, then immunized with rat peptides, and this sequential immunization did induce helper T-cell and antibody responses to rat PAP. Researchers believe that their ability to immunize females but not males is related to the peptides they used, which are far less abundant in females than in males; they are currently investigating this supposition.

Even when they succeeded in immunizing male rats, however, researchers found that there was none of the inflammation to the prostate that would have been expected. This suggests that tumor immunotherapy vaccination is very ineffective for inducing any antitumor response. Researchers suspect that it will be necessary to use T-cell therapy to get the precursor frequency high enough to support an immune response. The researchers have not yet tested or tried to elicit CTLs.

Researchers are currently trying to determine which proteins are most immunogenic in autoimmune prostatitis, and will focus in the future on those among them that are expressed by prostate cancer. Relatively little is known about autoimmunity and prostate in either humans or rats—only that prostate inflammation can be induced in rats immunized to prostate homogenate. Previous studies used multiple injections of homogenate with repeated use of complete Freund's, which is no longer allowed. This results in antibody response to a variety of different proteins, which are now being identified, but immunization with whole prostate doesn't get a response to PAP.

By selecting out the fractions of protein that induce the greatest antibody response, and then immunizing to these fractions alone, researchers were able to generate a very substantial, rapidly progressive, destructive autoimmune prostatitis. The researchers are now concentrating their efforts on (1) identifying the exact targets of this response and (2) learning how to induce this response prospectively and at will.

Considerable additional research will be needed before these results can be used for therapeutic benefits in human prostate cancer. Autoimmune prostatitis is an ill-defined syndrome, and none of the relevant antigens have been identified. Animal experiments may reveal how to maximize the destructive response, but it will still be necessary to identify the human proteins that are homologous to rat proteins, and verify that the homologous antigen is immunogenic in humans, before instituting human vaccine and T-cell therapy trials for prostate cancer.

In response to questions from the audience, Dr. Cheever added the following:

- Several strains of rats are used in these studies.
- Whole prostate homogenate appears to contain fractions that somehow suppress or block the immune response, as well as fractions that induce a response. Researchers use the Western blot test to determine which induce an antibody response, and then select for them.
- Ras and other oncoproteins still represent a valid approach, but it will apply only to a small subset of patients. The advantage of working on a protein like HER-2/neu is the greater likelihood of getting a response in every individual who has that very common protein.

CYTOKINES AND THEIR LOCAL ENVIRONMENTS[26]

Potential Energy Model. A certain threshold level of response against a particular tumor antigen is required for rejection of that tumor. The endogenous level of immunity against the antigen is below this threshold; vaccination must enhance existent immunity sufficiently to raise the response above this threshold level. This has implications for the choice of antigen and vaccine strategy:

- Even if the endogenous level of immunity to antigen A is close to the thre-shold, if the vaccine approach is weak, the response will not reach the threshold, and the vaccine fails.
- On the other hand, if the endogenous level of immunity to antigen B is much lower, even a strong vaccine may not be able to raise the response to the threshold, and the vaccine still fails.

An extreme example of the latter case is an antigen expressed in the thymus, with tolerance generated by clonal deletion; the endogenous immunity is negative, and no vaccine approach could hope to produce a therapeutic response.

Consequently, the ideal strategy is to identify a good antigen whose endogenous level of immunity is relative close to the threshold, along with a strong vaccine approach. This involves issues of endogenous self-tolerance, repertoire, and vaccine approaches. At the present time, however, there is almost an embarrassment of riches in terms of different approaches to cancer vaccines—peptides, recombinant adenovirus, pox virus, Listeria, BCG, etc. It may well be impossible to test each of them reasonably in patients unless there is first a concerted effort to compare them rigorously, in a head-to-head fashion, in the appropriate animal models.

Role of Cytokines. For many cancers these target antigens still aren't known, although it is assumed that tumor cells themselves are important—the

---

[26] Based on a presentation by Drew Pardoll, M.D.

antigens relevant to immune response are in there, somewhere. However, another avenue of research has concentrated on the lack of signal 2 as the missing ingredient in immune response against tumors. There was evidence from earlier studies that one way to activate T-cells against tumor antigens was to provide signal 1 and signal 2 on the same cell, and that an important signal 2 for CTLs was IL-2 (or lymphokines made by helper T-cells).

Based on this paradigm, researchers began introducing cytokine genes into tumor cells, beginning with IL-2, in order to produce a whole-cell vaccine that contained all of the antigens and presented peptide as MHC signal 1 and signal 2 on the same cell. Aided by the use of defective retroviral vectors, they inserted a wide range of cytokine genes into a weakly immunogenic tumor, vaccinated animals, and compared the resulting protection against challenge with wild-type tumor cells. The most effective vaccine involved tumor cells transduced with a GM-CSF gene.

This was a surprise at the time, but other groups soon reported that GM-CSF has the unique and interesting function of inducing hematopoietic progenitors to differentiate not only into granulocytes and macrophages, but also into dendritic cells. It may be that these high-potency APCs, differentiating locally in the presence of GM-CSF, have something to do with the enhanced systemic immune response to GM-CSF-transduced tumor cells. Subsequent research has tried to explain how this process works.

Paracrine Cytokine Adjuvant. What turned out to be important physiologically, in addition to the particular cytokine, is the elaboration of that cytokine *at the site of the antigen.* In a sense, the GM-CSF-transduced tumor cell actually represents a timed-release depot for two sets of molecules: its own antigens, and GM-CSF. Importantly, it also replaces the complex "black boxes" of conventional adjuvants (BCG, C. parvum, mycobacterium, TB) with a single molecule, and in doing so generated a systemic antitumor immune response that was more potent than mixing irradiated tumor cells with conventional adjuvants.

Researchers have learned that APCs that differentiated at the site of the vaccine, under control of GM-CSF, actually ingest antigens from tumor cells and process them into both the Class I and Class II pathways, an example of crosspriming. As the APCs are ingesting and processing antigens, they are travelling to the draining lymph node, where one can first identify activated Class I- and Class II-restricted CTLs and helper cells. Once activated, these cells leave the draining lymph node and circulate systemically.

An important implication is that effector-phase CD4 is very important, in addition to CD8-positive cells. Consequently, the best vaccines will involve epitopes that actually represent tumor antigens. For this reason, there should be concern over the use of "universal helper epitopes," which are not expressed by the tumor cell.

Clinical Trials. These results led researchers to initiate a Phase I trial in patients with metastatic renal cancer who had undergone nephrectomy to remove the primary tumor. They used a retroviral vector to transduce human GM-CSF gene into tumor cells, expanded these cells, irradiated them at doses that inhibited replication but not immunogenicity, and then vaccinated patients with three monthly injections at two different doses, half the dose intradermal and half subcutaneous. Researchers didn't expect and didn't find any toxicity; the important results were immunological.

In order to determine whether paracrine elaboration of GM-CSF generated human immune responses, patients were randomized in a double-blind fashion to receive either irradiated tumor cells or irradiated tumor cells transduced with the GM-CSF gene. DTH was chosen as the simplest and most reproducible assay for in vivo immune response. A total of 30 days after vaccination, 1 million nontransduced cells were injected at a distant site, and the diameter of induration, edema, and erythema was measured to determine DTH response.

When the blind was broken, the results indicated that the lower vaccine dose (4 million cells) did not induce significant immune responses. However, the higher dose (40 million cells) did produce some fairly impressive DTH responses in patients who had received the GM-CSF-transduced vaccine. Even more encouraging were the results of the biopsy analysis of infiltrates at the DTH site. In addition to the quantitative difference, roughly 50 percent of the infiltrating cells in GM-CSF-transduced patients were eosinophils, whereas no eosinophils were found infiltrating the DTH sites of nontransduced patients. This was the same result observed in animal tests.

Anecdotally, one of the three patients that received the higher dose of transduced vaccine showed a fairly significant clinical response. This patient had multiple pulmonary metastases from his renal cancer that had progressed very rapidly over the 2 months between surgery and initial vaccination. After 1 vaccination, there was evidence of regression, and after the third vaccination there was a 95-percent reduction in the volume of metastatic tumor. While anecdotal, this suggests that there may be a therapeutic correlate to the observed immune response.

Allogeneic Vaccines. In these renal cancer patients, as in the melanoma patients discussed above, the vaccine did not induce a response against normal tissue; patients showed no impairment or autoimmunity of their remaining kidney, just as melanoma patients did not develop vitiligo. This suggests that it should be possible to generate responses against them without generating a clinically prohibitive autoimmune disease. At the same time, there is mounting evidence that the immunorelevant antigens in tumors are shared, as was the case in the MAGE proteins (see above).

This may provide a rationale for using a genetically modified allogeneic vaccine. Tumor antigens are presented to T-cells not by the tumor but by APCs derived from host bone marrow. This implies that it may not be necessary to match HLA between the vaccine and the patient. Certainly, generic vaccines would be far less labor-intensive and less expensive than individualized vaccines, and—since quantities would no longer be limited by the growth potential of the individual's tumor—it would also be possible to vaccinate with higher doses.

Antigen-Specific Tumor Vaccines. Researchers also hope to use activated T-cells to identify the relevant antigens for antigen-specific vaccines. One group has been pursuing this concept in the mouse model using CT26, an NMU-induced colon cancer, in order to identify the repertoire of antigens that are being recognized by the CD8 arm of the immune response following vaccination with GM-CSF-transduced tumor cells. Their technique involves taking bulk T-cells from the draining lymph nodes (rather than tumor-specific CTLs), eluting peptides from Class I molecules, fractionating them with reverse-phase HPLC, and using surrogate targets to assay peptide fractions for bioactivity. The results indicated that there was only one bioactive fraction, suggesting that the majority of CD8-positive immune response was focused on a single peptide among the many presented by the CT26 tumor. These results have been repeated in 40 separate experiments.

This peptide, called AH1, had a molecular weight of 1,128 and was doubly charged. It sensitized surrogate target cells down to a concentration of 5×10^{-12} molar. Upon sequencing, it proved to be a peptide derived from an endogenous murine MuLV gene that is normally completely silent in the BALB/c genome but is reactivated by altered methylation, much like MAGE-1 (see above). (The latter finding has led to new interest in endogenous human retroviruses, which also seem to be reactivated in human tumors.)

AH1 is not expressed in normal tissues from BALB/c mice, including normal colon and small intestine epithelium, but it is turned on in a number of different tumors. Interestingly, if T-cells from vaccinated animals are stimulated for two rounds with AH1 plus IL-2 and then adoptively transferred back into animals with CT26 tumors, most of the animals are cured. However, there is no significant response when tumor-bearing animals are vaccinated with AH1-pulsed dendritic cells or other approaches.

Researchers believe that they should examine several other approaches for introducing these gene products in vivo, such as viruses that target them to both the Class I and Class III MHC pathways. In addition, there are some interesting recombinant viral and bacterial approaches that should be compared head-to-head with endogenous tumor antigen models before deciding which approaches will be taken to clinical trials, with their tremendous investment of time, effort, and expense.

In response to questions from the audience, Dr. Pardoll added the following:

• Although GM-CSF up-regulates B7 in macrophages, it does not do so in tumor cells and, hence, this cannot explain their increased immunogenicity. In fact, the major effect of transducing B7 into tumors is to provide a target molecule for NK cells to more actively lyse the tumor cells. A B7-transduced tumor cell isn't nearly as good an APC as a bone marrow progenitor that differentiates into a dendritic cell in the presence of GM-CSF.

- Researchers have compared paracrine GM-CSF (either by transduction or by time-release microspheres) with BCG and C. parvum in seven or eight different tumor models. The resulting systemic immune response generated by GM-CSF is between 1.5 and 4.0 logs more potent than either adjuvant.
- While researchers have learned a tremendous amount from their experiments, they are also certain that transducing autologous tumor explants is not feasible for large-scale application in the general patient population. Microsphere approaches obviate the need for GM-CSF transduction, and the question is moot if immunodominant tumor antigens are in fact shared.
- However, it may be 15 to 30 years before investigators identify the relevant antigens for all of the important tumors.
- GM-CSF significantly up-regulates both Th-1 and Th-2 lymphokines.
- A single vaccination with B7-transduced tumor cells does not evoke a measurable response that maps to the tumor's MHC type. There is a small response to a second vaccination.
- Tumor antigens will ultimately prove to be very important, but at present the best strategy for identifying immunorelevant antigens is to use whole-cell vaccines and let the immune system indicate which of the 50,000 or 100,000 antigens in that tumor it is capable of responding to.
- There is no data to support the assertion that viral sequences bind to MHC better than self-sequences. However, high-affinity binding generates a much more profound tolerance.
- A total of 10 percent or 15 percent of tumors turn off MHC Class I, in which case CTL response is irrelevant. In such cases, NK cells can be brought into the response to replace CD8 responses.
- Once the relevant antigens are defined, melanoma and cervical cancer are both logical targets for cancer vaccines. So, too, are cancers of dispensable tissues (e.g., ovary, prostate, breast). Eventually, tumor vaccines might be used prophylactically, to prevent tumors caused by viruses before they occur (e.g., human papilloma virus, hepatitis C virus).

APPENDIX 29

Questions Posed to Outside Experts and List of Responders

If possible, please list references for specific estimates.

1. What is your estimate of overall and age-specific incidence (rate or cases per year)?

OR

What is your estimated incidence of clinical disease, subclinical infection, latent infection, and chronic infection?

2. Is the incidence of the disease changing? In what manner and why?

3. What groups are at greatest risk of illness (e.g., by age, sex, ethnicity, socioeconomic status, immunologic competence, geographic area)?

4. What are specific risk factors for this illness?

5. Please describe **typical** patterns for the clinical course of this illness, inclu-ding variations in presentation, variations of patterns and severity, complications, case fatality, relapses and sequelae, duration of stages of illness and sequelae, and proportion of cases following each course.

6. Please describe typical forms of care and estimate their effectiveness and cost.

7. What strategies are currently available to prevent this condition (e.g., vector control, treatment of water supply, reduction of behavioral risks [IV drug use, unprotected sexual contact], etc.)?

435

8. How would you compare these strategies in terms of effectiveness, cost, and practicality to a likely vaccine?

9. What are the known components of immunity for this organism (antibody to what antigens, T-cells, B-cells, etc.)?

10. What are the critical determinants of an immune response associated with protection against infection?

11. What are the correlates of immunity (e.g., surrogates for protection) that may be useful or necessary for vaccine development?

12. To your knowledge, is vaccine development for this disease occurring now? If so, describe the type of vaccine (what antigen, live or killed, subunit, naked DNA, etc.).

13. Who (individual, group, company) is working on this vaccine?

14. How far has vaccine development progressed (preclinical, clinical trials: Phase I, II, or III)?

15. When could Phase III trials be expected to start for such a vaccine?

16. When could such a vaccine be expected to be licensed for use?

17. If a vaccine is not in development, what new knowledge is necessary to undertake vaccine development?

18. Who should develop it (e.g., industry, government, military)?

19. What are the barriers to success in developing a vaccine (money for research, scientific knowledge, correlates of immunity, lack of animal model, public perceptions, etc.)?

20. Please estimate future R&D funding (public and private) needed to achieve licensure of a vaccine and postmarketing costs.

21. Is this vaccine likely to be part of a combination vaccine (with other antigens)?

22. For an anticipated vaccine, please estimate its likely efficacy, likely cost per dose, and number of doses needed for complete immunization (initial series, frequency of boosters).

23. What would be the appropriate target population for a vaccine (e.g., all infants, adolescents, pregnant women, older adults [age 65+], residents of an endemic area)?

24. What would be the anticipated time interval between vaccination of an individual in the target population and the realization by that individual of the health benefits?

25. What would be the anticipated time interval between vaccination in a target population and realizing health benefits to unvaccinated individuals from "herd immunity"?

26. Would delivery of this vaccine incur special costs (e.g., form of administra-tion, education for providers or the public, etc.)? If so, please identify and esti-mate those costs.

27. What factors could be expected to influence acceptance of the vaccine?

28. If possible, please identify recent key articles on this condition/ organism or on development of a vaccine against it that you think represent the best current thinking.

29. If there is a recently published article with which you particularly disagree, please identify and explain.

30. Please identify any other experts who should be consulted.

LIST OF RESPONDERS

Ann M. Arvin, M.D.
Department of Pediatric Infectious
    Diseases
School of Medicine
Stanford University
Palo Alto, CA

Robert Baughn, Ph.D.
VA Medical Center
Houston, TX

Robert B. Belshe, M.D.
Department of Infectious Diseases
St. Louis University School of
    Medicine
St. Louis, MO

Robert Betts, M.D.
University of Rochester
Rochester, NY

Dr. Martin J. Blaser
Division of Infectious Diseases
Vanderbilt University, School of
    Medicine
Nashville, TN

Dr. Thomas Broker
Biochemistry Department
University of Alabama at
    Birmingham

Dr. Robert Brunham
Medicine - Microbiology
University of Manitoba
Winnipeg, Manitoba, CANADA

Dr. Francis V. Chisari
The Scripps Research Institute
Molecular and Experimental
    Medicine
La Jolla, CA

H. Fred Clark, D.V.M., Ph.D.
The Children's Hospital of
    Philadelphia

Frank M. Collins, M.D.
Mycobacteriology Laboratory
Division of Bacterial Products
Food and Drug Administration
Bethesda, MD

Robert Couch
Microbiology and Immunology
Baylor College of Medicine
Houston, TX

Christopher P. Crum, M.D.
Brigham & Women's Hospital
Boston, MA

Dr. Stephen J. Czinn
Department of Pediatrics
Case Western University
Rainbow Babies and Children's
    Hospital
Cleveland, OH

James B. Dale, M.D.
Veterans Administration Medical
    Center
Memphis, TN

George S. Deepe, Jr., M.D.
Division of Infectious Diseases
University of Cincinnati

Dr. Gail Demmler
Pediatrics
Baylor College of Medicine
Houston, TX

Floyd W. Denny, M.D.
Chapel Hill, NC

Peter Densen, M.D.
Department of Internal Medicine
University of Iowa
Iowa City, IA

Michele Estabrook, M.D.
Division of Pediatric Infectious
    Diseases
Rainbow Babies and Childrens
    Hospital
Cleveland, OH

Monica M. Farley, M.D.
Departments of Medicine and
    Infectious Diseases
Emory University School of
    Medicine and the VA Medical
    Center
Atlanta, GA

Mark Fendrick, M.D.
Department of Internal Medicine
University of Michigan Hospital
Ann Arbor, MI

Vincent A. Fischetti, Ph.D.
Rockefeller University
New York, NY

Stacey C. FitzSimmons, Ph.D.
Cystic Fibrosis Foundation
Bethesda, MD

Dr. Ian H. Frazer
Papillomavirus Research Unit
Lions Human Immunology
    Laboratory
University of Queensland
Princess Alexandra Hospital
Woolloongabba, AUSTRALIA

John N. Galgiani, M.D.
VA Medical Center
Tucson, AZ

Denise A. Galloway, Ph.D.
Departments of Microbiology and
    Pathology
University of Washington
Seattle, WA

Dr. Donald Ganem
Microbiology and Immunology
University of California
School of Medicine
San Francisco, CA

Lutz Gissmann, Ph.D.
Department of Obstetrics and
    Gynecology
Stritch School of Medicine
Loyola University Medical Center
Maywood, IL

Paul Glezen
Microbiology and Immunology
Baylor College of Medicine
Houston, TX

Emil Gotschlich, M.D.
Laboratory for Bacterial
    Pathogenesis/Immunology
The Rockefeller University
New York, NY

Dan M. Granoff, M.D.
Chiron Biocine
Emeryville, CA

John R. Graybill, M.D.
Audie L. Murphy VA Hospital
Division of Infectious Diseases
San Antonio, TX

Harry B. Greenberg, M.D.
Department of Medicine
Stanford University
Palo Alto, CA

Thomas L. Hale, Ph.D.
Department of Enteric Infections
Walter Reed Army Institute of
    Research
Washington, D.C.

Dr. Scott B. Halstead
Department of the Navy
Naval Medical Research and
    Development Command
National Naval Medical Center
Bethesda, MD

Sharon L. Hillier, Ph.D.
Magee-Women's Hospital
Pittsburgh, PA

Harold J. Jennings, Ph.D.
National Research Council of
   Canada
Division of Biological Sciences
Ottawa, Ontario CANADA

Dennis L. Kasper, M.D.
Channing Laboratory
Harvard Medical School
Boston, MA

Ben Z. Katz, M.D.
Northwestern University Medical
   School
Division of Infectious Diseases
The Children's Memorial Hospital
Chicago, IL

Theo Kirkland, M.D.
Veterans Medical Center
San Diego, CA

Dr. Robert Kurman
Johns Hopkins Hospital
Baltimore, MD

Dr. Myron M. Levine
University of Maryland School of
   Medicine
Baltimore, MD

Sheila A. Lukehart, Ph.D.
Department of Medicine
Division of Infectious Diseases
Harborview Medical Center
Seattle, WA

Kenneth McIntosh, M.D.
Division of Infectious Diseases
Children's Hospital
Boston, MA

Dr. Suzanne M. Michalek
University of Alabama
Birmingham, AL

Dr. Andrew J. Morgan
Department of Pathology and
   Microbiology
School of Medical Sciences
University of Bristol
Bristol, UNITED KINGDOM

Dr. Richard Moss
School of Medicine
Stanford University
Stanford, CA

Brian Murphy, M.D.
Division of RVS, NIAID
National Institutes of Health
Bethesda, MD

Dr. James Nataro
Center for Vaccine Development
The University of Maryland
Baltimore, MD

Kristin Nichol, M.D.
Veterans Medical Center
Minneapolis, MN

Demosthenes Pappagianis, M.D.
University of California School of
   Medicine
Microbiology and Immunology
Davis, CA

Peter R. Paradiso, Ph.D.
Lederle-Praxis Biologicals
West Henrietta, NY

Robert F. Pass, M.D.
Professor, Director, Pediatric
Infectious Disease
University of Alabama at
Birmingham

Gerald B. Pier, Ph.D.
Harvard Medical School
Boston, MA

Dr. Stanley Plotkin
Pasteur Merieux Connaught Co.
Marnes-la-Coquette, FRANCE

Alice Prince
Department of Pediatrics
Columbia-Presbyterian Medical
Center
New York, NY

Justin D. Radolf, M.D.
University of Southwestern Texas
Department of Medicine
Division of Infectious Diseases
Dallas, TX

Dr. Rino Rappuoli
Head, Research and Development
Vaccine Sclavo SA
Sienna, ITALY

Dr. Cliona Rooney
Department of Virology
St. Jude Children's Research
Hospital
Memphis, TN

Craig E. Rubens, M.D., Ph.D.
Division of Infectious Diseases
Children's Hospital and Medical
Center
Seattle, WA

Julius Schachter, Ph.D.

Professor of Epidemiology
University of California, San
Francisco
Chlamydia Research Laboratory
San Francisco General Hospital

Dr. Mark Schiffman
NIH-National Cancer Institute
Bethesda, MD

Dr. Richard C. Schlegel
Department of Pathology
Georgetown University School of
Medicine
Washington, DC

John Schrieber, M.D.
Pediatric Infectious Diseases
Rainbow Babies and Children's
Hospital
Cleveland, OH

Anne Schuchat, M.D.
Meningitis and Special Pathogens
Centers for Disease Control and
Prevention
Atlanta, GA

Keerti V. Shah, Ph.D.
Johns Hopkins School of Hygiene,
Immunology and Infectious
Disease
Baltimore, MD

Arnold L. Smith, M.D.
University of Missouri Medical
School
Columbia, MO

Fred Sparling, M.D.
Chair, Department of Medicine
University of North Carolina
Chapel Hill, NC

Walter E. Stamm, M.D.
Division of Allergy and Infectious
Diseases
University of Washington Medical
Center
Seattle, WA

Stuart Starr, M.D.
Allergy, Immunology, and
Infectious Diseases
Children's Hospital
Philadelphia, PA

Dr. Allen Steere
Tufts University
Boston, MA

David A. Stevens, M.D.
Santa Clara Valley Medical Center
Division of Infectious Diseases
San Jose, CA

Dennis Stevens, M.D., Ph.D.
Veterans Affairs Medical Center
Boise, ID

Dr. Lode J. Swinnen
Section of Hematology/Oncology
Loyola University Medical Center
Maywood, IL

Martin A. Taubman, D.D.S., Ph.D.
Department of Immunology
Forsyth Dental Center
Boston, MA

Dr. Ram P. Tewari
Department of Microbiology and
Immunology
Southern Illinois University
Springfield, IL

L. Joseph Wheat, M.D.
Wishard Memorial Hospital
Department of Medicine
Indianapolis, IN

Richard Whitley, M.D.
Pediatrics, Microbiology and
Medicine
University of Alabama at
Birmingham

Dr. Gary Wormser
Infectious Diseases
New York Medical College
Valhalla, NY

Peter F. Wright, M.D.
Pediatric Infectious Diseases
Vanderbilt University Medical
Center
Nashville, TN

Dr. T.C. Wu
Johns Hopkins Hospital
Baltimore, MD

Michael Yancey, M.D.
Maternal-Fetal Medicine
Department of the Army
Headquarters, Tripler Army Medical
Center
Tripler AMC, HI

Index

A

Acellular antigens, 11, 18, 20, 28, 30, 129, 446
Adenovirus, 29, 33
Adjuvants, 34–35, 372–377, 430
  animal models, 373–374, 375, 376
  defined, 372
  diabetes, 388
  Helicobacter pylori, 365–366
  hepatitis C virus, 336
  Histoplasma capsulatum, 358
  mycobacterium tuberculosis, 352–353
  papillomaviruses, 340
Administration of vaccines, *see* Delivery of vaccines
Adolescents, *see* Children
Adults, 23, 47–50, 100, 111, 112
  chlamydia, 149
  dengue virus, 345–346
  Epstein-Barr virus, 7, 88, 177
  hepatitis B, 18
  hepatitis C, 189
  herpes simplex virus, 196
  influenza virus, 21, 224
  papillomaviruses, 213
  pneumonococcal vaccines, 21
  polio, 24
  streptococus, group B, 6, 305–306, 307, 309

Streptococcus pneumoniae, 314
  see also Elderly persons; Men; Women
African Americans, 50
Age factors, 4, 435
  Coccidiodes immitis, 160, 359
  cost-effectiveness model, analytic approach, 60, 66, 68–69, 80–83, 84
  cost-effectiveness model, detailed review, 93, 95, 98–100, 101–103, 105
  diabetes mellitus, 233
  ethical issues, 112
  Helicobacter pylori, 181, 182
  herpes simplex virus, 197
  Histoplasma capsulatum, 207, 208
  influenza virus, 225–226
  melanoma, 239
  multiple sclerosis, 245
  mycobacterium tuberculosis, 252, 253
  parainfluenza virus, 275
  quality-adjusted life years, 58, 66, 68–69, 80–82, 84, 80–83, 84, 95, 98–99
  respiratory syncytial virus, 279, 280, 281
  rheumatoid arthritis, 285, 286
  streptococcus, group A, 299
  streptococcus, group B, 305, 306
  Streptococcus pneumoniae 313, 314
  see also Adults; Children; Elderly persons; Infants

443

Aggregation
  ethical issues, 117–118, 119
  quality-adjusted life years, 2, 56
AIDS, *see* Human immunodeficiency
  virus
American Academy of Pediatrics, 45, 126
American College Health Association, 49
Americans with Disabilities Act, 112–113
Animal models, 419, 423, 425, 426–427,
  436
  adjuvants, 373–374, 375, 376
  antigen delivery, 378–379, 380
  autoimmune diseases, 386–387, 388–
    395, 399–403, 404–407
  chlamydia, 349, 350–351
  cholera, 376
  Coccidioides immitis, 357, 358–359
  costimulation 408
  diabetes, 386–387, 388–395
  DNA vaccines, 382–383
  Epstein-Barr virus, 333–334
  gonorrhea, 368–369, 371
  Helicobacter pylori, 365–366
  hepatitis C virus, 335, 336, 337, 338
  herpes simplex virus, 328–329
  Histoplasma capsulatum 357–358
  papillomaviruses, 340–341
  programmed T-cell death, 397
  streptococcus, group A, 361–362, 363
Antigens, 18, 20, 26–27, 28, 29, 30, 31,
  35, 40, 377–381, 412, 417, 420–
  424, 432
  acellular, 11, 18, 20, 28, 30, 129, 446
  autoimmune disease, 35–38
  chlamydia, 350–351
  Coccidioides immitis, 358–359
  dengue virus, 346
  diabetes, 387–388
  DNA vaccines, 381–386
  gonorrhea, 368–371
  Helicobacter pylori, 367
  hepatitis B virus, 378
  hepatitis C virus, 337
  Helicobacter pylori, 364
  Histoplasma capsulatum 358
  influenza virus, 223
  multiple sclerosis, 399, 400

polio, 24
programmed T-cell death, 37, 395–
  399, 409, 410–411
streptococcus, group A, 360
see also B cells; T cells
Apoptosis, 37, 395–399, 409, 410–411
Attenuated live viruses, 19, 20, 379
  herpes simplex virus, 328–329
  mycobacterium tuberculosis, 352
  polio, 24–25
Attitudes
  physicians, 47
  public complacency and fear, 9, 46,
    73–74, 130
  vaccine acceptance, 11, 20
Autoimmune diseases, 1, 12, 35–38, 45,
  380, 399–407
  animal models, 386–387, 388–395,
    399–403, 404–407
  antigens, 35–38
  diabetes mellitus, 6, 35, 37, 37, 54,
    67, 87, 90, 233–238, 386–389, 391,
    392, 393–395, 403
  cancer therapy, 427–429, 431
  multiple sclerosis, 6, 35, 54, 87, 245–
    249, 397, 399–400
  programmed T-cell death, 397–399
  rheumatoid arthritis, 6, 35, 54, 67, 87,
    285–290, 403
  T cells, 35–38, 233, 245, 389–391,
    392–395, 399–406 (passim)

B

Barriers to research and development, 11,
  13, 90, 130–131
  see also Litigation; Market forces
B cells, 28, 32, 35, 380, 381, 436
  adjuvants, 372, 376
  autoimmune disease, 36, 37
  diabetes, 387, 391
  Epstein-Barr virus, 330, 332, 334
  Helicobacter pylori, 364
  streptococcus, group A, 362
  see also Mucosal immunity

Biotechnology, 26, 30, 33–34, 90, 379, 381–386
    attenuated live viruses, 19, 20, 24–25, 328–329, 352, 379
    Epstein-Barr virus, 332–333, 334
    hepatitis B virus, 18, 379
    hepatitis C virus, 337
    herpes simplex virus, 327–328
    Histoplasma capsulatum 358
    hybridoma, 30
    monoclonal antibodies, 29–30
    mycobacterium tuberculosis, 355
    papillomaviruses, 339–340
    risk capital, 125
    Salmonella, 31–32
    see also DNA; Genomes; RNA
Bordetella pertussis, 11, 18, 19, 20, 28, 30, 46
Borrelia burgdorferi ,7, 44, 54, 88, 91, 100, 143–148
Burkitt's lymphoma, 330, 331, 332, 333

C

Canada, 49, 62, 66, 68, 96, 99
Cancer, 1, 12, 185, 189, 190, 194, 213–219, 381, 411, 415–433
    autoimmune therapy, 427–429, 431
    Epstein-Barr virus, 330–333
    melanoma, 6, 54, 88, 89–90, 239–243, 421
    papillomaviruses, 338–342
Caribbean region, 343
Centers for Disease Control and Prevention, 14, 28, 50, 100, 125, 126
Central nervous system, 67, 399–403
    herpes simplex virus, 196–200 (passim), 202, 204, 328
    multiple sclerosis, 6, 35, 54, 87, 245–249, 397, 399–400
    see also Neisseria meningitidis
Children, 7, 8–9, 45–47, 60, 69, 72, 80–82, 91, 99, 100, 101, 111, 130, 377
    American Academy of Pediatrics, 45, 126
    CDC recommendations, 28
    chlamydia, 6, 88, 157
    combination vaccines, 9, 18, 38, 46–47, 75, 130
    contraceptive vaccines, health effects, 76
    cytomegalovirus, 6, 90, 167
    dengue virus, 343, 345
    Epstein-Barr virus, 7, 88, 177, 179, 330–331, 333
    gonorrhea, 6, 88
    Helicobacter pylori, 181
    herpes simplex virus, 6, 88, 196, 203, 329
    influenza virus, 223–224
    liability issues, 128–129
    meningitis, 267
    National Childhood Vaccine Injury Act, 20–21, 128–129, 258
    papillomaviruses, 6, 88, 219, 342
    pregnant, 51
    polio, 24
    record-keeping, 46, 47, 49
    respiratory syncytial virus, 88, 279, 280, 281
    rotavirus, 291–292
    school entry immunizations, 7, 8–9, 20, 49, 90, 130
    Shigella, 295
    streptococcus, group A, 299, 363
    streptococcus, group B, 6, 93, 310, 311–312
    Streptococcus pneumoniae 313, 314, 315
    Vaccines for Children Program, 47, 131
    see also Infants
Children's Vaccine Initiative, 127–128
China, 334
Chlamydia, 6, 54, 67, 88, 89–90, 97, 149–158, 347–351, 368
Cholera, *see Vibrio cholerae*
Clinical trials, 9, 19, 70, 105, 126, 406, 417, 424, 430–431, 436
    djuvants, 373, 374
    AIDS, 373, 379
    Bordetella pertussis, 30

Coccidiodes immitis, 7, 19
dengue virus, 345–346
diabetes, 387
Epstein-Barr virus, 329, 333
funding, 125
gonorrhea, 371
herpes simplex virus, 327
mycobacterium tuberculosis, 352,
  353–354, 355
papillomaviruses, 342
programmed T-cell death, 397–398
respiratory syncytial virus, 6, 19
streptococcus, group A, 362, 363
Cloning, 26, 36
Coccidiodes immitis, 7, 19, 44, 54, 88, 90,
  91, 159–164, 356–359
Cognitive impairments, 62, 64–65
Combination vaccines, 9, 18, 38, 46–47,
  75, 130, 436
  elicobacter pylori, 364, 366–367
  herpes simplex virus, 327
Computer technology
  committee's model, application of,
    13, 95
  Internet, IOM, 4, 323
  physician reminders, 48
Confidentiality, 47
Conjugate vaccines
  Haemophilus influenzae, 11
  varicella-zoster virus, 11, 18
Cost and cost-effectiveness analysis,
    general, 2–3, 11, 12, 17, 20, 435–
    436, 437
  age factors, analytic approach of
    model, 60, 66, 68–69, 80–83, 84
  age factors, detailed review of model,
    93, 95, 98–100, 101–103, 105
  aggregation, 2, 56, 117–118, 119
  children, 46
  combination vaccines, 47
  death rates, analytic approach of
    model, 61–62, 66, 68, 78–79, 80–
    83, 86
  death rates, detailed characterization
    of model, 95, 97–98, 100, 103–104
  defined, 56

discounting, 18, 60–61, 68–69, 74,
  80, 83, 85–86, 97–98, 99, 101–103,
  105–107, 114–115
ethical issues, 3–4, 58, 75, 109–122,
  128, 129
licensure possibilities, scope of study
  at hand, 39, 40, 43
licensure process, 19–20, 54–55, 58;
  see also Time factors
life expectancy, analytic approach of
  model, 57, 66, 68, 76, 120
life expectancy, detailed
  characterization of model, 95–96,
  98, 99, 101–102, 103, 104, 106–107
mathematical formulae, 94–97, 99,
  101–106 (passim)
model, analytical approach, 53–92
model, detailed description, 93–108
morbidity/morbidity scenarios,
  analytic approach of model, 61–66,
  67, 68, 69, 71, 76, 78–79, 80–85
morbidity/morbidity scenarios,
  detailed characterization of model,
  95, 96, 97, 98, 108
opportunity costs, 74, 115–116, 130
polio, 25–26
pregnant women, 22
ranking of vaccines covered, 5–8
reasons for, 57
sensitivity analysis, 3, 57
specific diseases/pathogens/vaccines,
  lists of, 54–55, 87–91
  review for each, 143–433; *see
  also diseases/pathogens/vaccines
  found in lists*
utilization of vaccines, analytic
  approach of model, 72–73, 75, 76,
  79, 80, 86, 88, 89, 91
utilization of vaccines, detailed
  characterization of model, 95, 107–
  108
see also Death rates; Efficacy of
  vaccines; Morbidity scenarios;
  Quality-adjusted life years
Contraceptive vaccines, 75–76
Costimulation, 372, 373, 375, 389, 398,
  399, 400, 401, 402, 407–412, 419

Court cases, *see* Liability issues;
Litigation
Cuba, 343
Cystic fibrosis, 33, 42
Cytokines, 27, 374, 409–411, 415, 429–
433
autoimmune disease, 36, 38, 389–392,
404–405
chlamydia, 348–349
dengue virus, 344
gonorrhea, 371
Interleukin, 27, 38, 348–349, 372,
373, 374, 388, 389, 390–394, 396,
402–403, 405–406, 409, 410, 411–
412, 420, 424, 430, 432
Cytomegalovirus (CMV), 6, 19, 20, 22,
54, 87, 89, 90, 165–171

D

Death rates, 377
as assessment criterion, 27
model, analytic approach, 61–62, 66,
68, 78–79, 80–83, 86
model, detailed characterization, 95,
97–98, 100, 103–104
chlamydia, 149
Coccidioides immitis, 159, 160, 162
dengue virus, 343
gonorrhea, 257
Helicobacter pylori, 181, 182
herpes simplex virus, 198
Histoplasma capsulatum, 207, 208
influenza virus, 225–226
malaria, 43
melanoma, 239
meningitis, 267, 268
mycobacterium tuberculosis, 252,
253, 351
parainfluenza virus, 273
polio, 24
papillomaviruses, 215
respiratory syncytial virus, 279, 281,
283
rheumatoid arthritis, 287
rotavirus, 291

streptococcus, group B, 305, 307, 309
Streptococcus pneumoniae 313, 321
see also Life expectancy; Quality-
adjusted life years
Dengue hemorrhagic fever, 342–347
Dental caries, 44–45
Delivery of vaccines, 130
adults, 47–50
antigens, various, 377–381
children, 45–47
DNA vaccines, 381–386
intranasal immunization
mycobacterium tuberculosis, 354
polio, 25–26
pregnant women, 50–51
see also Noninjection routes;
Utilization of vaccines; Vaccine
schedules
Demographic factors, 58
see also Age factors; Immigrants;
Men; Race/ethnicity; Regional
factors; Travelers; Urban areas;
Women
Dengue hemorrhagic fever, 8
Department of Health and Human
Services, 20–21
Centers for Disease Control and
Prevention, 14, 28, 50, 100
Food and Drug Administration, 14,
125, 126, 362, 367, 373, 374; *see
also* Licensure, vaccines
Health Care Financing
Administration, 71, 106
see also National Institutes of Health;
specific institutes
Developing countries, 1, 17, 127–128,
173, 355, 360
Diabetes mellitus, 6, 35, 37, 54, 67, 87,
90, 233–238, 386–389, 391, 392,
393–395, 403
Diptheria, 20, 28, 30, 46, 49
Disabilities, 63–66, 68, 78–79, 86, 89,
97–98
cognitive impairments, 62, 64–65
emotional impairments, 64–65
ethical factors, 111, 112–113, 114–
115

mobility impairments, 24, 25, 64,
126–127
sensory impairments, 62, 64, 64, 67,
236
Disability-adjusted life years, 63, 66, 111,
112
Discounting, 18, 60–61, 68–69, 74, 80,
83, 85–86, 97–98, 99, 101–103,
105–107
ethical issues, 114–115
quality-adjusted life years, 18, 60–61,
68–69, 114–115
time factors, 68–69, 86, 101
Disease burden, 7–8, 11, 12, 43–45, 86,
89, 126, 127, 129
cost-effectiveness analyses, specific
diseases, 24–25, 42–43, 143–437
(passim); *see also specific
pathogens*
ethical issues, 109, 117–118, 121
malaria, 42–43
polio, 24–25
waterborne pathogens, 42
workshop summaries, specific
diseases, 326–433 (passim)
see also Death rates; Disabilities;
Epidemiology; Incidence;
Morbidity
Disease scenarios, *see* Death rates;
Incidence; Morbidity scenarios;
Prevalence;
*Diseases of Importance in Developing
Countries*, 1, 11
*Diseases of Importance in the United
States*, 1, 11, 17
DNA, 33, 34, 90, 381–386, 418, 420, 421,
422
antigen delivery, 380, 395
chlamydia, 348
Coccidiodes immitis, 358–359
dengue virus, 346
Epstein-Barr virus, 330, 331
hepatitis B virus, 379
hepatitis C virus, 335, 336, 337
HIV, 382–383
papillomaviruses, 6, 54, 88, 213–221,
338–342, 384, 433

transfection, 32, 34
tuberculosis, 383–384
see also Genomes
Drug resistance, 131, 380
gonorrhea, 368
malaria, 43
mycobacterium tuberculosis, 252,
253–254, 351

E

E-coli, see Escherichia coli
Economic factors, 9
market forces, 9, 19, 125–126
see also Cost and cost-effectiveness
analysis; Funding
Efficacy of vaccines, 32, 71–72, 79, 80,
94, 95, 107–108
Borrelia burgdorferi, 145, 147
chlamydia, 157
Coccidiodes immitis, 163, 164
cytomegalovirus, 170
diabetes mellitus, 237, 238
DNA vaccines, general, 384
enterotoxigenic *E. coli*, 174, 176
Epstein-Barr virus, 179, 180
gonorrhea, 264, 265
Helicobacter pylori, 186–187
hepatitis C virus, 193
herpes simplex virus, 203, 204, 328,
329
Histoplasma capsulatum, 209, 210
influenza virus, 229, 230
melanoma, 242
meningitis, 271, 272
multiple sclerosis, 248
mycobacterium tuberculosis, 254,
255, 256, 351–352, 355
papillomaviruses, 219, 220
parainfluenza virus, 276
respiratory syncytial virus, 282, 283
rheumatoid arthritis, 289
rotavirus, 292–293
Shigella, 296–297
streptococcus, group A, 303–304
streptococcus, group B, 310–312

Streptococcus pneumoniae 320–321
see also Clinical trials; Quality-
adjusted life years
Elderly persons, 23, 47–48, 49, 80–82,
100, 112
Helicobacter pylori, 181
influenza, 48, 223–224
Medicare, 4, 49–50
parainfluenza, 6, 273, 275
rheumatoid arthritis, 285
respiratory syncytial virus, 279
streptococcus, group B, 6, 7, 47–48,
310
Streptococcus pneumoniae 313, 314,
316–317, 319–321
ELISA, *see* Enzyme-linked
immunosorbent assays
Emotional impairments, 64–65
Emergency departments, 49
Enterococci, 42
Enterotoxigenic *E. coli, see Escherichia
coli*
Enzyme-linked immunosorbent assays,
341, 342
Epidemiology, 12, 17, 26, 44, 435
dengue virus, 343
hepatitis C virus, 334–335
poliomyelitis, 23–26, 91–92
see also Death rates; Incidence;
Morbidity; Morbidity scenarios;
Prevalence
Epstein-Barr virus, 7, 54, 67, 88, 177–
180, 329–334
Equations, *see* Mathematical formulae
Escherichia coli, 7, 54, 67, 88, 91, 173–
176, 361, 365–366, 374, 379
Ethical issues, 3–4, 109–122, 128, 129
aggregation, 117–118, 119
committee membership, 14
confidentiality, 47
contraceptive vaccines, 75
incidence of disease, 117, 118
pregnant women, 22
quality-adjusted life years, 3–4, 58,
111, 112, 113, 114–115, 120–121,
129–130
transplants, 120–121, 122

worst-off/sickest persons, 119–120
see also Quality of life
Europe, 347, 367, 377
Expanded Programme on Immunization,
127–128
Expert judgment, 3, 12
committee membership, 14, 17
list of, 437–442
morbidity scenarios, 97
survey instrument, 435–437

F

Fairness, *see* Ethical issues
Federal Advisory Committee on
Immunization Practices, 45
Fertility, 62, 65, 151, 155, 259, 264
contraceptive vaccines, 75–76
Food and Drug Administration, 14, 125,
126, 362, 367, 373, 374
see also Licensure, vaccines
Foreign countries, 1, 5, 8, 11, 17, 39, 42–
43, 59, 110
dengue virus, 343
polio, 25
pregnant women, 21
see also Developing countries;
Immigrants; Travelers; *specific
countries*
Formulae, *see* Mathematical formulae
Funding, 8, 19, 123–126, 436
National Childhood Vaccine Injury
Act, 20–21

G

Gender factors, *see* Men; Women
Genetics, 233
Epstein-Barr virus, 330–332
Helicobacter pylori, 364–365
papillomaviruses, 339–340
see Biotechnology; DNA; Genomes;
RNA
Genomes, 32, 395
Epstein-Barr virus, 330–331, 333–334

hepatitis C virus, 335
herpes simplex virus, 327, 328
influenza, 223
Geographic factors, *see* Developing
countries; Foreign countries;
Regional factors; Urban areas
Glycopolymers, 374
Glycoprotein vaccines, 19, 20, 33, 223,
327, 336, 380, 382–383
Gonorrhea, *see Neisseria gonorrhea*
Group A streptococcus, 6, 43, 54, 67, 88,
299–304, 359–363
Group B streptococcus, 6, 19, 20, 54, 67,
87, 88, 89, 90, 129, 305–312
adolescent girls, 93
pregnant women, 7, 21, 22, 23, 93
Guillain-Barré syndrome, 21

H

Haemophilus influenzae (Hib), 11, 18, 19,
23, 28, 46–47, 114, 126
Health Care Financing Administration,
71, 106
Health care workers
hepatitis B, 18
hepatitis C virus, 337
see also Nurses; Physicians
Health departments, 46, 49
varicella-zoster virus, 18
Health insurance, 131
children, 47, 90
incentives to, 9
performance measures, 7
Health utility index (HUI), 62–68
(passim), 76, 96, 97, 98–99, 102
Borrelia burgdorferi, 143, 145, 146
chlamydia, 150, 151–152
Coccidiodes immitis, 161, 162
cytomegalovirus, 165–166, 167
diabetes mellitus, 234
enterotoxigenic *E. coli,* 173
Epstein-Barr virus, 177, 178
ethical issues, 117, 119
gonorrhea, 257, 258
Helicobacter pylori, 181, 182, 183

hepatitis C virus, 191
herpes simplex virus, 196, 200
Histoplasma capsulatum, 208
influenza virus, 227
melanoma, 239
meningitis, 267–268
multiple sclerosis, 246
mycobacterium tuberculosis, 252, 254
papillomaviruses, 214, 215–216
respiratory syncytial virus, 279
rheumatoid arthritis, 286
streptococcus, group A, 300, 301
streptococcus, group B, 305
Streptococcus pneumoniae 313
Heat shock proteins, 353
Helicobacter felis, 30
Helicobacter pylori, 6, 54, 67, 88, 181–
188, 363–367
Hepatitis A virus, 11, 18, 19, 334, 337
Hepatitis B virus, 11, 18, 19, 28, 30, 44–
44, 47–48, 114, 334, 337, 378, 379,
412–415
Hepatitis C virus, 6, 54, 88, 189–194,
334–338, 433
Herpes simplex virus, 6, 19, 22, 54, 67,
88, 195–205, 326–329, 384
Herpesvirus (Epstein-Barr), *see* Epstein-
Barr virus
Hispanics, 50
Histoplasma capsulatum 7, 44, 54, 67, 89,
91, 207–212, 356–359
Historical perspectives, 123–124
childhood immunizations, 46
hepatitis, 334
IOM studies, 1, 2, 11, 17, 123–124
litigation, 20–23
malaria, 42–43
quality-adjusted life years, 2, 56
polio, 23–26, 91–92
syphilis, 41
vaccine development, 12
Hodgkin's disease, 330, 331
Hospitals and hospitalization, 4, 48–49,
67, 106
cost-effectiveness, general, 59, 71
chlamydia, 153–156
Coccidiodes immitis, 161, 162

cytomegalovirus, 166, 167, 168–169
gonorrhea, 257–263 (passim)
Helicobacter pylori, 184–185
hepatitis C virus, 190, 192
herpes simplex virus, 202–203
Histoplasma capsulatum, 209, 211
influenza virus, 224, 227
melanoma, 240, 241
meningitis, 268, 269, 270
multiple sclerosis, 246, 247
mycobacterium tuberculosis, 252, 254, 255
nosocomial infections, 9, 18, 41, 42, 131
papillomaviruses, 214
parainfluenza virus, 274, 275
respiratory syncytial virus, 20, 281, 282
rheumatoid arthritis, 286, 288
streptococcus, group A, 301–302
streptococcus, group B, 306, 307, 308, 309
Streptococcus pneumoniae 318–320
HUI, *see* Health utility index
Human immunodeficiency virus, 2, 13–14, 22, 32, 42, 43, 44, 112, 119–120, 159–160, 165, 195, 330, 368, 373, 377, 379, 380, 382–383, 386
Human papillomaviruses, *see* Papillomaviruses
Humoral immunity, 41
adjuvants, 373
Coccidiodes immitis, 357
hepatitis C virus, 337
Histoplasma capsulatum 357
see also B cells; Mucosal immunity; T cells
Hybridoma, 30, 401–402, 404–405

I

Iceland, 378
Immigrants
Borrelia burgdorferi, 7, 88, 145
Coccidiodes immitis, 7, 88, 159, 161, 163

Histoplasma capsulatum, 7, 89, 207, 209
Immune system, general, 26–30, 377
Coccidiodes immitis, 358–359
chlamydia, 349–351
dengue virus, 345–346
gonorrhea, 368–369
hepatitis C virus, 336
herpes simplex virus, 327, 329
Histoplasma capsulatum 357–358
mycobacterium tuberculosis, 352–353
papillomaviruses, 339
pregnant women, 22–23
streptococcus, group A, 363
see also Adjuvants; Antigens;
Autoimmune diseases; B cells;
Macrophages; Mucosal immunity;
Peptide therapy; T cells
Immunoglobin, 27, 28, 29–30, 32, 33, 378, 379–380, 408, 426
Epstein-Barr virus, 334
Helicobacter pylori, 364, 366
streptococcus, group A, 362
transplacental transport, 22–23
Impairments, *see* Disabilities; Morbidity
Incidence, 3, 435
Bordetella pertussis, 143, 144
chlamydia, 149–152, 347
Coccidiodes immitis, 159, 160, 162, 356–357
cost-effectiveness model, analytic approach, 58, 68, 80–84 (passim), 87, 89
cost-effectiveness model, detailed review, 100
cytomegalovirus, 165–166
dengue virus, 343
diabetes mellitus, 233
enterotoxigenic *E. coli,* 173
Epstein-Barr virus, 177, 329–330
ethical issues, 117, 118
gonorrhea, 257, 367–368
Helicobacter pylori, 181, 182, 183, 363
hepatitis C virus, 189, 191, 334
herpes simplex virus, 196, 197, 326

Histoplasma capsulatum 207, 208, 356–357
influenza virus, 224, 225, 227
melanoma, 239, 240
meningitis, 267, 268
multiple sclerosis, 245
mycobacterium tuberculosis, 252, 253, 351
papillomaviruses, 213, 338
parainfluenza virus, 6, 273
polio, 24–25
respiratory syncytial virus, 279, 280
rheumatoid arthritis, 285
rotavirus, 291
Shigella, 295
streptococcus, group A, 299, 300, 360
streptococcus, group B, 305, 306
Streptococcus pneumoniae 313, 314
see also Death rates
Infants, 8–9, 23, 45–47, 60, 69, 84, 100, 101
Borrelia burgdorferi, 7, 88, 145
chlamydia, 152, 153, 156, 347–348
Coccidiodes immitis, 7, 88, 161, 163
cytomegalovirus, 165–166, 168, 170
enterotoxigenic *E. coli,* 7, 88, 173
Haemophilus influenzae, 11, 114
Helicobacter pylori, 88
hepatitis B virus, 18, 114
herpes simplex virus, 6, 88, 199, 201, 326, 327–328
Histoplasma capsulatum 7, 89, 209
meningitis, 7, 23, 89, 267
parainfluenza virus, 6, 273, 275
respiratory syncytial virus, 6, 19, 279, 280, 281, 282
rotavirus, 6, 88, 291–292
Shigella, 7, 89, 295, 296, 297
streptococcus, group A, 6, 88, 303
streptococcus, group B, 20, 23, 88, 305, 307, 308
Streptococcus pneumoniae 314
tuberculosis, 91
varicella-zoster virus, 18
see also Pregnant women
Infertility, *see* Fertility

Inflammatory response, 35, 36, 37, 385, 390, 397, 398, 411–412, 422, 423, 428
adenoviruses, 33
central nervous system, 399, 401, 402, 403
disbetes, 233, 386, 387
gastric, 363, 264
heat shock protein, 351
macrophage activation, 372, 373
multiple sclerosis, 245
pelvic inflammatory disease (PID), 150, 153, 257, 348
peptides, 403, 404, 405, 406
rheumatoid arthritis, 285
Influenza virus, 6, 11, 19, 22, 30, 34, 48–50, 54, 59–60, 67, 87, 89, 223–231, 382, 386
litigation, 21
see also Parainfluenza virus
Insert baculovirus system, 30
Insulin-dependent diabetes mellitus, *see* Diabetes mellitus,
Insurance, *see* Health insurance
Interferon, 351, 357, 373, 387, 388, 392, 393, 409
Interleukin, 27, 38, 348–349, 372, 373, 374, 388, 389, 390–394, 396, 402–403, 405–406, 409, 410, 411–412, 420, 424, 430, 432
International perspectives, *see* Foreign countries
Internet, IOM, 4, 323
Intranasal delivery, 9, 28, 29–30, 33, 34, 37, 47, 130, 355, 358, 361–362, 366, 378, 380

J

Japan, hepatitis C virus, 334

L

Legislation, general
pregnant women, 7

school entry immunizations, 7, 8–9, 20, 49, 90, 130
Legislation, specific
   Americans with Disabilities Act, 112–113
   National Childhood Vaccine Injury Act, 20–21, 128–129, 258
Less-developed countries, *see* Developing countries
Liability issues, 19, 128–129
   see also Litigation
Licensure, vaccines, 1, 4, 5, 11, 18–19, 39, 43, 89–91, 436
   Borrelia burgdorferi, 145
   chlamydia, 157
   Coccidiodes immitis, 20
   cytomegalovirus, 20, 167
   diabetes mellitus, 234, 237
   enterotoxigenic *E. coli,* 174
   Epstein-Barr virus, 179
   funding issues, 8
   gonorrhea, 6, 20, 264, 265
   Helicobacter pylori, 185
   hepatitis A, 18
   hepatitis B, 18
   hepatitis C, 190
   herpes simplex virus, 201
   Histoplasma capsulatum, 209
   influenza virus, 228
   length of process, general, 19–20, 54–55, 58, 60–61, 79, 80–82, 90, 95, 108, 121, 437
   melanoma, 240
   meningitis, 271
   multiple sclerosis, 246
   mycobacterium tuberculosis, 253
   papillomaviruses, 219
   parainfluenza virus, 20, 276
   polio, 25, 126–127
   respiratory syncytial virus, 20, 280
   rheumatoid arthritis, 287, 289
   rotavirus, 18, 292
   Shigella, 296, 297
   streptococcus, group A, 302
   streptococcus, group B, 20, 306–309
   Streptococcus pneumoniae 317, 321
   therapeutic vaccines, general, 45

varicella-zoster virus, 18
   see also Animal models; Clinical trials; Time factors
Life expectancy, general
   cost-effectiveness model, analytic approach, 57, 66, 68, 76, 120
   cost-effectiveness model, detailed characterization, 95–96, 98, 99, 101–102, 103, 104, 106–107
   ethical issues, 112, 113, 120
   see also Quality-adjusted life years
Litigation, 8, 20–23, 127, 128–129
   pregnant women, 21–23
   streptococcus, group B, 6
   see also Liability issues
Local government, *see* Health departments
Lymphocytes, *see* B cells; T cells

M

Macrophages, 27, 28, 246, 353, 357, 372, 373, 374, 375, 377, 378, 392, 393, 399, 401, 402–403, 409, 430, 432
Major histocompatibility complex (MHC), 26–27, 32–37 (passim), 344, 350, 358, 373, 381, 390, 399–400, 404, 406, 407, 410–422 (passim), 430, 432, 433
Malaria, 8, 42–43
March of Dimes, 24
Market forces, 9, 19, 125–126
Mathematical formulae, 94–97, 99, 101–106 (passim)
Measles, 20, 28, 49, 131, 386
Medicaid, 118
Medicare, 4, 49–50
Melanoma, 6, 54, 88, 89–90, 239–243, 421
Men, 68, 97, 98–99
   chlamydia, 97, 149–153 (passim), 155–156, 347
   gonorrhea, 257, 258, 260, 263, 264–265
   herpes simplex virus, 326
   papillomaviruses, 214, 216, 218–219

Meningitis, see *Neisseria meningitidis*
Microspheres, 378–379, 380
Migration, *see* Immigrants
Military personnel, 330, 356
Minority groups, *see* Race/ethnicity
Mobility impairments, 64
    polio, 24, 25, 126–127
    onoclonal antibodies, 29–30
    herpes simplex virus, 327
Mononucleosis, *see* Epstein-Barr virus
Monophosphoric lipid-A, 373
Morbidity, 61–66, 67, 68, 78–79, 108
    as assessment criterion, 27, 39, 80–
      82, 95, 96
    health utility index, general, 62–68
      (passim), 76, 96, 97, 98–99, 102
    scenarios, *see* Morbidity scenarios;
      specific diseases listed under Health
      utility index
    chlamydia, 347–348
    Coccidiodes immitis, 356
    dengue virus, 342–343
    Epstein-Barr virus, 330
    gonorrhea, 368
    hepatitis C virus, 334
    Helicobacter pylori, 363–364
    Histoplasma capsulatum 356
    malaria, 43
    papillomavirus, 338–339
    streptococcus, group A, 359–360
    see also Disabilities; Quality-adjusted
      life years
Morbidity scenarios, 69, 71, 78, 80–85,
    95, 96, 97, 98
    Bordetella pertussis, 143–144, 146
    chlamydia, 150, 151–152
    Coccidiodes immitis, 162
    cytomegalovirus, 165–166, 167
    diabetes mellitus, 234
    enterotoxigenic *E. coli,* 173
    Epstein-Barr virus, 177
    gonorrhea, 257, 259
    Helicobacter pylori, 182–183, 363–
      364
    hepatitis C virus, 190, 191
    herpes simplex virus, 196, 198–199
    Histoplasma capsulatum, 208, 210

influenza virus, 224, 227
melanoma, 239–240, 241
meningitis, 267–269
multiple sclerosis, 246
mycobacterium tuberculosis, 252, 254
papillomaviruses, 214, 215–216
parainfluenza virus, 273, 274
respiratory syncytial virus, 279, 281
rheumatoid arthritis, 285–286, 287
rotavirus, 291
Shigella, 295
streptococcus, group A, 299–300
streptococcus, group B, 305–306, 307
Streptococcus pneumoniae 313, 315–
    317
    see also Health utility index
Mortality, *see* Death rates
Mucosal immunity, 27, 28–30, 32, 33, 47
    adjuvants, 374–375, 376
    antigen delivery, 377, 378, 380
    autoimmune disease, 35, 37
    chlamydia, 348
    Epstein-Barr virus, 333
    Helicobacter pylori, 365
    papillomaviruses, 338–339, 341
    streptococcus, group A, 362
    see also B cells; Intranasal delivery
Multiple sclerosis, 6, 35, 54, 87, 245–249,
    397, 399–400
Mumps, 20, 28, 49
Mycobacterium tuberculosis, 6, 54, 88,
    89–90, 91, 100, 251–256, 351–355,
    383–384, 386

N

Nasal delivery, *see* Intranasal delivery
National Cancer Institute, 339–341
National Center for Health Statistics, 14
National Childhood Vaccine Injury Act,
    20–21, 128–129
National Foundation for Infantile
    Paralysis-March of Dimes, 24
National Health Interview Survey, 50

National Institute of Allergy and Infectious Diseases, 17, 18, 110, 124–125, 126
National Institute of Child Health and Development, 125
National Institute of Occupational Safety and Health, 356–357
National Institutes of Health
    hepatitis C virus, 334, 336
    HIV research, 13–14
    papillomaviruses, 339–341
    study at hand, methodology, 14, 110
National Vaccine Injury Compensation Program, 20–21, 128–129
Neisseria gonorrhea, 6, 20, 54, 67, 88, 100, 257–265, 367–372
Neisseria meningitidis, 7, 19, 23, 54, 66, 67, 89, 200, 251, 267–272
    streptococcus, group B, 20, 23, 88, 305, 307, 308–309
    Streptococcus pneumoniae 313–320 (passim)
Neonates, *see* Infants; Pregnant women
New Vaccine Development: Establishing Priorities, 1, 11, 17
Noninjection routes, vaccines, 9, 25, 29, 31–34, 47
    diabetes, 387–388
    intranasal administration, 9, 28, 29–30, 33, 34, 37, 47, 130, 355, 358, 361–362, 366, 378, 380
    oral administration, 9, 28, 29, 31–32, 37, 130, 378, 380
    polio, 20, 25–26, 28–29, 32
    tuberculosis, 354, 355
    particulate vaccines, 30–34
    rotavirus, 20–29
Nosocomial infections, 9, 18, 41, 42, 131
Nurses, 49, 255

O

Occupational health, *see* Health care workers
Older persons, *see* Elderly persons
Ontario Health Survey, 96

Opportunity costs, 74, 115–116, 130
Oral administration, 9, 28, 29, 31–32, 37, 130, 378, 380
    diabetes, 387–388
    Helicobacter pylori, 366
    mycobacterium tuberculosis, 354, 355
    polio vaccine, 20, 25–26, 28–29, 32
Organ transplants, *see* Transplants (organs)

P

Pain, 62, 65, 260–261
Pan-American Health Organization, 25
Panel on Cost-Effectiveness in Health and Medicine, 56, 85
Papillomaviruses, 6, 54, 88, 213–221, 338–342, 384, 433
Parainfluenza virus, 6, 19, 20, 54, 88, 273–277
Particulate vaccines, 30–34
Pasteur Institute, 340
Peptide therapy, 26–27, 33, 35–36, 37, 358, 395, 396, 410, 411, 412–432 (passim)
    adjuvants, 373, 374, 375
    autoimmune diseases, 399–401, 403–407
    chlamydia, 350
    dengue virus, 344
    Epstein-Barr virus, 333, 334
    gonorrhea, 369, 370
    hepatitis B virus, 412–415
    multiple sclerosis, 399, 300
    streptococcus, group A, 362
Pertussis acellular vaccine, 11, 18, 20, 28, 30, 129
Physicians, 17, 47–48
    Borrelia burgdorferi, 145
    chlamydia, 153–156
    Coccidiodes immitis, 161, 162
    cytomegalovirus, 166, 168–169
    diabetes mellitus, 234, 235–236
    enterotoxigenic *E. coli,* 174
    Epstein-Barr virus, 178, 179
    gonorrhea, 260–264 (passim)

Helicobacter pylori, 184
hepatitis C virus, 192
herpes simplex virus, 202–203
Histoplasma capsulatum, 211
influenza virus, 228
melanoma, 240, 241
meningitis, 270
multiple sclerosis, 246, 247
mycobacterium tuberculosis, 252, 255
papillomaviruses, 214, 215, 217–219
parainfluenza virus, 274, 275
respiratory syncytial virus, 282
rheumatoid arthritis, 286, 288
Shigella, 295–296, 297
streptococcus, group A, 302
streptococcus, group B, 306, 308, 309
Streptococcus pneumoniae 318–320
varicella-zoster virus, 18
Poliomyelitis, 20, 23–26, 28–29, 32, 91–
    92
Poverty
    ethical issues, 115–116, 118
    Medicaid, 118
    see also Developing countries
Pregnant women, 7, 21–23, 50–51, 69, 91,
    101, 128–129
    chlymadia, 154, 347–348
    contraceptive vaccines, 75–76
    fertility, 62, 65, 151, 155, 259, 264
    gonorrhea, 259, 368
    hepatitis C virus, 334
    herpes simplex virus, 326–327
    meningitis, 22
    parainfluenza, 88
    streptococcus, group B, 20, 90, 93,
        306, 307, 309, 310–311
    Streptococcus pneumoniae 22
    tetanus toxoids, 23
    time of delivery, 20, 23, 51
    various pathogens, 22
Prevalence
    cost-effectiveness model, analytic
        approach, 68
    cost-effectiveness model, detailed
        description, 100
    see also Incidence
Privacy, *see* Confidentiality

Private sector, 8, 19, 105, 125, 436
    market forces, 9, 19, 125–126
    papillomaviruses, 342
    streptococcus, group B, 6
    see also Health insurance; Litigation
Pseudomonas aeruginosa, 42, 44, 128
Psychological factors, *see* Attitudes;
        Cognitive impairments; Emotional
        impairments
Psychomotor impairments, *see* Mobility
        impairments
Puberty, *see* Children
Public Health Service, 56
Public opinion, *see* Attitudes

Q

Quality-adjusted life years, 2, 57, 58, 61–
    69, 76–89, 95–99 102–104, 106,
    107–108
    age and, 58, 66, 68–69, 80–82, 84,
        80–83, 84, 95, 98–99
    aggregation, 2, 56
    average population health states, 66,
        68
    definitional issues, 2, 56, 58, 61–62,
        86, 95
    disability-adjusted life years, 63, 66,
        111, 112
    discounting, 18, 60–61, 68–69, 114–
        115
    ethical issues, 3–4, 58, 111, 112, 113,
        114–115, 120–121, 129–130
    mathematical formulae, 95, 96, 99
    see also Life expectancy
Quality-adjusted life years, specific
        vaccines
    Borrelia burgdorferi, 147
    chlamydia, 157, 158
    Coccidiodes immitis, 163–164
    cytomegalovirus, 167, 170–171
    diabetes mellitus, 237, 238
    Enterotoxigenic *E. coli,* 174, 176
    Epstein-Barr virus, 179–180
    gonorrhea, 264–265
    Helicobacter pylori, 186–187

hepatitis C virus, 193–194
herpes simplex virus, 204
Histoplasma capsulatum, 210, 211
influenza virus, 229–230
melanoma, 241, 242–243
meningitis, 271, 272
multiple sclerosis, 248, 249
mycobacterium tuberculosis, 254, 256
papillomaviruses, 220
parainfluenza virus, 276, 277
ranking of vaccines covered, 5–7
respiratory syncytial virus, 282–283
rheumatoid arthritis, 289
rotavirus, 293
Shigella, 296, 297
streptococcus, group A, 301, 303, 304
streptococcus, group B, 307, 310–312
Streptococcus pneumoniae 315, 320–321
Quality of life, general, 15
Quality of Well-Being Scale, 63, 66

R

Race/ethnicity, 50
syphilis, 41
see also specific racial/ethnic groups
Receptor-centered regulation, 22, 26, 29, 30–31, 36, 37–38, 407, 418, 426
chlamydia, 349, 350
dengue virus, 343–344
gonorrhea, 369, 370–371
hepatitis B virus, 412–413
streptococcus, group A, 360
virus-like particles, 30–31
Record-keeping, 46, 47, 49
Regional factors, 7, 44, 71, 88, 89, 91, 93, 105, 128
Borrelia burgdorferi, 144, 145
chlamydia, 347
Coccidiodes immitis, 159
dengue virus, 343
gonorrhea, 257, 367–368
Histoplasma capsulatum 207, 209, 356–357
mycobacterium tuberculosis, 352, 355

see also Developing countries; Foreign countries; Immigrants
Respiratory syncytial virus, 6, 19, 20, 22, 23, 43, 54, 88, 90, 279–284
Rheumatoid arthritis, 6, 35, 54, 67, 87, 285–290, 403
RNA
dengue virus, 342–347
diabetes, 388
Epstein-Barr virus, 330
gonorrhea, 368
hepatitis C virus, 335, 336
Rotavirus, 6, 11, 18, 19, 22, 28–29, 54, 88, 291–294
Rubella, 20, 28

S

Salmonella, 31–32
Schedules, *see* Vaccination schedules
School entry immunizations, 7, 8–9, 20, 49, 90, 130
Sensitivity analysis, 3, 57
Sensory impairments, 62, 64, 64, 67, 236
Sex differences, *see* Men; Women
Sexually transmitted diseases, 7
chlamydia, 6, 54, 67, 88, 89–90, 149–158, 347–351, 368
hepatitis C virus, 334–335
herpes simplex virus, 6, 19, 22, 54, 67, 88, 195–205, 326–329, 384
gonorrhea, 6, 20, 54, 67, 88, 100, 257–265, 367–372
human immunodeficiency virus, 2, 13–14, 22, 32, 42, 43, 44, 112, 119–120, 159–160, 165, 195, 330, 368, 373, 377, 379, 380, 382–383, 386
papillomaviruses, 6, 54, 88, 213–221, 338–342, 384, 433
syphilis, 41
Shigella, 7, 43, 54, 100, 295–297, 379
Socioeconomic status, *see* Poverty; Race/ethnicity
Southeast Asia, 339, 343
Staphylococcus aureus, 42

State public health programs, *see* Health
    departments
Streptococcus, *see* Group A
    streptococcus; Group B
    streptococcus; *Streptococcus
    mutans; Streptococcus pneumoniae*
Streptococcus mutans, 44–45
Streptococcus pneumoniae 6, 21, 43, 47–
    48, 49, 54, 60, 88, 89, 313–322
Syncytial virus, *see* Respiratory syncytial
    virus
Syphilis, 41

T

Target populations, *see* Age factors;
    Immigrants; Men; Race/ethnicity;
    Women
T cells, 26–35, 408–409, 410, 415–433
    (passim), 436
    adjuvants, 372–373, 374, 376
    antigen-induced programmed cell
        death, 37, 395–399, 409, 410–411
    autoimmune disease, 35–38, 233, 245,
        389–391, 392–395, 399–406
        (passim)
    chlamydia, 348–349, 350
    cholera, 375
    Coccidiodes immitis, 357
    dengue virus, 344–345, 346, 347
    diabetes mellitus, 233, 387–389, 391,
        392, 393–395
    Epstein-Barr virus, 330, 331, 332, 333
    DNA vaccines, 378, 380, 381, 382,
        383, 385
    Helicobacter pylori, 364
    hepatitis B virus, 412, 413–415
    hepatitis C virus, 335, 337–338
    herpes simplex virus, 329
    Histoplasma capsulatum 357
    mycobacterium tuberculosis, 353–355
    papillomaviruses, 342
Tetanus, 20, 23, 28, 30, 46, 49
Time factors, 68–69, 79, 86
    Bordetella pertussis, 145
    chlamydia, 156

    Coccidiodes immitis, 161
    cytomegalovirus, 167
    development/licensure process, 19–
        20, 54–55, 58, 60–61, 79, 80–82,
        90, 95, 108, 121, 437
    diabetes mellitus, 234, 237
    enterotoxigenic *E. coli,* 174
    Epstein-Barr virus, 179
    gonorrhea, 264
    Helicobacter pylori, 185
    hepatitis C, 190
    herpes simplex virus, 201
    Histoplasma capsulatum, 209
    influenza virus, 228
    melanoma, 240
    meningitis, 271
    multiple sclerosis, 246, 248, 249
    mycobacterium tuberculosis, 252, 254
    papillomaviruses, 219, 220
    parainfluenza virus, 276, 277
    respiratory syncytial virus, 280, 282–
        283
    rheumatoid arthritis, 287, 289
    rotavirus, 292, 293
    Shigella, 296, 297
    streptococcus, group A, 302, 304
    streptococcus, group B, 306, 311
    Streptococcus pneumoniae 317, 321
    discounting, 68–69, 86, 101
    licensure possibilities, scope of study
        at hand, 39, 40, 43
    patient time costs, 74
    patterns of vaccine use, 60, 93–94
    pregnant women, 20, 23, 51
Tobacco, 379–380
Tourists, *see* Travelers
Transfection, 32, 34, 416, 418, 423–424
Transplants (organs), 391
    cytomegalovirus, 165, 169
    Epstein-Barr virus, 330
    ethical issues, 120–121, 122
    hepatitis C virus, 334
Travelers, 105
    E. coli, 7, 88, 173, 174
    malaria, 42–43
    Shigella, 7, 89, 295, 296, 297
Treponema pallidum, 41

Tuberculosis, *see Mycobacterium
  tuberculosis*
Tyler's murine encephalomyelitis, 399
Typhoid, 29, 30, 47

U

Urban areas
  influenza, 50
  syphilis, 41
Utilization of vaccines, 9, 39, 45, 130
  Borrelia burgdorferi, 147
  chlamydia, 157
  Coccidiodes immitis, 163, 164
  complacency and fear, 9, 46, 73–74
    [ALL]
  cost-effectiveness model, analytic
    approach, 72–73, 75, 76, 79, 80, 86,
    88, 89, 91
  cost-effectiveness model, detailed
    review, 95, 107–108
  cytomegalovirus, 170
  diabetes mellitus, 237, 238
  E. coli, 174, 176
  Epstein-Barr virus, 179, 180
  gonorrhea, 264, 265
  streptococcus, group B, 6
  Helicobacter pylori, 186–187
  hepatitis C virus, 193, 194
  herpes simplex virus, 204
  Histoplasma capsulatum, 210
  influenza virus, 229, 230
  melanoma, 242, 243
  meningitis, 271, 272
  multiple sclerosis, 248, 249
  mycobacterium tuberculosis, 253–
    254, 255, 256
  papillomaviruses, 219, 220
  parainfluenza virus, 276, 277
  respiratory syncytial virus, 281, 282,
    283
  rheumatoid arthritis, 289
  rotavirus, 292–293
  school entry immunizations, 7, 8–9,
    20, 49, 90, 130
  Shigella, 296–297

specific vaccines, various, 53
streptococcus, group A, 303–304
streptococcus, group B, 310–312
Streptococcus pneumoniae 320–321
  see also Attitudes; Barriers to
    research and development; Delivery
    of vaccines

V

Vaccine Injury Compensation Program,
  20–21, 128–129
Vaccine schedules, 45–46, 431–432
  Borrelia burgdorferi, 145, 147
  chlamydia, 157
  Coccidiodes immitis, 163
  cytomegalovirus, 170
  diabetes mellitus, 237
  enterotoxigenic *E. coli*, 174
  Epstein-Barr virus, 179
  gonorrhea, 264
  Helicobacter pylori, 186
  hepatitis C virus, 193, 336
  herpes simplex virus, 203, 329
  Histoplasma capsulatum, 209
  influenza virus, 229
  melanoma, 242
  meningitis, 271
  multiple sclerosis, 248
  mycobacterium tuberculosis, 254
  papillomaviruses, 219
  parainfluenza virus, 276
  respiratory syncytial virus, 282
  rheumatoid arthritis, 289
  rotavirus, 292
  Shigella, 296
  streptococcus, group A, 303
  streptococcus, group B, 310
  Streptococcus pneumoniae 320
Vaccines for Children Program, 47, 131
Varicella-zoster virus, 11, 18, 19, 28
Vector-borne pathogens, 8, 42–43, 342–
  347
Vibrio cholerae, 30, 31, 35, 374, 375–
  376, 378
Virus-like particulates, 30–34

Visting Nurse Assocations, 49

W

Waterborne pathogens, general, 42
World Bank, 63
World Health Organization, 21, 25, 63
Women, 68, 98–99
   chlymadia, 97, 149, 150–152, 153, 154
   contraceptive vaccines, 75–76

fertility, 62, 65, 151, 155, 259, 264
gonorrhea, 257, 258, 259–265
papillomaviruses, 214, 215, 217, 338–342
respiratory syncytial virus, 6, 280, 281
streptococcus, group B, 6, 88, 309, 307, 310
syphilis, 41
   see also Pregnant women
World Wide Web, *see* Internet